T0200138

Narrative and Mental Health

EXPLORATIONS IN NARRATIVE PSYCHOLOGY

MARK FREEMAN
Series Editor

BOOKS IN THE SERIES
Narrative Imagination and Everyday Life
Molly Andrews

Decolonizing Psychology: Globalization, Social Justice,
and Indian Youth Identities
Sunil Bhatia

Beyond the Archive: Memory, Narrative, and the Autobiographical Process
Jens Brockmeier

Speaking of Violence
Sara Cobb

Not in My Family: German Memory and Responsibility After the Holocaust
Roger Frie

Entangled Narratives: Collaborative Storytelling and
the Re-Imagining of Dementia
Lars-Christer Hydén

Narratives of Positive Aging: Seaside Stories
Amia Lieblich

The Ethics of Storytelling: Narrative Hermeneutics, History, and the Possible
Hanna Meretoja

Rethinking Thought: Inside the Minds of Creative Scientists and Artists
Laura Otis

The Narrative Complexity of Ordinary Life: Tales from the Coffee Shop
William L. Randall

A New Narrative for Psychology
Brian Schiff

Life and Narrative: The Risks and Responsibilities of Storying Experience
Brian Schiff, A. Elizabeth McKim, and Sylvie Patron

Words and Wounds: Narratives of Exile
Sean Akerman

The Transformative Self: Personal Growth,
Narrative Identity, and the Good Life
Jack Bauer

Navigating Cultural Memory: Commemoration and
Narrative in Postgenocide Rwanda
David Mwambari

Narrative and Mental Health

Reimagining Theory and Practice

Edited by

JARMILA MILDORF, ELISABETH PUNZI, AND
CHRISTOPH SINGER

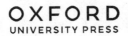

OXFORD
UNIVERSITY PRESS

Oxford University Press is a department of the University of Oxford. It furthers
the University's objective of excellence in research, scholarship, and education
by publishing worldwide. Oxford is a registered trade mark of Oxford University
Press in the UK and certain other countries.

Published in the United States of America by Oxford University Press
198 Madison Avenue, New York, NY 10016, United States of America.

Library of Congress Cataloging-in-Publication Data
Names: Mildorf, Jarmila, editor. | Punzi, Elisabeth, editor. |
Singer, Christoph, 1982– editor.
Title: Narrative and mental health : reimagining theory and practice /
edited by Jarmila Mildorf, Elisabeth Punzi, Christoph Singer.
Description: New York, NY : Oxford University Press, 2023. |
Series: Explorations in narrative psychology |
. Includes bibliographical references and index.
Identifiers: LCCN 2023000001 (print) | LCCN 2023000002 (ebook) |
ISBN 9780197620540 (cloth) | ISBN 9780197620564 (epub) | ISBN 9780197620571
Subjects: LCSH: Narrative therapy. | Psychotherapy and literature.
Classification: LCC RC489.S74 N359 2023 (print) |
LCC RC489.S74 (ebook) | DDC 616.89/165—dc23/eng/20230202
LC record available at https://lccn.loc.gov/2023000001
LC ebook record available at https://lccn.loc.gov/2023000002

DOI: 10.1093/oso/9780197620540.001.0001

Printed by Integrated Books International, United States of America

Contents

Contributors   vii

Narratives and Mental Health: An Introduction   1
  Jarmila Mildorf, Elisabeth Punzi, and Christoph Singer

PART I: THEORETICAL APPROACHES TO RESEARCHING NARRATIVES AND MENTAL HEALTH

1. Imagining an Alternate Psychology   15
   Brian Schiff

2. I Have Many Sick Hearts: Stories About Illness and Life   32
   Jens Brockmeier and Maria I. Medved

3. Narrative Practices in Mental Health: Narrative Therapy
   and the Fictive Stance   45
   Daniel D. Hutto

PART II: CURRENT NARRATIVE PRACTICES IN PSYCHOLOGY AND PSYCHOTHERAPY

4. The Art of Teaching the Art of Listening: An Interview
   Study with University Teachers in Clinical Psychology and
   Social Work   69
   Elisabeth Punzi and Malgorzata Erikson

5. The Aftermath of Silencing the Trauma: A Narrative Case Study   86
   Soly Erlandsson and Nicolas Dauman

6. Writing as Narrative Resource in Therapeutic Settings: Diaries,
   Sketches, Notes   104
   Jarmila Mildorf and Daniel Ketteler

7. What Constitutes Mad Behavior? Changes in the Grand
   Narrative of Disorder Delineated in Psychiatric Diagnoses
   Between 1832 and 1980   123
   Malin Hildebrand Karlén

PART III: NARRATIVES OF AGING, DEMENTIA, AND DEPRESSION

8. How to Narrate a Healthy Life: Life Stories and Mental
   Health in Interviews with the Elderly Aged 90+   153
   Mari Hatavara

9. Narrative Ethics and Dementia: Critical Comments
   and Modifications   174
   Daniela Ringkamp

10. Narrative Experiments with Medical Categorization and
    Normalization in B. S. Johnson's *House Mother Normal*   190
    Sara Strauss

11. Mental Illness Representations in the German Mass Media:
    The Case of Depression   207
    Marina Iakushevich

PART IV: MENTAL HEALTH, LIFE STORYING, TRAUMA, AND ARTISTIC EXPRESSION

12. Narrating Shame in Contemporary Mental Distress Memoirs
    by Female British Authors   231
    Katrin Röder

13. Psychic Relief and Nonnarrative Configurations in Graphic
    Memoirs About Mental Health   257
    Lasse R. Gammelgaard

14. Memory Is a Strange Thing: Science Fiction, Trauma,
    and Time in *Arrival*   273
    Christoph Singer

Index   291

Contributors

Jens Brockmeier
Department of Psychology, Health, and Gender
American University of Paris
Paris, France

Nicolas Dauman
Department of Psychology
University of Poitiers
Poitiers, France

Malgorzata Erikson
School of Public Administration
University of Gothenburg
Gothenburg, Sweden

Soly Erlandsson
Department of Social and Behavioral Studies
University West
Trollhättan, Sweden

Lasse R. Gammelgaard
Department of Communication and Culture
Scandinavian Studies
Aarhus University
Aarhus, Denmark

Mari Hatavara
History, Philosophy, and Literary Studies
Faculty of Social Sciences
Tampere University
Tampere, Finland

Malin Hildebrand Karlén
Department of Psychology
University of Gothenburg
Gothenburg, Sweden

Daniel D. Hutto
School of Liberal Arts
Faculty of Arts, Social Sciences, and Humanities
University of Wollongong
Wollongong, Australia

Marina Iakushevich
Department of German Studies
University of Innsbruck
Innsbruck, Austria

Daniel Ketteler
Department of Health Sciences
Medical School Berlin
Berlin, Germany

Maria I. Medved
Department of Psychology, Health, and Gender
American University of Paris
Paris, France

Jarmila Mildorf
Department of English and American Studies
Paderborn University
Paderborn, Germany

Elisabeth Punzi
Department of Social Work
University of Gothenburg
Gothenburg, Sweden

Daniela Ringkamp
Department of Geriatric Care
Caritas Association for the Diocese of Magdeburg
Magdeburg, Germany

Katrin Röder
Department of English and American
Studies
Humboldt-University Berlin
Berlin, Germany

Brian Schiff
Department of Psychology, Health,
and Gender
American University of Paris
Paris, France

Christoph Singer
Department of English
University of Innsbruck
Innsbruck, Austria

Sara Strauss
Department of English and American
Studies
Paderborn University
Paderborn, Germany

Narratives and Mental Health

An Introduction

Jarmila Mildorf, Elisabeth Punzi, and Christoph Singer

Creative Narrative Approaches to
Mental Health and Distress

This book investigates the nexus between narratives and mental health from an interdisciplinary perspective by staging a dialogue between psychology, social work, psychiatry, and other fields and disciplines such as linguistics, philosophy, and literary and cultural studies. It explores narratives of mental health as intertextual and as embedded in a constantly evolving and transforming web of narratives. The contributions address questions surrounding mental health and distress in individual as well as cultural stories, and also attend to their reciprocal influence. Within clinical mental health practice, it is increasingly emphasized that assessment and interventions need to be based in the clients' narratives. In the United Kingdom, a group of psychologists and users, supported by the British Psychological Society, has developed the Power Threat Meaning Framework (PTMF) (Johnstone et al., 2018). PTMF explicitly focuses on the personal narrative and is thereby an alternative to symptom-based psychiatric diagnostic systems. As such it has gained widespread attention. Moreover, the terms *narrative psychiatry* (Lewis, 2011) and *narrative social work* (Burack-Weiss et al., 2017) have been proposed for holistic mental health care in which creative expressions and meaning making as well as social and cultural contexts and background have a natural place. In this volume, we foreground not only the importance of narrative as a conceptual paradigm for understanding mental health issues but also the significance of literary stories and other artistic forms as alternative sources of knowledge and of expression in an area where humans are or should be at the center of attention. In our view, it is not only the personal narrative that seems important for human development; literature

Jarmila Mildorf, Elisabeth Punzi, and Christoph Singer, *Narratives and Mental Health* In: *Narrative and Mental Health.*
Edited by: Jarmila Mildorf, Elisabeth Punzi, and Christoph Singer, Oxford University Press.
© Oxford University Press 2023. DOI: 10.1093/oso/9780197620540.003.0001

and other creative forms provide opportunities for dealing with affects, relationships, and experiences through our imagination (Cole et al., 2014; Mar & Oatley, 2008). Fictional texts and poetry might support our capacity for empathy and for understanding complex social interactions (LeHunte & Golembiewski, 2014; Mildorf, 2019) because they present us with vicarious experiences of problems and issues surrounding mental health and distress. Literature might also facilitate self-change concerning, for example, affect regulation and self-perception (Djikic & Oatley, 2014). Such change occurs in unique individual ways, and it is not a result of explicit intentions to make the reader think or act in certain ways. On the contrary, the effects of literature and other art forms occur because of their nondirective influence, opening for change by transcending our current self and thus presenting a multitude of possible selves.

Conversely, this book is also interested in the limits and limitations of such an approach. What happens when narratives become normative and an inability to construct narratives is perceived as a somewhat deficient mode of communication? How do culturally dominant forms and genres of narrative structures shape a listener's perception of narratives that fail to adhere to these expectations? How do narratives translate in intercultural and transcultural contexts? All of these questions become especially pertinent in a globalized world where people and goods are constantly on the move, uprooted and relocated. Most importantly it is also their stories and their idea of what a "proper" story is supposed to be in the first place. Additionally, culturally specific ideas of what constitutes mental health and a lack thereof are equally permutable. Consequently, one needs to ask: How do narrative, mental health, and narrative representations of mental health intersect?

Narratives and Mental Health

As already mentioned, mental distress and, conversely, the promotion and sustenance of mental health and well-being pose great challenges in our globalized world. Economic, political, demographic, and cultural changes affect all societies and the individuals living in them. Each year, 38.2% of the population in Europe suffer from mental health problems (Wittchen et al., 2011). Millions of people worldwide experience various forms of mental distress. Some mental health problems are connected to increased longevity and old age, such as forms of dementia, and since there is an aging population in many parts of the world, such problems are also on the rise. Mental health is furthermore affected by trauma caused by disruptive and life-changing events. Global pandemics such as the swine flu that hit the world in 2009 (Davis & Lohm, 2020) or the more recent one caused by COVID-19 are cases in point. Similarly, traumatic experiences of refugees can lead to mental health issues. Their experiences of being uprooted and having to settle into new surroundings and new lives (Bhugra & Gupta, 2010) paradoxically often result in a perceived inability to narrate their disruptive and disrupting experiences (Rotter, 2015). Even though mental health problems are highly idiosyncratic and can manifest themselves in myriads of ways, the medicalization of psychological care as well as of mental health services more generally has led to research approaches that favor evidence-based procedures and to forms of treatment that focus on the application of standardized tests and the prescription of psychopharmacological drugs (Bschor & Kilarski, 2016).

In our economy-driven societies, clinical psychology is predominantly framed as a natural science, and clinical training is, to a greater extent than before, framed in the medical paradigm. Methods and instruments of quantification are privileged over dialogue and understanding (Elkins, 2004; Punzi, 2015, and Chapter 4 in this volume). Thus, questionnaires and diagnostic reference works such as the latest edition of the *Diagnostic and Statistical Manual of Mental Disorders* (DSM-5) or, to a lesser extent, the *International Classification of Diseases* (ICD) have become the standard tools for diagnosis in many countries. Rather than attending to individual persons and their idiosyncratic narratives, such manuals and approaches extrapolate from "typical," standardized cases (Kirschner, 2013). However, knowledge about subjective experiences, processes of meaning making, and lived psychological suffering are expressed through personal—and often disrupted or disorderly—narratives (Frank, 1995; Frie, 2010; Hollway & Jefferson, 2008; Schiff, 2017, and Chapter 1 in this volume). This calls for a change in thinking about mental health, especially by connecting it more assiduously with people's lived experiences. Open-ended approaches are therefore fundamental for understanding clients and their difficulties (Keaney, 2006; Punzi et al., 2014; Shedler et al., 1993).

This book champions and draws upon such open approaches by adopting narrative as a key paradigm. As Elisabeth Punzi and Malgorzata Erikson argue in their contribution (Chapter 4), narrative requires close listening, and professionals working in psychology and social work (both in teaching and clinical practice) consider it important to be given and to give opportunities for narratives to emerge in more dialogical set-ups. Jarmila Mildorf and Daniel Ketteler's case study (Chapter 6) shows the significance of alternative methods such as diary writing and artistic expression to complement more traditional psychotherapeutic methods. The narrative or person-centered interview as a prime methodological tool to learn about how people make sense about themselves and others (Hollan, 2001; Riessman, 2007)—above all in diverse cultural settings—is discussed by Jens Brockmeier and Maria I. Medved in Chapter 2 and underlies the materials analyzed in the chapters by Mari Hatavara (Chapter 8) and Soly Erlandsson and Nicolas Dauman (Chapter 5). Since the participants in this project also include literary and cultural studies scholars, this book goes beyond the purview of narrative psychology and social science disciplines interested in narrative by exploring literary texts (Sara Strauss in Chapter 10), film (Christoph Singer in Chapter 14), graphic memoir (Lasse R. Gammelgaard in Chapter 13), and autobiography (Katrin Röder in Chapter 12) as resources for broadening our understanding of issues surrounding mental health and distress.

Conceptualizations of Narrative

Theoretical approaches and respective new subdisciplines such as narrative psychology, narrative medicine, or the medical humanities have over the past decades also challenged the existing institutional frames of reference and practices in psychiatry, psychology, and medicine (Bleakley, 2015; Charon, 2006; Schiff, 2017, and Chapter 1 in this volume). They foreground especially the significance of narrative as a creative way of sense making and self-expression and its relationship to identity work, remembering, and human communication. Moreover, philosophical debates surrounding the ethical implications of biomedicine and questions concerning personhood, autonomy, and the "good life" have pinpointed the importance of self-reflection and a more critical stance (Ringkamp, Chapter 9 in this volume; Ringkamp & Wittwer, 2018).

The importance of narratives for understanding, treating, and communicating mental health issues also increasingly finds attention in a range of disciplines, not least in the areas of mental health care and mental health recovery (Launer, 1999; Llewellyn-Beardsley et al., 2019; Spector-Mersel & Knaifel, 2018). Indeed, it has been argued many times that narrative is intrinsic to human experience and to the creation of our identities

(Brockmeier & Harré, 2001). From a psychological perspective, it is acknowledged that as human beings we create and recreate a personal narrative that is essential for our capacity to understand ourselves, others, our life world, as well as our past and our future (Bruner, 1987, 1991; Crossley, 2000; Freeman, 2010; Lieblich et al., 1998; McAdams & McLean, 2013). Identity evolves through the personal narrative that the individual consciously and unconsciously creates, binding together many different aspects of the self (McAdams, 1993, 2006). And this narrative is constituted by the many smaller narratives or anecdotes that emerge from our daily experiences and that we tell our friends and family about or simply circulate in our own minds. Thus, narratives bring a sense of order to our world. However, this sense-making function of narrative has also been criticized because not everyone may feel that their life trajectories are narrative in nature (Strawson, 2004). Especially in the context of mental distress or other "disruptions," aspects of linearity and coherence need not necessarily be taken for granted (see Goldie, 2012; Hydén & Brockmeier, 2008; and Chapters 2, 10, and 14 in this volume). The role of silence, of what is not mentioned or verbalized, in narratives about mental distress must also be taken into account (see Chapters 5 and 12 in this volume).

Narratology as an epistemic tool and a heuristic for exploring meaning making has the potential to offer new insights for mental health care. And yet, there is little agreement what precisely constitutes narrative even in narratology (Abbott, 2014), let alone across other disciplines (Hyvärinen, 2017). Ryan (2007) and Jannidis (2003) have called narrative a "fuzzy concept," and Ryan (2005, p. 6) suggested that one needs to distinguish between an artifact "being a narrative" and "possessing narrativity" and thus to focus on *degrees of narrativity* instead, which has also made the concept transferable to many other areas of study. While the minimal definition in narratological inquiry involves a temporal sequence of events that brings about some change ("the king died, and then the queen died"), many narratologists find this unsatisfactory because this resembles merely a report. They therefore add at least questions of cause and effect, motivation, or some other logical connection into the equation ("the king died, and then the queen died of grief") (Forster, 1927; Herman, 2002). Fludernik (1996) introduced the notion of *experientiality* as a key defining feature of narrative—that is, that narratives must offer a perspective that orients the action and that gives recipients a sense of how the story world is experienced. Herman (2009), in his *Basic Elements of Narrative*, resumes this idea and links it to the cognitive-psychological term of *qualia* or "what it is like," while also talking about story world disruption as one key feature.

To view narrative as an essential means to get across to others an idea of what certain experiences were like is useful for applications in mental health care because it is often incisive life experiences that lead to mental health problems. Likewise, having narrative at one's disposal to talk about what one's mental health difficulties feel like is of equal importance although, as we saw, mental distress may precisely make it difficult or even impossible to access seemingly paradigmatic narrative structures. Moreover, the role of narratives can be extended to include not only a wider social and cultural perspective that emphasizes narratives as a basic form for human communication and action (Habermas, 1986; Ricoeur, 1992) but also as a cultural-ideological tool used for the creation and perpetuation of dominant master narratives (Lyotard, 1984). This is particularly relevant when thinking about how mental distress is classified, perceived, and dealt with in any given society.

It is important to acknowledge that the current paradigm in Western psychology/psychiatry is also subject to a master narrative prevalent at this historical juncture and that it has called forth counternarratives such as alternative methods for treatment. Such master narratives are subject to change over time, and so are definitions of mental distress as well as approaches to their treatment (see Chapter 7 by Malin Hildebrand Karlén in this volume). In fact, even notions of narrative do change over time and in different cultural contexts. So, when looking at it from one's current (temporal and cultural) vantage point, there is a danger of reducing the concept of narrative to a static theoretical frame rather than acknowledging its dynamic and historically changeable nature. The volatility and mutability of narratives of mental health become especially interesting when we regard the reciprocal interplay between individual and cultural narratives of mental health.

Chapter Outline

This book, while anchored in the field of psychology, thus offers a forum for cross-disciplinary and interdisciplinary debate regarding the nexus between narratives and mental health. The sections of this book provide different angles, and the thematic structure of the anthology is as follows.

Part I, "Theoretical Approaches to Researching Narratives and Mental Health," comprises three chapters by eminent scholars in the fields of psychology and philosophy who explore theoretical questions concerning narrative methodologies in psychology and psychotherapy today. In Chapter 1 Brian Schiff discusses the importance of a paradigm shift in psychology towards an even stronger narrative psychology. He highlights the misunderstanding that is inherent in quantitative approaches: that they can contribute to explanations of what mental health problems or distress are like for individuals. Focusing on generalizability and mean values, such approaches suggest that they capture real phenomena, while in fact they abstract from lived experience. It is a qualitative and especially a narrative approach that allows room for the exploration of an individual person's actual experience of mental distress, Schiff argues, expanding work from his book-length study (Schiff, 2017).

In Chapter 2 Jens Brockmeier and Maria I. Medved take the narrative interview under closer scrutiny, arguing for more cultural sensitivity concerning people's narrative practices. Their examples of stories about health and illness told by indigenous women in a Canadian reservation show that beliefs about causes of illness are steeped in cultural ways of living and world making and are also negotiated in narratives about self. To understand such processes of meaning making, one needs to attend to the cultural narratives feeding into the personal ones.

In Chapter 3 Daniel D. Hutto discusses narrative approaches to psychotherapy and, more specifically, Australian-based Narrative Therapy from a philosophical perspective and demonstrates its conceptual conundrums and potential shortcomings because it is based on the expectation that clients tell the "truth" and that the therapy can offer alternative narratives that are sometimes resented by clients. To address these challenges, Hutto suggests to "go fictive"—that is, to recognize the creative potential in narratives and thus to allow for more flexibility in expectations concerning what narratives represent and "do" in therapy.

Part II, "Current Narrative Practices in Psychology and Psychotherapy," discusses current approaches in psychological and psychiatric practice and offers specific case studies. In Chapter 4 Elisabeth Punzi and Malgorzata Erikson explore the views of psychology and social work teachers about their own teaching and clinical practices and their endorsement of dialogical approaches that allow for narratives to emerge. Their findings suggest that more room for dialogue and narrative is seen as desirable by psychologists and social workers and is experienced as helpful in teaching contexts but that this view is sometimes not verbalized openly because of the predominance of evidence-based, quantitative approaches in clinical practice and research.

In Chapter 5 Soly Erlandsson and Nicolas Dauman present a case study of an elderly woman suffering from tinnitus who, in the course of her psychotherapy, managed to open up about being raped as a young woman. Their case study demonstrates how giving time and room for narratives can allow clients to reinterpret physical manifestations of trauma and to come to terms with difficult situations that may even be perceived as life-threatening.

In Chapter 6 Jarmila Mildorf and Daniel Ketteler explore the usefulness of diaries and notes in psychotherapeutic treatment in the specific case of a client who overcame a severe state of depression and now continues to use his diary as a means of self-expression and self-exploration.

In Chapter 7 Malin Hildebrand Karlén offers a detailed diachronic outline of how the perception and conceptualization of "mad" behavior changed from the nineteenth to the twentieth century. She critically reflects on psychiatric diagnoses from a meta-perspective, reminding us that any cultural practice—and psychiatric treatment can also be considered one such practice—is determined by what is considered "normal" and "deviant" at any given time. She thus also analyzes the underlying cultural narratives that eventually shape treatment and client care.

In Part III, "Narratives of Aging, Dementia, and Depression," Mari Hatavara (Chapter 8) investigates self-narratives told by elderly people as part of a Finnish research project exploring living to an old age. Her contrastive narratological analysis of two narratives shows that there may be discrepancies between the "story" and "discourse" sides of those narratives (i.e., the *what* and the *how*), suggesting that storytellers' narrative *practices* may be part and parcel of their resilience or lack thereof when it comes to mental distress and well-being.

Daniela Ringkamp's contribution (Chapter 9) follows on from Hutto's philosophical discussion to look at the usefulness and applicability of narrative as a philosophical concept. Her focus is on narrative and personhood in connection with dementia, and she critically addresses the suggestion that someone's life story may be continued by family and caregivers.

Old age and representations of mental health issues like dementia are also at the center of Sara Strauss' chapter (Chapter 10). She discusses B. S. Johnson's novel *House Mother Normal*, showing how evaluations of mental "illness" and "normality" are subtly inverted and called into question by this text.

In Chapter 11 Marina Iakushevich discusses both master or "grand" narratives and narratives of personal experience surrounding mental health and distress in Germany by looking specifically at narrative discourses about depression as can be found in newspapers and other media. Applying linguistic analysis to metaphorical language and grammatical constructions, the chapter illustrates the extent to which conceptualizations of depression are subject to culture-specific imagery and convey an ideology about mental health and well-being currently prevalent in Western societies.

Part IV, "Mental Health, Life Storying, Trauma, and Artistic Expression," brings together chapters that highlight the contribution that artistic or imaginative narrative forms of expression such as literary illness memoirs, novels, and graphic novels can make to discourses on mental health and distress. The chapters in this section illustrate how these art forms offer unique insights into mental distress by providing perspectives that are not otherwise available in real life or by using their aesthetic-affective potential to indirectly point to underlying, hidden, or simply "inexpressible" aspects.

In Chapter 12 Katrin Röder investigates the complex dynamics of presentations of shame in Joanne Limburg's *The Woman Who Thought Too Much* and Amanda Green's *My Alien Self: My Journey Back to Me*. These autobiographical texts offer their authors spaces of freedom for expressing in quasi-literary form what would otherwise be exceedingly difficult to verbalize. The article is particularily interested in the role of mental distress memoirs in the problematization and questioning of stigma related to mental distress.

In Chapter 13 Lasse R. Gammelgaard discusses graphic memoirs of mental distress and shows how they offer means of expression not only through narrative but also through their nonnarrative or poetic features. He thus broadens the view of the potential healing powers of artistic expression in *any* shape and format, while also implicitly criticizing the dominance of a narrative paradigm in disciplines such as the medical humanities.

Christoph Singer closes the volume with Chapter 14, a discussion of the science fiction film *Arrival*, which uses unconventional presentations of time to accommodate a trauma narrative. Singer argues that in challenging viewers, this and other films like it stimulate reflection on the impossibility of narrating traumatic experience. Like Gammelgaard, Singer thus also offers a critical perspective on a narrative paradigm that champions coherence and linearity.

Generally speaking, the volume brings together contributions that address broader narrative discourses and discursive constructions of mental well-being and mental health issues in public arenas (i.e., at the societal and cultural levels) as well as individual and personal stories of narrative distress. It demonstrates that those micro and macro levels must be considered in tandem and must be understood as conglomerations of mutually influential and dynamic processes if we want to form a better idea of what constitutes mental health and distress and how people make sense of their often conflicting experiences. Mental health and distress are not opposite poles but often overlap in the course of a person's lifetime. They are also extremely subjective categories that are negotiated in various contexts. Narrative, by attending to individual lived experience and by allowing multiple perspectives, and other forms of expression, including artistic or creative ones, are therefore best suited to explore the complexities in mental health and distress and the interplay between the culture and the individual therein.

References

Abbott, H. P. (2014). Narrativity. In P. Hühn, J. Pier, W. Schmid, & J. Schönert (Eds.), *The living handbook of narratology*. Hamburg University. https://www-archiv.fdm.uni-hamburg.de/lhn/node/27.html

Bhugra, D., & Gupta, S. (Eds.). (2010). *Migration and mental health*. Cambridge University Press.

Bleakley, A. (2015). *Medical humanities and medical education: How the medical humanities can shape better doctors*. Routledge.

Brockmeier, J., & Harré, R. (2001). Narrative: Problems and promises of an alternative paradigm. In J. Brockmeier & D. Carbaugh (Eds.), *Studies in narrative. Narrative and identity: Studies in autobiography, self and culture* (pp. 39–58). John Benjamins.

Bruner, J. (1987). *Actual minds, possible worlds*. Harvard University Press.

Bruner, J. (1991). The narrative construction of reality. *Critical Inquiry, 18*, 1–21.

Bschor, T., & Kilarski, L. L. (2016). Are antidepressants effective? A debate on their efficacy for the treatment of major depression in adults. *Expert Review of Neurotherapeutics, 16*, 367–374.

Burack-Weiss, A., Lawrence, L. S., & Mijangos, L. B. (2017). *Narrative in social work practice: The power and possibility of story*. Columbia University Press.

Charon, R. (2006). *Narrative medicine: Honoring the stories of illness*. Oxford University Press.

Cole, T. R., Carson, R. A., & Carlin, N. S. (2014). *Medical humanities: An introduction*. Cambridge University Press.

Crossley, M. L. (2000). *Introducing narrative psychology: Self, trauma and the construction of meaning*. Open University Press.

Davis, M., & Lohm, D. (2020). *Pandemics, publics and narrative*. Oxford University Press.

Djikic, M., & Oatley, K. (2014). The art in fiction: From indirect communication to changes of the self. *Psychology of Aesthetics, Creaticity, and the Arts, 8*, 498–505.

Elkins, D. N. (2004). The deep poetic soul: An alternative vision of psychotherapy. *The Humanistic Psychologist, 32*, 76–102.

Fludernik, M. (1996). *Towards a Natural Narratology*. Routledge.

Forster, E. M. (1927) *Aspects of the novel*. Edward Arnold.

Frank, A. W. (1995). *The wounded storyteller*. University of Chicago Press.

Freeman, M. (2010). *Hindsight: The promise and peril of looking backward*. Oxford University Press.

Frie, R. (2010). A hermeneutics of exploration: The interpretive turn from Bingswanger to Gadamer. *Journal of Theoretical and Philosophical Psychology, 30*, 79–93.

Goldie, P. (2012). *The mess inside: Narrative, emotion, and the mind*. Oxford University Press.

Habermas, J. (1986, 1991). *The theory of communicative action, Vol. I–II*. Polity Press.

Herman, D. (2002). *Story logic: Problems and possibilities of narrative*. University of Nebraska Press.

Herman, D. (2009). *Basic elements of narrative*. Wiley.

Hollan, D. (2001). Developments in person-centered ethnography. In C. C. Moore, H. F. Mathews, & N. Quinn (Eds.), *The psychology of cultural experience* (pp. 48–67). Cambridge University Press.

Hollway, W., & Jefferson, T. (2008). The free association narrative method. In L. Given (Ed.), *The Sage encyclopedia of qualitative research methods* (pp. 296–315). Sage.

Hydén, L. C., & Brockmeier, J. (Eds). (2008). *Health, illness, and culture: Broken narratives*. Routledge.

Hyvärinen, M. (2017). Foreword: Life meets narrative. In B. Schiff, A. E. McKim, & S. Patron (Eds.), *Life and narrative: The risks and responsibilities of storying experience* (pp. ix–xxv). Oxford University Press.

Jannidis, F. (2003). Narratology and narrative. In T. Kindt & H.-H. Müller (Eds.). *What is narratology? Questions and answers regarding the status of a theory* (pp. 35–54). De Gruyter.

Johnstone, L., Boyle, M., Cromby, J., Dillon, J., Harper, D., Kinderman, P., Longden, E., Pilgrim, D., & Read, J. (2018). *The Power Threat Meaning Framework: Towards the identification of patterns in emotional distress, unusual experiences and troubled or troubling behavior, as an alternative to functional psychiatric diagnosis*. British Psychological Society.

Keaney, F. (2006). Assessment and screening. *Psychiatry, 5*, 431–436.

Kirschner, S. R. (2013). Diagnosis and its discontents: Critical perspectives on psychiatric nosology and the DSM. *Feminism & Psychology, 23*, 10–28.

Launer, J. (1999). A narrative approach to mental health in general practice. *British Medical Journal, 318*, 117–119.

LeHunte, B., & Golembiewski, J. A. (2014). Stories have the power to save us: A neurological framework for the imperative to tell stories. *Arts and Social Sciences Journal, 5*, 73–76.

Lewis, B. (2011). *Narrative psychiatry: How stories can shape clinical practice*. John Hopkins University Press.

Lieblich, A., Tuval-Mashiach, R., & Zilber, T. (1998). *Narrative research: Reading, analysis, and interpretation*. Sage.

Llewellyn-Beardsley, J., Rennick-Egglestone, S., Callard, F., Crawford, P., Farkas, M., Hui, A., Manley, D., McGranahan, R., Pollock, K., Ramsay, A., Sælør, K. T., Wright, N., & Slade, M. (2019). Characteristics of mental health recovery narratives: Systematic review and narrative synthesis. *PLoS One, 14*(3), e0214678.

Lyotard, F. (1984/1979). *The postmodern condition*. Manchester University Press.

Mar, R. A., & Oatley, K. (2008). The function of fiction is the abstraction and simulation of social experience. *Perspectives on Psychological Science, 3*, 173–192.

McAdams, D. P. (1993). *The stories we live by: Personal myths and the making of the self*. Guilford.

McAdams, D. P. (2006). The problem of narrative coherence. *Journal of Constructivist Psychology, 19*, 109–125.

McAdams, D. P., & McLean, K. C. (2013). Narrative identity. *Current Directions in Psychological Science, 22*(3), 233–238.

Mildorf, J. (2019). Why poetry matters: Defamiliarization and perspective in poetry. In F. Steger & K. Fürholzer (Eds.), *Lyrik und Medizin* (pp. 199–212). Winter.

Punzi, E. (2015). "These are the things I may never learn from books": Clinical psychology students' experiences of their development of clinical wisdom. *Reflective Practice, 16*, 347–370.

Punzi, E. H., Tidefors, I., & Fahlke, C. (2014). Excessive sexual activities among male clients in substance abuse treatment: An interview study. *Mediterranean Journal of Clinical Psychology, 2*, 1–16.

Ricoeur, P. (1992). *Oneself as another*. Chicago University Press.

Riessman, C. K. (2007). *Narrative methods for the human sciences*. Sage.

Ringkamp, D., & Wittwer, H. (Eds.) (2018). *Was ist Medizin? Der Begriff Medizin und seine ethischen Implikationen*. Karl Alber.

Rotter, R. (2015). Waiting in the asylum determination process: Just an empty interlude? *Time and Society, 25*(1), 1–22.

Ryan, M.-L. (2005). On the theoretical foundations of transmedial narratology. In. J.C. Meister (Ed.), *Narratology beyond literary criticism: Mediality, disciplinarity* (pp. 1–23). De Gruyter.

Ryan, M.-L. (2007). Toward a definition of narrative. In D. Herman (Ed.), *The Cambridge companion to narrative* (pp. 22–35). Cambridge University Press.

Schiff, B. (2017). *A new narrative for psychology*. Oxford University Press.

Shedler, J., Mayman, M., & Manis, M. (1993). The illusion of mental health. *American Psychologist, 48*, 1117–1131.

Spector-Mersel, G., & Knaifel, E. (2018). Narrative research on mental health recovery: Two sister paradigms. *Journal of Mental Health, 27*(4), 298–306. doi:10.1080/09638237.2017.1340607

Strawson, G. (2004). Against narrativity. *Ratio, VII*, 428–452.

Wittchen, H. U., Jacobi, F., Rehm, J., Gustavsson, A., Svensson, M., Jönsson, B., Olesen, J., Allgulander, C., Alonso, J., Faravelli, C., Fratiglioni, L., Jennum, P., Liebe, R., Maercker, A., van Os, J., Preisig, M., Salvador-Carulla, L., Simon, R., & Steinhausen, H-C. (2011) The size and burden of mental disorders and other disorders of the brain in Europe 2010. *European Neuropsychopharmacology, 21*, 655–679.

PART I

THEORETICAL APPROACHES TO RESEARCHING NARRATIVES AND MENTAL HEALTH

1

Imagining an Alternate Psychology

Brian Schiff

In this chapter I present what I view to be the essential argument for how a narrative perspective on psychology can contribute to our understanding of mental illness. The argument pivots on the conceptual problem posed by studying experience using the standard research practices of quantitative psychology. However, my ambitions are not methodological but, in fact, theoretical—arriving at dynamic, process-oriented descriptions of mental illness in which meaning making is central.

Of course, method and theory are intertwined and our theoretical understanding of a particular phenomenon can be enhanced or constrained by the methodological tools that we employ. A useful, nuanced, and complex understanding of the experience and meaning of illness, mental or physical, must rely upon grounded observations and descriptions of the phenomenon itself, which can only be provided through the theoretical and methodological tools of narrative.

The Conceptual Problem

In the discipline of psychology, theory has always been a contested space. An easy illustration of this fact is that the world's largest association of psychologists, the American Psychological Association, houses a stunning array of divisions—54 in total. Although there is overlap and conversation across many divisions, several distinct and, indeed, incommensurable ontological positions on human beings can be discerned that essentially function as disciplines in their own right, what are sometimes referred to as perspectives on psychology.

Interestingly, this absence of an overarching theoretical understanding of human psychology actually masks a deeper variety of unity—a unity in the methods that psychologists use in their research. Psychologists, often, do not

Brian Schiff, *Imagining an Alternate Psychology* In: *Narrative and Mental Health*. Edited by: Jarmila Mildorf, Elisabeth Punzi, and Christoph Singer, Oxford University Press. © Oxford University Press 2023.
DOI: 10.1093/oso/9780197620540.003.0002

share the same theories about why persons act, think, or feel the way they do or even a common conception of the nature of human nature. However, they are quite clear about the kinds of methods that should count as psychological research.

Curiously, mainstream psychology is methodologically unified around so-called psychological variables. Abstract and quantified measures intended to depict and fix psychological phenomena, variables are the main preoccupation and product of academic psychology. Our journals are filled with variables, strategies for measuring them, descriptions of their properties, and sophisticated statistical analyses of their relationship with other variables. Institutionalized in the mid-twentieth century and established throughout the whole of the discipline, variable-centered research is the common metric for studying *all* psychological problems (Danziger, 1997).

For those outside of the discipline, it is especially important to stress this point, which is the exact opposite of psychology's commonsense representation: Disciplinary psychology is not concerned with the study of persons, their experience, or how they understand the world. Above all else, psychologists are concerned with variables. For the mainstream, variable-centered research is the *standard practice*. It is the one and only way of doing psychological science.

I want to stress that there is nothing inherently wrong with studying variables. For certain research questions, such as those focused on population-level preferences or the effectiveness of an experimental manipulation, variable-centered methods are often the most appropriate and efficient choice. The problem is that not all psychological questions, or even the most crucial ones, are answerable using variable-centered methods. Strangely enough, psychology's method of choice is not equipped to observe how psychological phenomena play out in the thoughts, experiences, and reflections of persons (Schiff, 2017).

In the standard practice, researchers begin from the premise that they are investigating psychological attributes or qualities—how persons think, feel, or interpret action—but quickly move to the formulation of variables in order to represent how these qualities work at the psychological level of analysis. The procedures for defining and measuring variables are rigorously outlined in the researcher's operational definitions, which follow strict protocols to achieve acceptable reliability and validity. Variables are then, usually, measured on individuals—persons fill out surveys or are observed in experimental settings. After data collection, their responses are analyzed statistically at the level of the group.

As a description of the group, there is no conceptual problem—indeed, group-level patterns are exactly what such analyses are designed to describe. The trouble begins when researchers attempt to move back from the group to the level of the person and their psychological experience. But, going back to the person is impossible: Group-level statistics, describing the relationship between variables in the group, are not and cannot be a model for a person's psychological experience (Lamiell, 2003, 2019).

Yet, habitually, and incorrectly, researchers imbue variables with agency *as if* they exist in a psychological relationship in the person rather than a statistical relationship in the group and *as if* these variables interacted with or affected each other. They don't. The relationship between variables is merely a statistical one observed in the pattern of results across the group. But, researchers make the specious move of applying the findings from the group level to the person. If the relationship exists at the level of the group, then, in some measure, it is fallaciously supposed to exist in the person (Lamiell, 2003, 2019). However, we have no basis for knowing *if* they are related on the psychological level because we have not observed it. The method of analysis did not probe into the connective fiber of how persons tie together thoughts and experiences that might have led to the scores discovered on this variable and that variable. This is a succinct description of the profound conceptual problem at the heart of psychology.

It is important to note that the problem is not remediable with the introduction of mediating and moderating variables or more complex methods of statistical analysis. It is trenchant and represents the most devastating logical oversight of contemporary psychology, affecting survey and experimental work in all branches of the discipline. Rather than dealing with the workings of psychological phenomena, researchers are left with decontextualized and disembodied fragments without a good sense of how psychological life actually functions.

This is exactly where narrative methods can make a substantial contribution to psychological knowledge. Narrative methods can, indeed, reach the psychological level and can do so in a way that is scientifically credible, offering the opportunity for the development of complex theories about how persons interpret experience, self, and world.

Delusional Variables

I want to go beyond an abstract discussion of psychological methods and get to a concrete case. This is the best way to appreciate the conceptual problem in mainstream psychology and the unique contribution that a narrative perspective can make to the understanding of psychological phenomena such as mental illness. As a concrete example, I want to compare and contrast a quantitative approach to the study of delusions in schizophrenia (Phalen et al., 2017) with a personal account of the experience of delusions (Zelt, 1981).

Before critiquing Phalen et al.'s (2017) research, it is important to note that I am criticizing the form of the argument and not the research itself. The problems that I document are ubiquitous in psychological research. In fact, the high quality of Phalen et al.'s (2017) research, including the accessibility of the writing and analysis, actually makes such a critique possible.

Conceptually, Phalen et al.'s (2017) study is interested in the functioning of persons diagnosed with schizophrenia and, specifically, the consequences of persecutory delusions on aspects of their social functioning. Although it is logical to suppose that false and intrusive paranoid beliefs would decrease the ability to form and sustain social relationships, Phalen et al. (2017) note that across several studies, this relationship has been inconsistent. As they write: "One possible explanation for this paradox is that persecutory delusions do influence social function, but only under certain conditions. In other words, it may be that persecutory delusions only affect social functioning when there are other deficits present" (p. 66).

Their answer to this "paradox" is that some other factor, Theory of Mind (ToM), moderates (in plain language, partially stands in between) persecutory delusions and social functioning. In other words, more sophisticated and elaborate methods of reasoning about the thoughts and motives of other persons could serve to soften the negative impact of damaging persecutory thinking on social relationships.

> There would seem to be negative synergy between ToM deficits and persecutory beliefs such that persecutory beliefs might deeply impact social functioning when individuals lack the ability to come up with any kinds of ideas about the intentions and mental states of others which might at least partially titrate persecutory ideation. (Phalen et al., 2017, p. 66)

One should note that their theoretical model addresses the psychological level of analysis. Their theory pertains to how persons reason about others and how this reasoning might be related to other aspects of their functioning. Perhaps the theoretical model is simplistic, but it is interesting and does, as the researchers note, point to potential concrete clinical applications treating schizophrenic patients. But, as we will see, they never get there, and it is simply impossible to do so given the design of their research into the problem.

In a sample of 88 persons diagnosed with schizophrenia and schizoaffective disorder during a nonacute phase of their illness, Phalen et al. (2017) operationally define and measure a number of variables designed to test their theory. I will concentrate on the three central variables that they measure: Persecutory Delusions, ToM, and Social Functioning.

Persecutory Delusions was assessed with an item from the Positive and Negative Syndrome Scale (PANSS) on suspiciousness/persecution. The item, like the scale, is based upon both observer ratings and an interview. The item is rated "from (1) an absence of any indication of unusual suspiciousness of other people to (7) a network of systematized persecutory delusions that dominate the patient's thinking, social relations and behavior" (p. 67). *ToM* was measured with the Hinting Test, a measure "that presents participants with a brief story and then instructs the participant to make a judgment about the intentions of one of the fictional characters on the basis of 'hints' embedded within the story" (p. 66). Finally, *Social Functioning* was assessed with the Social Functioning Scale, a self-report measure that asks participants to respond to questions about their engagement and activities in a variety of settings including friendships, family, work, and their ability to live independently.

It is important to note that each of these variables was assessed separately and that statistical relationships were calculated at the level of the group. Their statistical analysis of the relationship between these variables, in the form of a regression analysis, showed that Persecutory Delusions are strongly, and negatively, related to Social Functioning ($\beta = -20.83$, $t = -3.94$, $p < 0.0002$). Also, they find that, when predicting Social Functioning, there is a significant interaction between Persecutory Delusions and ToM ($\beta = 2.43$, $t = 2.33$, $p < 0.02$). In a follow-up analysis, they document that for those participants with the most developed ToM, measured by the highest scores on the Hinting Task (the top 22nd percentile), Persecutory Delusions were unrelated to Social Functioning. The analysis leads Phalen et al. (2017) to conclude:

> Consistent with predictions, mental state reasoning—an aspect of theory of mind pertaining to the ability to detect or infer others' knowledge or desires . . . *attenuated the effect* of persecutory delusions on social functioning. For participants with poor mental state reasoning abilities, more severe delusions of persecution were associated with significant deficits in social functioning. However, for participants with relatively strong mental state reasoning abilities, persecutory delusions *did not negatively impact* social functioning. (p. 68, my emphasis)

Phalen et al.'s (2017) conclusion is warranted if we remain on the level of the statistical relationship in the group. Although far from perfect, the research provides convincing evidence of a statistical relationship between the variables.

But, as I have italicized above, we are likely to interpret these statistical relationships in ways unwarranted by the analysis. Has ToM "*attenuated the effect*" (p. 68) of persecutory delusions on social functioning? Yes, in a statistical sense. But we read this finding *as if* these two variables have interacted on the psychological level, which the research does not comment upon.

Participants were rated on the extent of their Persecutory Delusions. They were also rated on their performance on the Hinting Task. Similarly, they filled out a questionnaire on Social Functioning. Then, looking at the group as a whole, the researchers discovered a statistical relationship in the patterns of results. In a statistical sense, the variable, ToM, attenuated the effect of a second variable, Persecutory Delusions, on a third variable, Social Functioning. But we have no idea how or *if* it attenuated anything on the psychological level of analysis for any given person. And there is no evidence in this regard and no possible conclusions that can be drawn.

What about those participants with the highest scores on the Hinting Task—in other words, those participants with the most sophisticated understandings of others' intentions and beliefs? Can we say, as Phalen et al. (2017) do, that "persecutory delusions did not negatively impact social functioning?" (p. 68). Once again, yes, if we confine ourselves to the statistical relationship on the level of the group. At best, we can say that those participants who performed well on the Hinting Task also rated their Social

Functioning as high. However, on the psychological level, one variable did not impact another variable.

It is us, the interpreters and readers of this research, who, on the basis of the group-level analysis, (mis)place these abstract variables together on the psychological level and begin to weave together a story. Certainly, it is a plausible story: One would suppose that persons with a more complex and accurate reading of other people's mental states would be more prepared to handle schizophrenic delusions when they come along. But there is nothing in the data that actually connects these concepts together psychologically.

Indeed, we should ask: What are the lines that bring together, in the psychological experience of persons, Persecutory Delusions, ToM, and Social Functioning? The connective fiber is missing precisely because we have not studied it. In order to understand how (and *if*) they are connected, we need to bring our research to the level of the person.

In the variable-centered frame, there is no pathway out of this conceptual quagmire toward meaning. But there are viable alternatives to variable-centered research. In particular, a narrative perspective allows us to bring problem and method in direct conversation in order to make observations about how basic psychological phenomena work. By studying persons, one at a time, and closely listening to how they make connections between various aspects of their life experience, researchers can observe the kinds of basic psychological phenomena that Phalen et al. (2017) are interested in but are unable to access and, on that basis, to develop rich theories of the phenomena at play.

First-Person Delusions

The only route to answering the question "How do persecutory delusions influence functioning?" is to focus our attention on a single person in order to discover this person's experience. Narrative research is centered on making visible and open for analysis the interpretations that persons make about self, life, and world.

Although the focus is on interpretations, analysis goes beyond "what" was said and "how" it was said. The job of the researcher is to question and open up the text before us in order to grasp the context of production. Inquiry includes a consideration of the speaker's life circumstances and experience ("who" is speaking) but also questions aspects of developmental and historical time ("when") and the social and cultural space ("where") that frame every interpretative action. Such questions are not a final destination but rather serve as useful starting points into uncovering and describing the dynamics of interpretation and developing theories of "why."

In order to get to the psychological level, I want to take a close look at a single case, David Zelt's (1981) first-person account, "The Messiah Quest," published in *Schizophrenia Bulletin*. His account of a blossoming delusional world in an acute episode of schizophrenia can provide some insight into delusions and functioning. And, it can do so in a way that remains squarely on the psychological level of analysis in order to see the manner in which David presents and manages the development and meaning of his delusions. How do David's persecutory delusions unfold? What are the connections that David makes? What effect does this experience have on his life?

It is important to note that David's narrative is a published account, not an interview—my preferred method of investigation. I didn't have the opportunity to ask David questions and frame the conversation myself. Thus, my analysis is less complete than I might like. But, there are important clues, marked in the text itself, that can be interpreted.

Structurally, the space of David's "first person account" is a fascinating study in itself. David's illness narrative is framed by a bolded "preface" from *Schizophrenia Bulletin*'s editors and an afterword, "comments," from two therapists. The article opens with the words:

> The article that begins below is the fifth in a series of personal accounts to be published in the *Schizophrenia Bulletin*. In describing his account, the author commented: "The viewpoint is solely my consciousness. The substance of every statement and the specific words in many statements actually occurred to me. The third person narrative was chosen to convey a sense of my psychological distance from the experience. This distance was essential for accomplishing growth. I have described my emotions and thoughts as exactly as possible, and in sufficient detail for the reader to follow the sequence of change in thought form and content. In spite of certain passages in the text, I had never previously felt fervently about any religion, religious figure, or telepathy, and I had never felt harassed by the Central Intelligence Agency. The experience described followed many extreme stresses—death of a parent, end of a longtime romantic relationship, and a career change. Before these events, my emotional and social adjustment had been good . . ."

Brief comments by two clinicians who saw the author during different phases of the experience described are appended to his account.

> The *Bulletin* welcomes other contributions from patients, ex-patients, or family members. Our major editorial requirement is that such contributions be clearly written and organized and that a novel or unique aspect of schizophrenia be described, with special emphasis on points that will be important for professionals. Clinicians who see articulate patients, with experiences they believe should be shared, might encourage these patients to submit their articles to the *Bulletin's* new section, *First Person Accounts.*—The Editors (p. 527)

David's story is public and specifically addressed to a group of readers—those of *Schizophrenia Bulletin*—who, one would suppose, are principally researchers in the field of psychiatry. But, as framed by the preface and the name of the section, "First Person Accounts," David's narrative stands outside of the scholarly, scientific voice of the rest of the journal. To their credit, the editors have carved out a space for persons with schizophrenia to make-present and make-known their life experiences of living with mental illness. But it does lead one to wonder: How does the scientific voice of the journal coalesce with the experiences of people living with schizophrenia? What merit does the narrative of David's experience have for the "science" of mental illness? In any case, David's narrative needs to be understood within this context.

We should be aware that, temporally, the reader is given insight into the retrospective nature of the narrative that follows. The story was not written at the height of David's illness but is a polished reconstruction—after the fact. It is also possible that David is not the sole author or editor.

Distance is doubly marked in the text. One lamination is David's choice of the third person for a "first" person account. However, David promises us that he is faithful to the experience itself, he writes, "The substance of every statement and the specific words in many statements actually occurred to me" and further "I have described my experiences as exactly as possible" (p. 527). David is writing from a position later in time. A period of time has passed between the acute phase recounted in the narrative and the time of reflection and writing. His choice of the third person marks the distance between the David then and the David now.

Distance is also marked in the use of a pseudonym, David Zelt. The only footnote in the text reads, "David Zelt is a pseudonym" (p. 527). A critical question for our interpretation is murky: "Who" is David Zelt? The answer can only be partially inferred from the text itself.

After the preface, David begins his story with a key event in his illness narrative—his attendance at a psychology conference:

> A drama that profoundly transformed David Zelt began at a conference on human psychology. David respected the speakers as scholars and wanted their approval of a paper he had written about telepathy. A week before the conference, David had sent his paper "On the Origins of Telepathy" to one speaker, and the other speakers had all read it. He proposed the novel scientific idea that telepathy could only be optimally studied during the process of birth. He believed that the mother and infant have a telepathic bond that begins during delivery and should be studied before stimuli in the outer world significantly influence it. The paper described his observation, in an obstetrics clinic, of the mother and infant's facial expressions. They smiled or cried in parallel during delivery and for several minutes afterward... He hoped this correlate, consistently present at seven births, would be verified for all humans. *David knew that the paper, in reflecting engagement with an esoteric subject, was a signpost of his growing retreat from mundane reality.* (p. 527, my emphasis)

The narrative beginnings of what becomes a full-blown delusional episode are telling. David sends a paper to a psychologist who will be speaking at a conference. Then, David attends the conference. Although we cannot be certain, these seem to be actual events. His paper, on telepathy at birth, David notes, is "esoteric" and he has a sense that it "was a signpost of his growing retreat from mundane reality" (p. 527). One wonders: Is this his retrospective voice, writing the ending into the beginning? Or should we believe David that these were thoughts that "actually occurred" to him at the time? Was he aware of moving away from reality, as he states?

Although the framing of mother–infant relations as "telepathy" is "esoteric," one should note that the thesis of mother–infant attunement is not. There is some fantastical reasoning behind David's proposals, which are one step removed from observable reality. But to say that mothers and babies communicate with each other nonverbally is hardly esoteric; it is a part of mainstream literature in psychology and psychiatry (cf. Stern, 1985). This move, from reasonable to demonstrably less reasonable, from common knowledge to esoteric knowledge, is important because David's account as a whole is one of over-reading or hyper-reading of mundane reality, which moves, in some ways, sensibly from one reasonable premise to the next, but becomes much less reasonable in the process.

Interestingly, in the above passage, the reader is also given some clues for understanding "who" David is that, potentially, orient him professionally in the world of psychology, psychiatry, or the helping professions. The text provides no definitive response to the question of "who" the author is, but we might understand David as an aspiring student in mental health or the medical sciences.

The narrative continues:

> David's paper was viewed as a monumental contribution to the conference and potentially to psychology in general. If scientifically verified, his concept of telepathy, universally present at birth and measurable, might have as much influence as the basic ideas of Darwin or Freud. Each speaker focused on David. By using allusions and nonverbal communication that included pointing and glancing, each illuminated different aspects of David's contribution. Although his name was never mentioned, the speakers enticed David into feeling that he had accomplished something supernatural in writing the paper. (pp. 527–528)

The scene of the taleworld (Young, 2004), where the events are taking place, is still the conference. In that space, David begins to believe that the speakers (at least one of whom he might have sent his paper to) are talking about him. He knows this through "allusions and nonverbal communication," and he also knows that they greatly esteem David's intellect and his work. When reflecting upon the logic of David's thinking, I read this leap as moving one step further along the same pathway of the nonverbal communication of mothers and babies. Mothers and babies communicate telepahtically; therefore, others must too. Furthermore, this communication is directed at him.

Researchers know these false beliefs quite well. Diagnostically, we could say that delusions of reference and delusions of grandeur are taking hold. But, for David, these are logical steps. He is entranced with the idea that there are things said by other—nonverbal—channels. Once again, this is a reasonable idea and one of the classic arguments from Erving Goffman's (1959) seminal work *The Presentation of Self in Everyday Life*. But David becomes wrapped up in the idea and, indeed, overextends and overapplies it, seeing much more than what is there. And these overextensions lead to a series of deductions with only the most tenuous connections underlying them:

> David's sensitivity to nonverbal communication was extreme; he was adept at reading people's minds. His perceptual powers were so developed that he could not discriminate between telepathic reception and spoken language by others. He was distracted by others in a way that he had never been before. It was as if the nonverbal behavior of people interacting with him was a kind of a code. Facial expressions, gestures, and postures of others often determined what he felt and thought. (p. 528)

Once again, nonverbal information can be important information about what people really think. But David begins to believe that he can see and understand a hidden, deeper, meaning—beyond and behind the ordinary—and that these signs can be and, in fact, must be, deciphered. David calls this "the code."

Reading the signs, given off by persons or the environment, feels wonderful when the signs are positive. David is exalted by the world's attention on him as the savior:

> During the next few weeks David came to believe that he was the reborn figure of Jesus Christ and that their spirits were identical. Like Christ, he was constantly in touch with the infinite and the eternal, and lived with a halo around his head that represented unity with God. David believed that he was the only person who could prevent the impending war that would end the world. He would prevent it by loving all humans and never qualifying or compromising his love. (p. 528)

But such signs are extremely painful when read as negative or abusive or accusatory:

> David began to suspect and then perceive that a federal agency was observing him. From a moment of insight explaining many peculiar, recent events in his life, he knew that he had been accused of treason for slandering Americans during his psychotherapy. (p. 529)

David comes to believe that the CIA is observing even his private thoughts and tormenting him "by playing his thoughts aloud and also by making comments and criticisms about his thoughts" (p. 529). Once again, there is a tortured logic to David's thinking, which is fixated on the idea that there are secret messages that need to be deciphered. The signs all point to such a conclusion.

Still, for a period of time, he says that he is able to hold on to a sense of reality.

> David's thought processes and communication with others occurred in two basic ways: One was adapted to the rational realities of others, and the other way—the code—was magical, poetical, and fantastical. The code was used in his continuous struggles with the CIA and sometimes in communication with God. As time went on, the code came to dominate the functioning of his psyche. David never told anyone about the code. (p. 529–530)

It is important to highlight the process—the unfolding descent to these "magical, poetical, and fantastical" ways of interpreting others and his social environment. Until he succumbs. One thought leads to the next thought, which leads to the next:

> Eventually, all aspects of his life came to be influenced by the code. Ordinarily unimportant information from external reality took on new dimensions for him. For example, colors powerfully influenced him. At any given moment wherever David went, colors were used to express judgments about his spirituality. People used the colors of their clothes or cars to express positive or negative views of him . . . David was engulfed by an intrigue on the largest possible scale. Except for the presence of God and the CIA, though, he was lonely and isolated. No one else knew about the code. (p. 530)

In his interpretation, David's ability to hold on to reality disappears. The delusional logic, written on persons and into the environment, is too powerful, and he is left "lonely and isolated" in his fantasy world. He takes on the full-time job of the Messiah—the interpreter of code for the good of all humanity:

> As the Messiah, his psyche mirrored humanity's problems. He struggled against profound powers—Nazism, the CIA, and the self-destructive tendencies of humanity—but he knew that the power of God would

ultimately triumph. David's duty was to fulfill God's ultimate goal—to turn the Earth into a heavenly kingdom. He wanted to do everything he could to reach this goal. In heart and mind, David gave himself fully to his Messiah quest. (p. 531)

These are David's last words in the text.

Structurally, David's version of the story begins with the onset of this acute episode and leaves him at the height of his symptoms. David does not provide further information about his experience after the episode. But comments from two therapists provide additional information, from their positions, about the course of David's illness and a coda—letting us know the outcome. The "First Therapist" comments:

> In time, his critical faculties did work effectively, and one must acknowledge that the outcome has been favorable. The fact that he is well-endowed with high intelligence has, I think, played a vital part in his capacity to steer his episode toward growth and development. (p. 531)

After stating that she met with David on a daily basis, the "Second Therapist" comments:

> There were few people with whom he could share his feelings and ideas. Our meetings, an open exchange between two people, seemed to ameliorate the loneliness of his struggle and perhaps were helpful in the resolution of his struggle. Despite intense involvement with his inner life, he was able to function in the world on a simplified level. Besides taking care of himself, he went out and did things with people and also read. His writing is a demonstration of the usefulness of the experience and reflects his change for the wiser. (p. 531)

From the perspective of these two therapists, we vaguely learn that David's mental state did improve. We also learn, vaguely, that, in the opinion of the first therapist, restoring David's "critical faculties" was part of the resolution. There is also a contrast between David's portrayal of abject isolation during his acute episode and the opinion of the second therapist that he was able to maintain a relationship with her and that "he was able to function in the world on a simplified level" (p. 531).

Conclusions

Admittedly, the end result of my analysis is rather untidy. This is not unexpected. Paying close attention to a single life, we find that psychological phenomena are multifaceted, complex, dense, and, oftentimes, inconsistent. This is not some quirk of schizophrenic narratives but is found in all life stories. Bizarre as David's narrative is, inconsistencies are common features to all life stories and all lives.

Still, the narrative analysis captures a psychological level of human experience that is entirely absent from a variable-centered one, bearing no resemblance to the easily digestible categories and statistics in variable-centered research. Rather, we have a sense of a full-fledged person reflecting on and interpreting their life experience and can better describe in vivid detail the dynamic process of how this person interprets self, world, and others. I hope that is strikingly apparent in the contrasting analyses.

Although David's narrative is truncated and there are many questions that I would like to ask him, he does provide us with access to the unfolding nature of his illness during its acute phase and how he retrospectively understands his illness in the here and now of the early 1980s. His words, albeit imperfectly, show the logic and process of his descent into a complicated structure of delusions, how he arrived at the depths of his delusions, and the consequences of this experience on his life.

In David's narrative, we would be hard pressed to separate Delusions from Persecutory Delusions or Persecutory Delusions from his theory of other minds or from Social Functioning. These concepts, which are so neatly, and artificially, distinct in Phalen et al.'s (2017) research, blend into a complicated and untidy process of human interpretation. In David's narrative, in many ways, they are part and parcel of the same psychological process.

David's delusions begin somewhat innocently. There is some, convoluted, logic behind it. David seems to say that he gets stuck on the idea of extra-real communication. He is enchanted by this idea's magic, and comes to overapply and overextend it to new realms. At the beginning, he says that he has a sense that he is doing this. However, one overextension follows from the previous one, and he loses his sense of being able to manage the flow of ideas. His understanding of others' beliefs and intentions evolves and changes as he steps away from the "rational realities of others" (p. 530).

His delusions become persecutory but do not begin as such. As the code comes to dominate David's reading of the world, he feels increasingly isolated and lonely. David's interpretations provide a detailed model for understanding how he descends into delusional beliefs and the resultant feelings of loneliness and isolation.

For the mainstream, such observations are considered outside the bounds of scientific psychology. At best, they are beginning points that can serve as hunches when moving to a variable-centered model. But it is simply not possible to study the fundamental problems of human psychology (how persons think, feel, and interpret their actions) as statistical relationships between variables. In contrast, this is exactly the level at which a narrative analysis operates, describing how persons, in context, go about the business of making sense of their life experience.

I believe that such rich descriptions, no matter how untidy, can be of enormous scientific value. Effectively employed, narrative analysis can provide the means for observing, as close to the action as possible, the core questions of the discipline. The only way to disclose these fundamental psychological phenomena is to study them by listening to how persons, in their own words, make interpretations connecting aspects of their life experience. In regard to what is most central to the discipline of psychology, narrative can do this, and variable-centered research cannot.

It is true that studying a single person does not permit the kinds of generalizations that psychologists aspire to. Furthermore, I would not submit that my analysis of David's brief first-person account is more than a demonstration of the textured nature of self-interpretation and the theoretical value of closely attending to such interpretations. I cannot say that this is how the delusional world of some or all schizophrenics unfolds. Rather, this is how, according to David, his delusions *did* unfold.

But, more encompassing, nuanced, theories are possible by starting with a single person and adding comparisons and refinements—to discover common interpretative strategies—one by one by one. We could well imagine a more comprehensive study that builds upon this analysis, moving onto other persons, to make visible common ways that persons with schizophrenia describe the onset and course of their delusions and human relationships or other questions on other topics that progress in such a fashion in order to develop more far-reaching theories about psychological experience.

This is the challenge that we have in front of us: to describe and understand the workings of human psychology, one person at a time, and to build a veritable psychology of meaning. In my view, this is the way that scientific psychology is done and the unique contribution that a narrative perspective can make to our understanding of human beings.

References

Danziger, K. (1997). *Naming the mind: How psychology found its language.* Sage.

Goffman, E. (1959). *The presentation of self in everyday life.* Doubleday.

Lamiell, J. T. (2003). *Beyond individual and group differences: Human individuality, scientific psychology, and William Stern's critical personalism.* Sage.

Lamiell, J. T. (2019). *Psychology's misuse of statistics and persistent dismissal of its critics.* Palgrave Macmillan.

Phalen, P. L., Giancarlo, D., Popolo, R., & Lysaker, P. H. (2017). Aspects of Theory of Mind that attenuate the relationship between persecutory delusions and social functioning in schizophrenia spectrum disorders. *Journal of Behavior Therapy and Experimental Psychiatry, 56,* 65–70.

Schiff, B. (2017). *A new narrative for psychology.* Oxford University Press.

Stern, D. N. (1985). *The interpersonal world of the infant: A view from psychoanalysis and developmental psychology.* Basic Books.

Young, K. (2004). Frame and boundary in the phenomenology of narrative. In M. L. Ryan (Ed.), *Narrative across media: The languages of storytelling* (pp. 76–107). University of Nebraska Press.

Zelt, D. (1981). First person account: The Messiah quest. *Schizophrenia Bulletin, 7*(3), 525–531.

2

I Have Many Sick Hearts

Stories About Illness and Life

Jens Brockmeier and Maria I. Medved

What is an "illness story" in contrast to, say, a "normal story" or an "everyday story"—or, shall we say, in contrast to a "health story" or a "healthy story"? Obviously, such distinctions never work when matters are as complex and thorny as narrative and illness, whether biological or psychological, physical or mental. We live in cultural worlds that abound with stories of health and sickness and the many shades in between. Illness, as Susan Sontag (1978) famously remarked, is not *the other*; it is the "night-side of life"; everyone who is born, she went on to say, "holds dual citizenship, in the kingdom of the well and in the kingdom of the sick. Although we all prefer to use only the good passport, sooner or later each of us is obliged, at least for a spell, to identify ourselves as citizens of that other place" (p. 3). We want to argue that the relationship between these two kingdoms and their narrative cultures is even more intricate, so much so that this otherwise compelling picture of the two different realms becomes blurry. Whatever else illness is, it is always interwoven with people's life, experience, and emotion; it is endowed with meaning and sense making and this, as we know, hardly stops at any border. And so are stories, and this is why most of the time both of them, illness and narrative, are too messy to fit clear-cut definitions. This is not a terrain where we can easily draw up demarcations and borderlines.

Illness, Narrative, and the Border Zone in Between

Take the following short narrative. Told by a person we will call Ms. Kelly, it speaks of the life of an Indigenous woman in her forties from Manitoba, one of Canada's provinces. These extracts are from an interview Ms. Kelly gave us when we visited her. We were engaged in a research project studying the ways

Jens Brockmeier and Maria I. Medved, *I Have Many Sick Hearts* In: *Narrative and Mental Health.* Edited by: Jarmila Mildorf, Elisabeth Punzi, and Christoph Singer, Oxford University Press. © Oxford University Press 2023. DOI: 10.1093/oso/9780197620540.003.0003 in which Indigenous women living on reserve experienced their cardiac problems, an issue in the gray zone between the physical and the psychological. Of course, each element of the information just given—Indigenous people, women, living on reserve, cardiac problems, border zone—needs context and explication, which we will provide in a moment. But first consider this.

INTERVIEWER (I): . . . You said that you thought your anxiety problems are related to your childhood, and you know, when you mentioned it, it sounds like it was really difficult at least until seven or eight [years]. Um, how was that connected? Why would that link to anxiety?

MS. KELLY (MS. K): Um, because, um, it all, it all comes together like a puzzle because I've been to a lot of workshops. Like, Dr., was it, Peter Smith, did some workshops here [on reserve] on children and anxiety. So I got to learn through that, how there can be a connection.

I: What was the connection for you?

MS. K: For me? You mean anxiety, and um, the childhood, um, experiences? [. . .] I, I guess I've never thought of it that way. Like I've never really thought about that very, very much, but let me think about it. I think that, um, there were probably fears that I would have had that I can't directly remember, but I could, I could, I could remember a lot of situations we were put in where as a child, a normal child, a child would be afraid.

I: Can you give me one example?

MS. K: Yeah. Um, let me see. My dad, okay, um my dad, drinking, no he, I'm not sure if he was drinking because he didn't go to jail for it. Drinking and driving, no, he wasn't drinking and driving because he didn't go to jail for it. But we were driving down the road, it was late at night. We shouldn't have been driving down the road, we should have been in bed. And, um, there was three people, from what I remember, walking on the road, they were drunk, in the middle of the road, and we ran them over and killed them [laughs]. So, as a child, I think that would be very traumatic.

For many researchers, the genre of the stories they investigate appears as pregiven even before the start of the inquiry. It is a priori defined, narratologically (as a kind or type of story), discursively (as a particular "talk-in-interaction," such as a medical examination or research interview), contextually (through the situation or type of encounter, such as personal, clinical, journalistic, or academic), or paratextually (by the material surrounding the encounter, such as a medical record, recorder, video camera, or notepad). This beforehand definition comprises the genre of illness narratives, a genre somewhere in Sontag's kingdom of the sick. Likewise preset are the subjects and characters of these stories: There are patients, doctors, nurses, and other caregivers and health workers. In classic studies of illness narratives—by Oliver Sacks (1985), Arthur Kleinman (1988), Arthur Frank (1995), and Rita Charon (2006), to only name a few—the four defining criteria mentioned (narratological, discursive, contextual, and paratextual) are complemented by a fifth. This is the clearly marked poor health status of at least one of the protagonists—that is, the patient or sick person. Countless novels, reports, reportages, and accounts on health and illness clearly identify the type of sickness they deal with, as well as the genre in which the story is told. Another classic case is the medical doctor who translates wide-ranging experiential and phenomenological accounts of the patient into a medical text that constitutes the person as a patient (Aaslestad, 2009). Even the stated objective of the traditional case history, often more open to experiential and narrative detail, revolves around the diagnostic identification of the disease or disorder that is supposed to underlie the surface of symptoms and the patient's subjective narrative version of it (Abel, 2021; Hurwitz, 2017). Moreover, if we take into account the increasing institutionalization of illness narratives as a genre in medical training and education, it is not surprising that the at first sight successful application of the narrative turn to the world of health and illness (as demonstrated, e.g., in much detail in Charon et al., 2017), has tended "toward standardization and reductionism" of the very idea of illness narrative (Le et al., 2017).

Unmistakably, Ms. Kelly's narrative represents a different genre. In fact, it also reflects a different narrative environment, as narrative sociologists Jaber Gubrium and James Holstein (2008) call it. In this context, illness appears more as an aspect, a concomitant phenomenon, as one element (and not necessarily the most crucial one) of a life—more than this, of a community. Taken in isolation, it might not even be clear if the phenomenon at stake (at stake, that is, for the researcher) is to be called illness at all, let alone a specific illness.

It is, in fact, a problem for the treatment of many Indigenous women that they do not conceive of their heart issue as a specific and well-defined disease for which there exists established medical treatments; many women, for example, reportedly do not take their medication regularly (Garro, 1988). It is even questionable whether they themselves view and label their stories as illness narratives. Of course, this phenomenon is also known from other cultural communities; patients' narratives and the findings of medical diagnostics are interpreted quite differently by involved protagonists; these might include, besides the patient, medical personnel and other caregivers, family members, friends, social networks, and researchers.

The stories Ms. Kelly told about her heart issue are stories of this messy kind. Instead of an illness narrative, she shared with us stories about her life and her life world, everyday stories about psychological, social, and political events, experiences from all registers of life. Ultimately, as we will later explain, she told us stories about the consequences of colonialism, past and present, but not illness narratives in any strict sense—although this was the original focus of our research, a rather narrow focus for what she had to tell us, as we finally came to understand. For her, the drama of her illness was inextricably fused with the drama of her life, with no inherent borderline in between.

Illness and the Dramas of Life

It is true that there was the ongoing theme of the sick heart or "my many sick hearts," as Ms. Kelly put it at one point, which, however, was not least due to the questions she was asked. The interview—and even earlier, the lengthy process of getting in touch with her, being allowed to go onto the reserve, the preparatory conversations and arrangements—started out with a well-outlined idea of cardiac disease, and it was this idea that we, the researchers, imposed on the entire narrative environment, including the interview itself, of which we quoted a few turns. What Ms. Kelly brought up as her "anxiety problem" was an attempt to answer the question of what, in her view, were the factors that might have caused or influenced her cardiovascular troubles. And even this answer, as she indicated, was one suggested to her by a certain Dr. Smith, the psychologist or psychiatrist who in the past "did some workshops here on children and anxiety." Before those workshops—and, we might assume, before our visits to her reserve—she "never really thought about that very, very much," as she put it.

From a critical point of view—that is, an interview-critical point of view—it is perhaps less remarkable that Ms. Kelly, a member of the Cree First Nation, in talking about herself uses common Western narrative models and storylines that have little to do with traditional aboriginal ideas of life and illness (like in the extract about the psychotherapeutic models of Dr. Smith). The interesting point is, rather, that these models do not keep her from describing the troubles of her life, including her heart disease, as embedded in the drastic reality of living on reserve. Independently from the Western distinction between the sick and the healthy, these dramas unfold in a reality in which "illness" is inseparably intermingled with life—both in terms of the strength and resilience of the community and in terms of a life lived and experienced under degrading living conditions, with poverty, alcoholism, death, and deadly crime, as the stunned interviewer learns almost in passing, in a brief clause. An amalgam of illness, its social and cultural roots and consequences, and the attempt to cope with it, this story challenges all apparent experiential and conceptual borderlines.

Whereas Ms. Kelly sticks to her wide social and cultural perspective, her interviewer continues to pursue her clinical interests that, in the quoted sequence, revolve around the connection of heart disease to anxiety and childhood. The tension between these two perspectives, that of Ms. Kelly and that of the researcher, marks the various parts of the interview as well as the discursive or conversational dynamics of the entire encounter. It also underlies the layered structure of Ms. Kelly's narratives. What are these layers? To begin with, the interviewer, as already noted, has a clear monothematic idea of what she wants to hear: the narrativized experience of the interviewee's cardiac problems, an experience that reflects, to put it in Western medical terms, the fact that Ms. Kelly has high blood pressure and is on the cusp of having a heart attack; in other words, she is at high-risk with all elements of metabolic syndrome—including a mother who died from a heart attack. Also, she suffers from anxiety episodes, being often under the impression that her heart is failing. However, with this diagnostic picture in mind, what the interviewer gets is stories that interlace various kinds of experiences reaching far beyond her concept of illness and her related research focus. These stories speak about experiences of a life that is lived, in many respects, under tough conditions.

Talking about her cardiovascular issues, Ms. Kelly locates them on several layers of experiences and reflection. As we were trying to understand these layers, we were reminded of "dream narratives" that are common in traditional communities like Cree First Nations, weaving together multiple strata of action and imagination that are not ordered as chronological, linear, and experiential narrative sequences (e.g., McLeod, 2007). In sorting out these layers and the different contexts of reality they bring into this interview, we were amazed by the capacity of narrative to capture and synthesize multiple experiences at once. This capability of stratification, the arrangement of simultaneous layers of action, experience, and reflection, might be viewed as one of the most sophisticated constructive achievements of narrative discourse—in fact, of human language. Of course, this is not an individual ability of Ms. Kelly: Humans seem to be able to juggle these constructions without any apparent effort; it is a cognitive capacity people learn, much like they come to know how to tell a story. It appears that in the very act of narrating and communicating, multilayered scenarios are transformed into a synthesis, something that escapes our attention most of the time. "I don't really know what happened, but I can tell you this," remarked Ms. Kelly at another moment to her interviewer; and she went on to offer one of her pointed syntheses. Let us for a moment dwell on the question of how the act of narrating can evoke such multiple-order scenarios like those offered in our extract.

A crucial role is played by the "zooming together" of different time levels. There is the present in which the interview takes place, which is interlaced with the immediate past (when Ms. Kelly suffered from various cardiovascular problems) and the time when she attended the psychological workshops. These layers are interspersed with another layer of autobiographical memories from her early childhood. Although there seem to be many memories—"I could remember a lot of situations"—she zooms in on two. Both are related to her parents' alcoholism and its consequences. One singles out the horrendous car accident; the other refers to experiences not less dreadful:

> Yeah. So, you know, and just, lots of other things related to probably my parents drinking. Not protecting children. Like, I know my one brother was really sexually abused, and the pedophile, I call him a pedophile, would come right to the door and it was my dad's friend and just take him. I didn't know at the time what that was, but you find out later, you know. And just, um, being around a lot of drunk people when you're small. And, you know, I learned that as a child from, is it 1 to 3 or 1 to 5, whatever happens to you in that timeframe is going to set the pattern of how you're going to function as an adult. It's just so ingrained.

The events Ms. Kelly remembers from her childhood are not further specified in terms of how long they went on. Their narrative presentation is, like that of the car accident, not plot-oriented. There is no beginning and no end. There is no high point or turning point, nor development. The scenario cannot be sketched more scarcely. There are some episodes foregrounded in an opaque space of time. There is only a door; the pedophile "would come right to the door" and slip in—again, all said in a short and quick clause, in passing, like the pedophile dropping in. The narrative's shift from the past to the generalized present links a sense of timeless ongoingness with a traumatic presence, evoking what it means to live on reserve, "being around a lot of drunk people when you're small."

Living on Reserve

Let us change at this moment the point of view from which we undertake to understand the stories of Ms. Kelly, this time by highlighting the cultural landscape out of which her purported narratives of illness emerge. Ms. Kelly is a middle-aged woman who lives, as already mentioned, on a First Nations reserve in western Canada. Winter is harsh and long in this part of the world, and her reserve is far from other cities, villages, or First Nations. She is a foster mother and she has her own children. Her husband helps out at home while she works full-time.

That she lives on a reserve is one of the results of colonial violence. There is a long history of such acts by the Canadian government: lands, lakes, and rivers stolen, generations forcibly sent to remote "reserves," children "scooped" and committed to faraway residential schools (called boarding schools in the United States), cultural traditions and languages outlawed. In many First Nations the legacies of colonialization live on not only as generalized societal structures intersecting with imperatives of capitalism, class, ethnic descent, and gender, but also in specific ways in Ms. Kelly's community. Unemployment, poverty, low education attainment, and high rates of violence are prominent. Mental health problems such as alcoholism, substance abuse, and suicidality are rife (Gall et al., 2021; Mota et al., 2012; Nelson & Wilson, 2017; Ross, 2014; for a discussion see Bryant et al., 2021). Likewise, rates of chronic physical health problems are significantly higher in Indigenous peoples than in all other Canadians (Bruce et al., 2014).

Against this background it is no surprise that Indigenous women also have the highest rate of heart disease of any population in Canada. We took this fact as our point of departure. We wondered how First Nations women experienced and understood that they embody what is often referred to as White man's disease. It is called this because it is a disease that arrived alongside the intrusion of settler culture into Indigenous worlds and the concomitant loss of traditional bush life (Boston et al., 1997; Gone, 2013; on the meaning of "bush life" see Kulchyski, 2013). We set out with our Indigenous community partners to research what we originally thought were the illness narratives of women with cardiovascular problems, an approach that was in contrast to the mainly epidemiological research in the field.

The results were lengthy interviews, conversations, and observations "at the scene," to use Clifford Geertz's (1983) expression (e.g., Medved & Brockmeier, 2015; Medved et al., 2013; Medved & Sinclair, 2010). In our work we attempted to respect the original storytelling format characteristic of many Indigenous communities (Cruikshank, 1998; Sekwan Fontaine et al., 2019). And we also attempted to respect the clinical maxims of narrative medicine regarding how to listen to a storyteller within what Rita Charon (2017) calls an open-ended and nondirectional clinical conversation. To mention just one important element of such conversation, the beginning: "An open beginning, met with however pure an intention one can achieve, lets the listener hear the patient uninterruptedly speak"; this presumes a listener who is attentive and reflexive, and knows how to understand open-ended answers to his or her questions (p. 294).

In our investigations we learned, as already pointed out, that we could not just pull well-formed illness narratives out of the stew of illness, health, memories, and everyday life narratives. In fact, it was challenging to identify both specific stories about illness and classically defined narratives at all. The constant presence of broader cultural narratives permeating the narrative mix made it even more evident that this errand, if truth be told, was a folly.

While the gist of this chapter is not to delineate our cultural narratology or cultural narrative studies approach (on this approach see Brockmeier, 2012), it is essential to be aware of some notions of Indigenous health to gain a fuller understanding of the cultural picture. Many traditional Indigenous views of health and illness are grounded in the idea of balance, as reflected, for example, in the medicine wheel. Illness is thought to reflect and enact imbalance(s) in and with the community; at the same time, indigenous ways of understanding sickness and healing are interlaced with holistic spiritual environmental and community-based perspectives (Doetzel, 2018; Henderson, 2000). Although we do not consider Indigenous and Western ways of knowing and being as binary, we have nevertheless come to see the traditional Indigenous community orientation as substantially different from Western biomedical views of health that localize sickness within individual bodies and, often enough, individual minds.

Not surprisingly, the accumulative effect of colonialism has severely disrupted the cultural continuity of conventional Indigenous structures and "wisdom," as well as many spiritual bonds with the environment. Against this backdrop, many First Nations people equate sickness with colonialism, which in turn can help us to comprehend the finding that Indigenous women often resent the promotion of individualized heart-healthy lifestyle activities, as they resent to being told yet again how to live by settler cultures, this time in the name of "health" and proper "lifestyle" (Medved et al., 2013). This often-practiced approach of Western health care is obviously distinct from traditional Indigenous modes. But it also is distinct from contemporary postcolonial approaches (e.g., Duran, 2006; Stewart et al., 2017) that emphasize the (re)establishment of a communal sense of balance and cultural continuity (e.g., Iwasaki et al., 2005; Snowshoe et al., 2017; Walters & Simoni, 2002) as a prerequisite for the healing of physical and mental health problems.

Beyond differences in terms of health and illness, storytelling and narrative structures and techniques are also impacted by specific cultural traditions. Whereas typical Western illness narratives are first-person accounts that revolve around the "I" as their experiential and narrative center, in many of the stories Indigenous women told us about their heart problems, the agentive kernel is "we" or "us." In general, a first-person singular perspective is not in line with Indigenous experience, as explained by Rain Prud'homme-Cranford (2019); nor is it, by extension, in line with the experience of health and illness.

Lastly, to further complicate matters one must not forget that all our exchanges took place in English. English is the language of colonialism, imperialism, power, forced education, and Christian churches (which ran the residential school system and programs of "reeducation"), and it is also the language of the academic apparatus that, often enough, has been viewed as assuming the role of an inquisitor (Rosaldo, 1986). Some critical and Indigenous psychologists refer to forms of traditional academic research as "epistemic violence" (e.g., Held, 2019).

In sum, negotiating the meanings of all of the above factors contributes additional layers to the interview with Ms. Kelly, which, in turn, requires us to conceive of these increasingly multilayered narratives within an even larger epistemological frame.

Illness, Narrative, and the Cultural Fabric of Life

In previous work we have pointed out in more general terms why it is not possible to understand complex narratives like those of Ms. Kelly about the experience of her heart disease without being aware of the sociocultural context both of the stories and of the life of the teller (Medved & Brockmeier, 2015). Here, this is the life of a Cree woman living on reserve, and this situation permeates all of her narratives. We have approached her stories from various vantage points that we view, however, as complementing each other. Employing perspectives from postcolonial cultural anthropology (including native studies), cultural psychology, social medicine, narrative medicine, and narrative studies, we believe that only in this way can we live up to the multilayeredness, the laminarity of these stories. We have argued that with regard to the medical problems of our participants—Ms. Kelly is only one of the women with whom we worked—it is problematic to draw a clear borderline between stories dealing with illness and stories dealing with everyday life dramas, with what we dubbed at the beginning of our chapter, slightly ironically, as "everyday stories" or "health stories." The problematic of such a borderline, as noted, is also known from the more familiar Western labeling of a specific genre of illness narratives; but it deepens in view of the fundamentally different cultural traditions of Indigenous people who understand and cope with individual sickness by viewing it as an inherent part of communal life and its imbalances, rather than confining it to the individual as in Western medicine and psychology.

Drawing on these observations, we have explained that imposing the categorical distinction of illness narrative on the stories told by Ms. Kelly and our other participants fails the very phenomenon at stake. After all, these are stories that locate putatively individual sickness and its healing in the middle of the community. We therefore have suggested viewing these narratives as cultural forms of life. Storytelling, as demonstrated by Ms. Kelly, is particularly sensitive to the multilayered intricacies of life and illness. Two frontrunners of the approach we have tried to advance in our work, cultural psychologist Jerome Bruner (1993) and cultural anthropologist Clifford Geertz (1983), pointed out that there is no story that is not both a cultural representation and an enactment of culture. There is not a word, a syllable, not even the absence of all of this in the form of silence, that do not have meanings to be understood within the symbolic fabric of a cultural world. Most of the time, this is even the fabric of several cultural worlds coexisting simultaneously. In fact, the interview with Ms. Kelly is particularly interesting because she combined narrative resources from Indigenous traditions (e.g., in rejecting Western medical treatment programs as not communal, not in line with traditional Indigenous healing practices that comprise the entire community) and Western traditions of medical thinking (e.g., in using individual-centered psychodynamic models to describe her childhood experiences). In this way, this interview gives a pointed example of the well-known cultural hybridity of life lived on indigenous reserve within a settler culture. We leave it open whether this hybridity ultimately is a form of one-way assimilation to a "White man's world" and thus represents an identity problem for Ms. Kelly and her Indigenous community (Bell, 2014).

We suggested understanding the complexity of these forms of life and the many challenges they reflect—we have especially looked at one of these challenges, sickness—as the simultaneous presence of various, in fact many, strata of experience, culture, and practical life. Although these layers represent a broad range of the distinct experiences, which Ms. Kelly describes in tropes such as "I have many sick hearts," it is the act of narrating that creates a livable synthesis of her various lives and hearts. Reading Ms. Kelly's stories as unfolding such multiple structures has led us to conceive of each individual narrative or narratological investigation as inevitably turning itself into a multilayered cultural enterprise. Once more, the epistemological gap between researcher and researched people tends to disappear the more the researcher comprehends his or her practice as a cultural practice.

References

Aaslestad, P. (2009). *The patient as text: The role of the narrator in psychiatric notes, 1890–1990*. Radcliffe.

Abel, E. (2021). *Sick and tired: An intimate history of fatigue*. University of North Carolina Press.

Bell, A. (2014). *Relating Indigenous and settler identities: Beyond domination*. Palgrave MacMillan.

Boston, P., Jordan, S., MacNamara, E., Kozolanka, K., Robbish-Rondeau, E., Isherhoff, H., Mianscum, S., Mianscum-Trapper, R., Mistcheesick, I., Petawabano, B., Sheshamush-Masty, M., Wapachee, R., & Weapenicappo, J. (1997). Using participatory action research to understand the meanings aboriginal Canadians attribute to the rising incidence of diabetes. *Chronic Diseases in Canada, 18*, 5–12.

Brockmeier, J. (2012). Narrative scenarios: Toward a culturally thick notion of narrative. In J. Valsiner (Ed.), *Oxford handbook of culture and psychology* (pp. 439–467). Oxford University Press.

Bruce, S., Riediger, N., & Lix, L. (2014). Chronic disease and chronic disease risk factors among First Nations, Inuit, and Metis populations of northern Canada. *Chronic Diseases and Injuries in Canada, 34*(4), 210–217.

Bruner, J. (1993). *Acts of meaning.* Harvard Press.

Bryant, J., Bolt, R., Botfield, J. R., Martin, K., Doyle, M., Murphy, D., Graham, S., Newman, C. E., Bell, S., Treloar, C., Browne, A. J., & Aggleton, P. (2021). Beyond deficit: "Strengths-based approaches" in Indigenous health research. *Sociology of Health & Illness, 43*(6), 1405–1421.

Charon, R. (2006). *Narrative medicine: Honoring the stories of illness.* Oxford University Press.

Charon, R. (2017). Clinical contributions of narrative medicine. In R. Charon, S. DasGupta, N. Hermann, C. Irvine, E. R. Marcus, E. R. Colon, D. Spencer, & M. Spiegel (Eds.), *The principles and practice of narrative medicine* (pp. 227–309). Oxford University Press.

Charon, R., DasGupta, S., Hermann, N., Irvine, C., Marcus, E. R., Colon, E. R., Spencer, D., & Spiegel, M. (Eds.) (2017). *The principles and practice of narrative medicine* (pp. 227–309). Oxford University Press.

Cruikshank, J. (1998). *The social life of stories: Narrative and knowledge in the Yukon territory.* University of Nebraska Press.

Doetzel, N. A. (2018). Cultivating spiritual intelligence: Honouring heart wisdom and First Nations ways of knowing, *Interchange, 49*, 521–526.

Duran, E. (2006). *Healing the soul wound: Counselling with American Indians and other Native people.* Teacher's College Press.

Frank, A. W. (1995). *The wounded storyteller: Body, illness, and ethics.* University of Chicago Press.

Gall, A., Anderson, K., Howard, K., Diaz, A., King, A., Willing, E., Connolly, M., Lindsay, D., & Garvey, G. (2021). Wellbeing of indigenous peoples in Canada, Aotearoa (New Zealand) the United States: A systematic review. *International Journal of Environmental Research and Public Health, 18*(11), 5832–63. https://doi.org/10.3390/ijerph18115832

Garro, L. C. (1988). Explaining high blood pressure: Variation in knowledge about illness. *American Ethnologist, 15*, 98–119.

Geertz, C. (1983). *Local knowledge: Further essays in interpretive anthropology.* Basic Books.

Gone, J. (2013). Redressing First Nations historical trauma: Theorizing mechanisms for indigenous cultural as mental health treatment. *Transcultural Psychiatry, 50*(5), 683–706.

Gubrium, J. F., & Holstein, J. A. (2008). *Analyzing narrative reality.* Sage.

Held, B. (2019). Epistemic violence in psychological science: Can knowledge of, from, and for the (othered people) solve the problem? *Theory and Psychology, 30*(3), 349–370. doi:10.177/095935431983943

Henderson, J. (2000). Ayukpachi: Empowering Aboriginal thought. In M. Battiste (Ed.), *Reclaiming indigenous voice and vision* (pp. 248–278). UBC Press.

Hurwitz, B. (2017). Narrative constructs in modern clinical case reporting. *Studies in History and Philosophy of Science, 62*, 65–73.

Iwasaki, Y., Bartlett, J. G., & O'Neil, J. (2005). Coping with stress among Aboriginal women and men with diabetes in Winnipeg, Canada. *Social Science & Medicine, 60*, 977–988. doi:10.1016/j.socscimed.2004.06.032

Kleinman, A. (1988). *The illness narratives: Suffering, healing, and the human condition.* Basic Books.

Kulchyski, P. (2013). *Aboriginal rights are not human rights: In defense of indigenous struggles.* Arbeiter Ring.

Le, A., Miller, K., & McMullin, J. (2017). From particularities to context: Refining our thinking on illness narratives. *American Medical Association Journal of Ethics, 19*(3), 304–311.

McLeod, N. (2007). *Cree narrative memory.* Purich Publishing Press.

Medved, M. I., & Brockmeier, J. (2015). On the margins: Aboriginal realities and "White man's research." In R. Piazza & A. Fasulo (Eds.), *When identities are marked: Narrating lives between societal labels and individual biographies* (pp. 79–97). Palgrave.

Medved, M. I., Brockmeier, J., Morach, J., & Chartier-Courchene, L. (2013). Broken heart stories: Understanding Aboriginal women's heart problems. *Qualitative Health Research, 23*(12), 1613–1625. doi:10.1177/1049732313509407

Medved, M. I., & Sinclair, S. (2010). Vom Leben in zwei Welten [Life in two worlds] In C. Dege, M. Dege, T. Grallert, & N. Chimirri (Eds.), *Können Marginalisierte (wieder) sprechen? Zum politischen Potenzial der Sozialwissenschaften* [Can the marginalized speak? On the political potential of the social sciences] (pp. 113–134). Psychosozial Verlag.

Mota, N., Elias, B., Tefft, B., Medved, M. I., Munroe, G., & Sareen, J. (2012). Correlates of suicidality: Investigation of a representative sample of Manitoba First Nations adolescents. *American Journal of Public Health, 102*(3), 1353–1361.

Nelson, S., & Wilson, K. (2017). The mental health of indigenous peoples in Canada: A critical review of research. *Social Science & Medicine, 176*, 93–112.

Prud'homme-Cranford, R. (2019, May 29). Personal communication.

Rosaldo, R. (1986). From the door of his tent: The fieldworker and the inquisitor. In J. Clifford & G. E. Marcus (Eds.), *Writing culture: The poetics and politics of ethnography* (pp. 77–97). University of California Press.

Ross, R. (2014). *Indigenous healing: Exploring traditional paths.* Penguin Books.

Sacks, O. (1985). *The man who mistook his wife for a hat.* Summit Books.

Sekwan Fontaine, L., Wood, S., Forbes, L., & Schultz, A. (2019). Listening to First Nations women' expressions of heart health: Mite achimowin digital storytelling study. *International Journal of Circumpolar Health, 78*, 1630233. doi:10.1080/22423982.2019.1630233

Snowshoe, A., Crooks, C., Tremblay, P., & Hinson, R. (2017). Cultural connectedness and its relation to mental health wellness for First Nations Youth. *Journal of Primary Prevention, 38*, 67–86.

Sontag, S. (1978). *Illness as metaphor.* McGraw-Hill Ryerson.

Stewart, S., Moodley, R., & Hyatt, A. (Eds.) (2017). *Indigenous cultures and mental health counselling: Four directions for integration with counselling psychology.* Taylor and Francis.

Walters, K., & Simoni, J. M. (2002). Reconceptualizing Native women's health: An "indigenist" stress-coping model. *American Journal of Public Health, 92*(4), 520–524.

3

Narrative Practices in Mental Health

Narrative Therapy and the Fictive Stance

Daniel D. Hutto

Narrative practices can support mental health—or so this chapter will argue. On the face of it, the way we narrate our lives—how we make sense of who we are and why we do what we do—matters to our mental health and well-being. The way some people narrate their lives can empower them and help them to cope resiliently when it comes to dealing with specific challenges and overcoming certain impediments. Contrariwise, the way others narrate their lives can contribute to those lives going in the opposite direction, sometimes dramatically, leading to depression, despair, and, in the worst cases, death. Either way, it seems that our narrative practices matter to the upkeep of positive mental health and the quality of our social interactions.

It would be incredible to suppose that *only* narrative practices matter to mental health—that our narrative practices, alone and on their own, are all that matter to mental health. Yet a more modest proposition is, prima facie, more warranted: Narrative practices can make a difference, and sometimes a pivotally important difference, to mental health.

For example, to focus on a case that this chapter will look at in more detail, McConnell (2016a) defends the view that "first-hand accounts of addiction suggest that the agent's self-narrative also has an influence" (p. 307). The reason that our narrative practices are influential to the mental well-being of addicted individuals, according to McConnell, can be put down to the fact that the narratives we weave about ourselves can significantly impact our capacities for self-governance. In particular, he maintains that "a self-understanding *that goes beyond one's intentions* is an independent factor relevant to self-governance" (McConnell 2016a, p. 308, emphasis added). Accepting this modest thesis about the importance of self-narratives in the domain of mental health is perfectly consistent with acknowledging that there are other fundamental factors at play in recovery from addiction.

Daniel D. Hutto, *Narrative Practices in Mental Health* In: *Narrative and Mental Health*. Edited by: Jarmila Mildorf, Elisabeth Punzi, and Christoph Singer, Oxford University Press. © Oxford University Press 2023.
DOI: 10.1093/oso/9780197620540.003.0004

A great many clinicians, therapists, and mental health practitioners believe in the importance and efficacy of narrative practices. Moreover, some go further, adding a necessity clause to the importance of self-narratives in achieving mental health in some cases. Thus McConnell (2016a) reports that "most clinicians and people in recovery believe that the agential effort of the person trying to recover is *a necessary ingredient* for successful recovery" (p. 307, emphasis added).

These practitioners' beliefs explain why narrative practices feature—pride of place—in an array of therapeutic interventions that are designed to support, protect, and enhance mental health. Some prominent examples include Narrative Exposure Therapy, which has been used to treat the effects of trauma in refugees and to prevent psychiatric illness (Gwozdziewycz & Mehl-Madrona, 2013; Wilker et al., 2020); Mentalizing interventions used in the treatment of borderline personality disorders, which make use of narratives in training affected individuals in how to make sense of themselves and others (Allen et al., 2008; Bouchard et al., 2008.); and Social Stories interventions, as developed by Carol Gray, which use narratives to assist individuals with autism to develop greater social understanding (Gray & Garand, 1993).

Looking closely at McConnell and Snoek's (2018) valuable philosophical analysis of addiction recovery, this chapter focuses on another widely used and popular narrative-based approach to improving mental health, Australian-based narrative therapy (see Hutto & Gallagher, 2017).[1] Narrative therapy distinguishes itself from other "talking cures" in that it seeks to empower individuals and groups by getting them to alter their habits of self-narration so as to tell new stories about their individual or collective lives. Its re-authoring techniques are used to help people deal with a wide range of mental health problems, including addiction, anorexia, bulimia, depression, and other traumatic psychiatric illnesses (White & Epston, 1990).

There is limited scientific evidence of the efficacy of narrative therapy. Nevertheless, it enjoys a positive reputation as providing an attractive means of supporting people from diverse backgrounds (Denborough, 2014). Narrative therapy seeks to help people get beyond reliance on thin "off-the-shelf" narratives and to instead enable them to tell richer stories about their lives (Denborough, 2014, p. 49). The aim of such re-storying efforts is to increase "response-ability." The goal of the therapy is to equip clients to do the requisite narrative work and build up their narrative skills so that they become "more able to respond" (Denborough, 2014, p. 36). This equates to enabling people to see expanded possibilities and, thereby, to improve their practical know-how and life skills (White, 2004, pp. 39–40).

Despite its existing popularity among clients and practitioners, narrative therapy faces a trio of philosophical challenges—challenges that can induce skepticism about narrative-based approaches to mental health in general depending on standard interpretations of the aims of such approaches and how they are assumed to work. These philosophically motivated concerns stand in the way of narrative-based therapies being taken seriously more widely within and beyond the academy. Taken together, the trio of challenges threaten to undermine the theoretical credibility, universal applicability, and ethical credentials of narrative-based approaches to mental health.

This chapter offers a way of defending at least some narrative-based therapies from these challenges. Its action unfolds as follows. Section 1 considers, in detail, a particular philosophical analysis of the aims of narrative therapy and how it is assumed to work. It gives close attention to McConnell and Snoek's (2018) account of how narrative interventions might positively influence the prospects of recovery from addiction. Section 2 details three skeptical challenges that threaten to cast doubt on the acceptability of the aims and methods of narrative therapy, as depicted by McConnell and Snoek (2018), as well as, potentially, casting doubt on the acceptability of other, similar narrative-based approaches to mental health. Finally, Section 3 makes an effort to show that it is possible to address this trio of challenges by recasting certain assumptions about the core aims and methods of narrative therapy. It is proposed that by focusing on the "fictive" rather than the "factual" character of certain narrative practices, it is possible to rethink how narrative therapy might work in practice in such a way that protects it from the three skeptical challenges outlined in Section 2. To achieve this outcome, it is proposed that we adjust the way we understand the aims and methods of narrative therapy, and potentially other narrative-based approaches to mental health.

In the end, it is concluded that there is a way to see off the three skeptical challenges identified in this chapter and thus improve the philosophical credibility of narrative-based approaches in mental health, opening the path for their wider uptake.

Section 1: Narrative Therapy's Role in Addiction Recovery

In a series of articles McConnell and co-authors give significant attention to the role narrative practices could play in assisting with recovery from addiction (McConnell, 2016a, 2016b; McConnell & Snoek, 2018). These philosophical analyses of how narrative practices might make a difference to mental health rest on some standard philosophical assumptions about the way we use narratives both to understand ourselves and to constitute who we are. The standard assumptions about the role of narratives in self-understanding and self-constitution provide these authors with the basis for their account of how narrative therapy might work to help those seeking to recover from addiction.

It is well known that attempts to recover from addiction yield mixed results in the general populace. Most people fail to recover, often suffering repeated relapses over long tracts of time. The sad truth is that many never fully recover. Others are more successful: Some recover robustly and quickly. What could account for this difference?

McConnell and Snoek (2018) propose an answer. They maintain that an addicted person's self-narratives play a critical part in whether or not that person is able to successfully recover from addiction. Although these authors admit that self-narratives are not the only or primary causal factors at play in making successful recovery possible, they argue nonetheless that it would be a mistake to think of self-narratives as mere epiphenomenal outcomes of the recovery process.[2] If they are right, how we make sense of ourselves through narratives can matter pivotally to our mental health. Their analysis of what helps and hinders recovery from addiction reveals that a person's self-narrative practices are a significant factor: not the only factor to be sure, but in some cases such narrative practices can prove crucial.[3] In the end, McConnell and Snoek (2018) conclude "that existing forms of addiction treatment will tend to be more effective and efficient if they are complemented by narrative-focused interventions" (p. 41).

The philosophical analysis of recovery prospects offered by McConnell and Snoek (2018) gains some apparent empirical support from the findings of a qualitative study of 69 substance-dependent people that they conducted at a detox and opioid replacement treatment facility in Sydney. Their study involved follow-up interviews with a selection of the participants at years one, two, and three from baseline, resulting in 145 interviews in total.

Based on their analysis of the findings from those interviews, McConnell and Snoek (2018) propose a general explanation of why certain individuals as opposed to others do better or worse in their recovery efforts. Their explanation of this difference focuses on aspects of the narrative practices of different classes of individual. On their analysis, they distinguish two broad classes of individual: those who are most likely to recover from addiction and those who are unlikely to recover. These authors hypothesize that those in the first class are more successful at reliably managing conflicts that arise between those threads in their self-narratives that highlight their recovery goals and other threads in their self-narratives that highlight their proneness for continued drug use.

The explanation McConnell and Snoek (2018) advance holds that a person's recovery prospects are affected by their ability to accommodate and smooth out conflicts that arise between competing threads in their self-narratives. The kind of dissonance that arises from such competition occurs, say, when threads of a recovery-oriented self-narrative and an established drug-using self-narrative conflict.

The broader explanation that McConnell and Snoek (2018) propose builds on earlier work by McConnell (2016a) in which he defends the thesis that "given a certain self-narrative, some futures make more sense than others, and we *are inclined to enact our self-narratives so that they make sense*" (p. 308, emphasis added). Call this McConnell's Sense-Maximizing Thesis about what drives us to enact certain narratives. McConnell's thesis predicts that we will prefer self-narratives that best fit what we take to be the pattern of our lives and, in a mutually reinforcing way, we will tend to enact narratives in our lives that better fit those dominant self-narratives. The Sense-Maximizing Thesis offers the following explanation of why some people fail to recover from addiction, despite sincere and concerted efforts to achieve that end. It holds that such people are "inclined to continue their disvalued drug-using lifestyle because it nevertheless *makes the most sense* given who they understand themselves to be" (McConnell, 2016a, p. 308, emphasis added).

Other people in our lives play a big part in determining which of our self-narratives become the most dominant and established. Central to McConnell's analysis is the idea that creating and testing out which self-narratives make most sense of who we are is not a solo or solitary project. For one thing, we draw on ambient sociocultural archetypes in order to make sense of our lives, actions and experiences (Hutto, 2008, 2016a). Yet apart from providing inherited narrative frames with which we tend to operate, others also play a more direct role in determining which self-narratives we find credible. This is because we look to others to confirm which narratives they think best and most accurately apply to us. Thus, McConnell and Snoek (2018) stress that "[e]ven when we develop novel self-narrative content, we look to others to verify that content and we reconsider and often revise that content when it is challenged" (p. 33; see also McConnell, 2016b).

Echoing McIntyre (1984), the type of influence that others have on our self-narrating efforts can be understood as a kind of co-authoring of who we are. Co-authoring is at work whenever individuals come to "strongly identify with the aspects of their self-narratives that are consistently verified by others" (McConnell & Snoek, 2018, p. 31).

According to McConnell and Snoek (2018), the trouble for some who are trying to recover from addiction is that the continual influence of others on self-narrating efforts can push individuals to conservatively stick with and identify with established if disvalued self-narratives. This kind of conservative outcome is likely to be the case when addicted persons and their co-authors "treat those disvalued narratives *as factual*" (McConnell & Snoek, 2018, p. 32, emphasis added).

The addicted person's best chance of success in recovery is to find more factually credible threads to weave in with the older threads, thus creating a stronger new, preferred overall narrative. Accordingly, it needs to be the case that any new thread even if it "initially felt alien is *actually sufficiently plausible* . . . to integrate in her self-narrative" (McConnell & Snoek, 2018, p. 34; emphasis added). Failure to find new yet divergent self-narrative threads that are reasonable and plausible enough to integrate into a self-narrative that would aid recovery can be exacerbated by a person's general, background philosophical beliefs. For example, a general belief that selves have fixed essences will work against the very idea that is possible for a person to change and enact a new self-narrative. Essentialist assumptions about the nature of selves would likely lead an addicted individual to wonder how someone of their type—someone with their apparently fixed tendencies—could ever hope to change and recover. Background beliefs of this stripe can fuel debilitating and disempowering negative cycles of self-doubt.[4]

Putting all this together, the crux of McConnell and Snoek's explanation of the role that self-narratives play in failed recovery is ultimately put in terms of a conflict of values. Thus, they write: "[N]o matter how much one explicitly values recovery, one also values the things implicitly represented by the established self-narrative—diachronic agency, self-knowledge, and social inclusion" (McConnell & Snoek, 2018, p. 34).

Their explanatory proposal can be illustrated by appeal to an example. Drawing on findings from their Sydney studies, McConnell and Snoek (2018) discuss the case of Nicole, who suffered a major relapse two years from baseline. According to the interview data, Nicole claimed that her relapse was brought on by her having failed an important examination in her university course. McConnell and Snoek (2018) give the following report of her explanation:

> [T]his incident at her practical examination seriously *challenged the truth* of her recovery-directed narrative. This time, she did not have the mental resources to continue to try and convince herself and others that her recovery narrative was still true of her. She could much more easily explain her failure by incorporating it in her more established addiction self-narrative, her "old self." (p. 39)

If we accept this explanation, it is clear that Nicole would have had a better chance of staying the course with her recovery if she had managed to connect and weave together her two narratives, anticipating and smoothing out any conflicts between them.

On McConnell and Snoek's (2018) analysis, the only positive way forward for addicted people is to find ways of integrating the various conflicting threads in their overall self-narrative.[5] This might require mastering special techniques. But whatever the precise solution, the prospects of successful integration depend, fairly directly, on the addicted person's ability to deal with and defuse the inertia and momentum of the established narrative. Thus, as these authors are quick to point out, "whether a new narrative thread is ultimately integrated more permanently in the wider self-narrative *depends on successfully enacting it and convincing others of its truth*" (p. 35; emphasis added).

Addicted individuals seeking to change and recover need special narrative strategies and tactics. They could, for example, include drawing on classic narrative tropes and archetypes, such as "the redemption script," when telling their stories. Use of such devices would enhance their potential to contend with and break not only their own settled narrative habits and tendencies but also those of their co-authors. Only if such habits and tendencies can be held at bay will new narrative threads have any chance of being endorsed and enacted.

Crucially, McConnell and Snoek (2018) conceive of the core processes by which a person becomes persuaded of a self-narrative as everywhere truth-sensitive, belief-mediated processes. An agent and their co-authoring partners come to believe in the plausibility of certain self-narrative threads because those threads make the best and most coherent sense of the person's actions as compared to rival narrative threads. The overall self-narrative that makes the most sense carries the day: It is the one that is accepted and endorsed as capturing a truth about who the person is. Only after such endorsement is it enacted.

As is clear from the above descriptions of the processes involved, as McConnell and Snoek (2018) see it, the enterprise of endorsing a self-narrative is fundamentally intellectual in character. By their lights, crafting, testing out, and endorsing a self-narrative is not unlike crafting, testing out, and endorsing a scientific theory.

Any particular narrative thread must cohere with a person's established global self-narrative in order to be accepted, just as any given theory must cohere with a wider set of established theories in order to be accepted. It is for this reason that the narrative threads that get endorsed are those that

> are consistently intersubjectively *verified* and entrenched within a network of other verified threads. The agent and her peers then take these established threads to represent *facts* about who the agent is and who she can hope to become. (McConnell & Snoek, 2018, p. 33; emphases added)

These authors describe the process of evaluation of rival and conflicting self-narrative possibilities as an evaluation of their relative coherence and truth. Thus, McConnell and Snoek (2018) assume that the evaluation process requires asking if the existing threads of the overall narrative can support the new threads and if the new threads stand up to the facts (p. 34).

To be sure, McConnell and Snoek's (2018) proposal leaves room for feelings to play a part in the endorsement process. Thus, we are told that "any new self-narrative content that fails to cohere with the established self-narrative will feel alien to the addicted person and seem to be implausible both to herself and her peers" (McConnell & Snoek, 2018, p. 32). The less plausible one's self-narrative, the greater one's feelings of alienation. And, it is these feelings that "generate the intuition that the narrative projection under consideration 'just isn't me'" (McConnell & Snoek, 2018, p. 34).

Still, even so, the core of the evaluation process is clearly cognitively driven on this account. Negative emotions and feelings arise only if one goes against an established self-narrative, especially one that has strong support from others. It is this going against the narrative grain that gives rise to the uneasy feelings that can sap the person's motivational force and scupper their capacity for self-governance. Yet the feelings only follow in the wake of cognitive dissonance that arises from the failure to successfully integrate certain narrative threads in a plausible overall self-narrative.

Given all of the above, narrative therapy will seem especially attractive as a means of helping to promote the mental health and positive outcomes sought by this class of individuals. Narrative therapy holds out the possibility that a person might master techniques that would allow them to re-author their lives and weave a new overall self-narrative by establishing its alethic credentials.

Narrative therapy's re-authoring approach is designed to help people to revise detrimental aspects of existing self-narrative and, working with therapists, co-author more positive and productive self-narratives. Highlighting one key technique, McConnell and Snoek (2018) observe that narrative therapy might enable a person to reflect on their past to find "an alternative interpretation that can also make sense of events (e.g., one was not a victim but a survivor)" (p. 34).

In the best cases, when the therapy works, the result is that a person's revised and preferred self-narrative becomes credible and dominant. It takes hold. Once readily endorsed and enacted, the new self-narrative can enable a person to better further pursue their stated values precisely because the new self-narrative "provide[s] some basis for *imagining realistically achievable projections*" (McConnell & Snoek, 2018, pp. 32–33; emphasis added). Narrative therapy, it seems, has great potential to help people to "develop their belief in an open future by reinterpreting their past so that more valued projections become more plausible" (McConnell & Snoek, 2018, p. 38).[6]

Section 2: Three Skeptical Challenges

Despite its apparent promise, there are at least three challenges that skeptics and critics have raised about narratives that might make us concerned about the stated aims and methods of narrative therapy, at least as they are presented by McConnell and Snoek (2018).

Simply stated, the first challenge, call it the Explanatory Challenge, is this: Narrative therapy aims for people to operate with true and verifiable self-narrative accounts of who they are and why they do what they do, but it simply cannot achieve that ambition. Or, even more simply stated, to the extent that narrative therapy is understood as a truth-seeking enterprise, then it must fail. The basic reasoning motivating this challenge is as follows: To the extent that narrative therapy requires people to give true self-narrative accounts of who they are and what they do, then it is in trouble because, as a general rule, narratives—including factual narratives offered by historians—are incapable of getting at the truth of things.

A comparison may prove illuminating. Consider that every patient has a story about what underlies their mental health problems. Yet, if so, what should we make of the status of such stories? Launer (1999) puts his finger on the trouble:

> There is *a tension between the complex narrative that a patient brings* into the consulting room *and a doctor's understanding of what is really going on* as formulated in a diagnosis or an idea about pathology. Which is a "truer" account of reality: the patient's or the doctor's? Can both be true? If so, how? (p. 117, emphases added)

Elaborating on this worry, Rosenberg (2018) remarks on history's ambition to explain

> the past and the present by narrative: telling stories—*true ones*, of course; that's what makes them history, not fiction. Narrative history is not just an almanac or a chronology of what happened in the past. It is an *explanation* of what happened in terms of the motives and the perspectives of the human agents whose choices, decisions, and actions made those events happen. (Rosenberg 2018, p. 2, emphases added)

Assuming Rosenberg (2018) accurately captures history's explanatory ambitions, there are grounds for a serious complaint and challenge. He argues that, to the extent that history relies on narratives, it is simply unable to supply explanations that meet the required standards of truth. The putative narratives of history, he holds, systematically fail to meet their promises. By his lights, what such narratives supply is "not enough to understand any-thing . . . let alone the best or only way, to understand anything" (Rosenberg, 2018, p. 5).

On Rosenberg's analysis, the root trouble with all narrative explanations is that "they fail to identify the real causal forces that drive events" (Rosenberg, 2018, p. 6). Because of this congenital failing, narratives provide us with no genuine explanatory or predictive grip. Causal explanations and well-grounded predictions are the preserve of theories offered up by the natural sciences. It is only hard-won scientific theories, never homespun narratives, that are able to deliver predictive and explanatory power.

It is well known that interpretive disciplines—at which Rosenberg takes aim and of which narrative history is the chief exemplar—offer up narrative accounts of human action that never deliver definitive, incontestable accounts of what someone thought or why they did what they did. When we make sense of the actions of ourselves or others, there is no conclusive way to eliminate countless other rival yet coherent narrative possibilities, no way to conclusively eliminate alternative competing accounts and interpretations of those same actions. There is no empirically established method for choosing between rival narrative possibilities and, hence, no scientific basis for deciding between them once and for all.

Interpretative disciplines have no prospect and should make no pretense of supplying anything like the kind of theory-driven predictions and explanations that are the hallmark of the hard, natural sciences. The explanatory successes of the hard, natural sciences, at least according to the received wisdom, can be put down to the fact that their offerings compete and survive a winnowing process. There is nothing comparable to that process at work in interpretative domains. This is shown by the fact that we do not put rival narratives about someone's reasons for action through anything like such empirical tests and trials. Thus, we are in no position to assess rival narratives for their explanatory power in the same way that we assess rival theories for theirs, even if we wished to do so.

In short and in sum, according to this line of argument, if we are interested in the truth about how things stand with the world, then we have no choice but to look only to the well-established products of the natural sciences. And, when we look to the natural sciences, we discover that "Science is not stories; it's theories, laws, models, findings, observations, experiments" (Rosenberg, 2018, p. 4).

For Rosenberg (2018), when it comes to evaluating their truth-revealing prospects, the inevitable conclusion is that "*all* narratives are wrong—wrong in the same way and for the same reason" (p. 3; emphasis added). On this view, at best, "stories fan emotional flames rather than confer understanding" (p. 5). If we follow Rosenberg's reasoning and assume that narrative therapy is the truth-seeking, understanding-conferring business, as McConnell and Snoek (2018) argue, then it is the wrong business.[7]

But some critics do not stop there. Taken together, the above arguments not only give us reason to think that narrative therapy will prove futile in the final analysis but also give us reason to think that using its narrative practices in mental health may be positively dangerous. Rosenberg (2018) speaks of the broader perils of storytelling in the following terms:

> [N]arratives . . . have been harmful to the health, well-being, and the very lives of most people down through the chain of historical events. Stories . . . are deeply implicated in more misery and death than probably any other aspect of human culture. . . . it's the nature of the most compelling stories they tell that's responsible for the trail of tears, pain, suffering, carnage, and sometimes extermination that make up most of human history. (p. 3)

The stakes are high. But, for Rosenberg, the solution is not to tell better stories but to stop telling stories altogether. He acknowledges we are deeply addicted to narratives, noting that we have an "insatiable hunger for stories" (Rosenberg, 2014, p. 41). Indeed, he acknowledges that we take to narratives in the same way babies take to mother's milk. Yet he holds that narratives are "more like heroin than milk" (Rosenberg, 2018, p. 6).

This is because, he maintains, narratives unavoidably blind us to the truth. He holds that the best descriptions of reality "don't come in the form of stories with plots" (Rosenberg 2014, p. 41). For this reason, he contends that "our demand for plotted narratives is the greatest obstacle to getting a grip on reality" (Rosenberg, 2014, p. 41).

In Rosenberg's final reckoning, narratives are never any good for us. We are addicted to narratives to such a degree and extent that we are blocked from seeing the truth of our situation clearly.[8] On his analysis, the only way to escape the illusions that narratives create for us is to rid ourselves of the tendency to weave and receive narratives altogether. Against the recommendations of narrative therapy, he does not recommend coming up with more functional self-narratives; rather, he thinks that the only way to block the harmful effects of our addiction to narratives is give up storytelling and to embrace science, completely and totally.

Another major challenge targets the idea that the techniques of narrative therapy are universally applicable to all people, even if only as a necessary complement to other treatments, as McConnell and Snoek (2018) propose. Call this the Scope Challenge. It goes as follows: Narrative therapy is inappropriate for treating certain individuals and populations, and it is potentially dangerous insofar as it fails to recognize this fact. Narrative therapy is vulnerable to this challenge just in case it commits, as its philosophical champions propose it should, to "an account of narrative self-constitution" (McConnell, 2016a, p. 308).

Narrative accounts of self-constitution embrace the narrativity thesis, which holds that experiencing our lives narratively—even if only implicitly—is the basis of our selfhood. The narrativity thesis has proved incredibly popular: It has an impressive list of supporters both inside and outside the academy (MacIntyre, 1984; Rudd, 2012; Schechtman, 1996, 2007, 2011).

Strawson (2004, 2020) rejects it in both its descriptive and normative variants. He objects to its universalizing assumptions that all humans make sense of themselves through the lens of narratives and that doing so is always desirable. Against the narrativity thesis, he insists that there are nonnarrative individuals—people who do not naturally experience themselves or their lives in a narrative way. Further, he claims there are also antinarrative individuals—people who actively resist experiencing themselves or their lives in a narrative way. Strawson (2020) cites Montaigne, for example, as being "allergic to sequential order" and "suspicious of biographical coherence."

The central premise in Strawson's case against the narrativity thesis is that not all remembering operates in a narrative way; hence, people can differ profoundly in the way they experience and handle memory. If Strawson is correct, then to the extent that narrative therapy commits to the narrativity thesis its use would be inappropriate and, perhaps, potentially harmful for significant swathes of the population.

Finally, there is also the Manipulation Challenge. It goes as follows: The re-authoring techniques of narrative therapy risk, potentially unethically, manipulating people by encouraging them to re-narrate past events in ways that may be truth-distorting. This risk arises because others, including therapists, can have a strong influence on the way we narrate events in our lives.

Effectively, narrative therapists may act as revisionary co-authors. Co-authoring, in general, can present problems in that others "may contribute content to our narratives that we disvalue and/or leave us without content that we need" (McConnell, 2016b, p. 30). In this vein, McConnell (2016b) warns of both excessively dominant as well as apathetic co-authors creating problems in our ability to understand ourselves properly.

Yet narrative therapy is especially vulnerable to the dangers of manipulation through its guided imagination exercises in that it prompts clients to revisit significant events from their pasts with the intent to re-author them. Consider how McConnell and Snoek (2018) describe the practice:

> Briefly, clients are *asked to recall a situation in which they handled their addiction in a self-controlled way*, for example, successfully resisting an episode of craving. The counselor then *encourages the client to elaborate* on why this attempt was successful, *to develop an alternative narrative* in which their capacities to control their substance use is made central. (p. 41)

Assuming this description of its practice is accurate, narrative therapy, however well intentioned, runs a risk of installing false memories by directing people to revisit and re-author their pasts.

Elizabeth Loftus raised this exact concern about related practices in psychotherapy based on her seminal memory research (Loftus, 1979; Loftus & Ketcham, 1994). She highlighted the very real possibility that the use of guided imagination in psychotherapy might create false memories of complete, emotional, and self-participatory experiences in adults. This can happen, she proposed, because "some mental health professionals encourage patients to imagine childhood events as a way of recovering supposedly hidden memories" (Loftus, 1997, p. 73).

The risk is real. Recent findings "confirm earlier studies that many individuals can be led to construct complex, vivid and detailed false memories via a rather simple procedure" (Loftus, 1997, p. 75). The process is likely to work by means of "imagination inflation" (Loftus, 1997, p. 74). The person is asked to imagine childhood experiences that did not happen to them, and the mere act of imagining the detailed episode increases confidence that it actually occurred. Thus, "investigators found that the more times participants imagined an unperformed action, the more likely they were to remember having performed it" (Loftus, 1997, p. 74).[9] We can expect this effect to be enhanced based on the detailed richness of the imagined episode (see Hutto, 2016b).

The main lesson to draw from the memory data is that "mental health professionals and others must be aware of how greatly they can influence the recollection of events and of the urgent need for maintaining restraint in situations in which imagination is used as an aid in recovering presumably lost memories" (Loftus, 1997, p. 75). Narrative therapy appears especially open to this risk.

Section 3: Telling a Different Story
About Narrative Therapy

Is it possible to update the official story about narrative therapy's aims and methods so as to avoid the trio of skeptical challenges outlined in the preceding section? On the face of it, the answer is "yes." In the space remaining, I sketch what may prove to be an elegant solution that answers all three challenges. The proposal is that narrative therapy should "go fictive." The philosophical recommendation on the table is that narrative therapy would benefit from officially adopting what Goldie (2012) calls the "fictive stance." Within the fictive stance a narrative is regarded as fictional but not "in virtue of its content being false, but in virtue of its being narrated, and read or heard, as part of a practice of a special sort" (pp. 52–53).

The fictive stance is the stance we adopt when we treat what is purported to occur in a narrative as items of make-believe, as we do when pretending or in certain storytelling practices, such as reading a fairy tale. Philosophers take special interest in the question of how to make sense of truths within such fictions (see, e.g., Currie, 2010; Sainsbury, 2010). However, what is important for our purposes is that adopting the fictive stance within particular practices allows us to explicitly frame stories so that the question of their truth or falsity is explicitly bracketed and, hence, does not arise. As a result, it is simply inappropriate to evaluate such stories according to standards of accuracy, consistency, or empirical adequacy in anything remotely in the same manner that truth-seeking theories are evaluated by such criteria.

It has been proposed, by Gerrans (2014), that deluded individuals may be adopting a fictive stance without necessarily noticing they are doing so. On Gerrans's analysis, rather than understanding delusions as arising from false, recalcitrant beliefs, what is going on in cases of delusions is that a deluded person's imaginative tendencies drive them to tell and re-tell particular narratives, even though such narratives do not warrant credence. Thus, Gerrans (2014) says of one such patient that he is

> telling a story. The story is consistent with his experience (though not with his knowledge about the nature of reality) but from the point of view of a third person it is unbelievable. Nonetheless he cannot abandon that story, or revise it to fit with his wider empirical knowledge, and continues to act according to it. Hence his ambivalence when pressed about its empirical adequacy when treated as a description of reality. (p. 7)

What is being proposed here is that there may be special advantages of thinking of the narrative practices that confer therapeutic benefit as operating in an explicitly fictive mode. The suggestion that narrative therapy might benefit from explicitly endorsing the fictive stance is in effect to suggest that it can take a leaf out of the Solution-Focused Brief Therapy (SFBT) playbook so as to avoid the skeptical challenges presented in the preceding section without loss of therapeutic power.

SFBT is a future-oriented approach to therapy that stands apart from most other therapeutic approaches in that it "spends very little or even no time on the origins or nature of the problem, the client's pathology, or analysis of dysfunctional interactions" (de Shazer & Dolan, 2007, p. 2). A core assumption of SFBT is that "solutions *need not necessarily be related to the problems* they resolve" (de Shazer & Dolan, 2007, p. ix, emphasis added). Reversing a familiar therapeutic polarity, SFBT insists that it is preferable to focus on "constructing a future trajectory rather than achieving past accuracy" (Graham, 2010, p. 14).

A key device in SFBT is that it asks clients to imagine a future in which their problem has miraculously dissolved. It then presses them to describe, in increasing detail, what would be different for them and about them in that imagined future scenario as they develop their reply to the so-called miracle question. The client is asked questions in order to measure degrees of noticed change in the imagined scenario.

Given its explicit orientation towards the future and the character of the "miracle question," there is simply no question of being concerned about the accuracy of the imagined scenario. Questions of whether the imagined event is a plausible, let alone factually accurate, depiction of a future happening do not arise at all.

The proposal on the table here is that narrative therapy might make adopting the fictive stance explicit in its practices in just the same way when asking clients to look back and think about their pasts. Thus, rather than asking people to provide accurate, verifiable accounts of episodes in their lives where they coped successfully in their past history so as to weave new threads into a new overall self-narrative, they might simply and explicitly imagine such episodes in order to put them in a stronger position to imagine, as Singer (2001) poignantly puts it, "new endings to painful and repetitive stories" (p. 389). Narrative therapy, so understood, can shape our thinking without aiming to provide accurate, factual self-narratives about who we are or to establish new beliefs in us about our past doings.

Going fictive in the core practices of narrative therapy would allow it to deal with and defuse the trio of challenges raised in the foregoing section. Both the explanatory and manipulation challenges disappear immediately once the question of the truth of the narratives deployed in the therapy is bracketed and no longer arises.

An advantage of making fictive bracketing explicit is that it puts to rest tricky questions about how it might be possible to establish the truth about such past events. For as Loftus notes in her discussion of autobiographical remembering, in any case, "without corroboration, there is little that can be done to help even the most experienced evaluator to differentiate true memories from ones that were suggestively planted" (Loftus, 1997, p. 75).

Although the scope challenge is not immediately answered by going fictive, it is important to note that it is only a challenge to narrative therapy so long as that therapy makes a strong philosophical commitment to "an account of narrative self-constitution" (McConnell, 2016a, p. 308). McConnell and Snoek (2018) recommend making such a commitment based on their analysis of what is involved in attempts to recover from addiction. Their recommendation is bound up with their reasons for thinking that "self-narration is necessary for self-governance" (p. 32). Narratives are necessary for self-governance if specifying the meaningful connections that are needed to reason practically can only be achieved by means of self-narration. Thus, it is because McConnell and Snoek (2018) take this to be the case that they hold "*all* exercises of agency are influenced by the established self-narrative context" (p. 40).

Yet if the core practice of narrative therapy is framed, explicitly for all, as only making use of the fictive stance, then it is compatible with more modest philosophical commitments that need not provoke the scope challenge. In particular, construing the aims and methods of narrative therapy along fictive lines is perfectly compatible with softening the aforementioned necessity claims about self-governance and rejecting strong narrative self-constitution views (see Hutto, 2016a, for an independent discussion of why we should favor a more modest self-shaping account of the role that narratives play in making us who we are). In short, if narrative therapy is taken to operate only with a fictive stance, then there is no conflict at all in recognizing that there can be nonnarrative ways of experiencing and, perhaps, governing one's life.

It helps to understand how narrative therapy might operate in an explicitly fictive mode if we recognize that not all of our narrative practices subscribe to the same epistemic norms that apply in our scientific pursuits. To better understand the norms of fictive storytelling in the context of therapy it may be worthwhile investigating and comparing Western truth-focused, narrative practices with, say, the storytelling practices of other cultures, such as Australian Aboriginal narrative practices, especially when those practices aim at promoting mental health and well-being (Klapproth, 2004; Wingard et al., 2015).[10]

There is a larger question looming in the background: How can any therapy that adopts the fictive stance explicitly be effective? What work could such a therapy do to yield beneficial outcomes?

To a first approximation, exploring possibilities—whether in one's imagined past or future—by constructing personal narratives requires imagining, "rich, particularized, and unified . . . cycles of thoughts, actions and contingencies" (Currie, 2010, p. 36). Though narratively driven, this sort of process will enlist our emotionally charged imaginations of the sort that typically operate and come into play below our full-fledged narrative capacities. As defended in Hutto (2015, 2016b) and Hutto and Myin (2017), such experientially and emotionally charged imaginative episodes can be understood "as narrative elements or fragments" (Gerrans, 2014, p. 101).[11] In this light, to more fully understand how a narrative therapy that only adopts a fictive stance might work would require getting clearer about how the construction of the relevant narratives is supported and fueled by the nonnarrative activity of imagining and experiencing specific episodes.

Importantly, narratively driven acts of imagining can be assumed to be fully embodied—visceral and hot—and, hence, deeply motivational. There are reasons to favor the enactivist idea that people are complex, dynamical systems (see Hutto & Myin, 2013, 2017; see also Gallagher, 2017, 2020). If that idea is along the right lines, then any changes wrought in us through motivationally charged acts of imagination can have many more, downstream and possibly long-lasting, effects for which possibilities for action we see. For "once a small change has been made, it will lead to a series of further changes, which in turn lead to others, gradually resulting in a much larger systemic change" (de Shazer & Dolan, 2007, p. 2).

In the end, there is reason to think that narrative therapy could yield important results even if it restricted itself to operating explicitly with the fictive stance in something like the way SFBT does. Doing so would allow it to deftly avoid all three of the aforementioned challenges by bracketing questions about the truth of its narratives and the universality of its application in one fell swoop. Yet, even if it set aside concerns about the accuracy, consistency, and empirical adequacy of its narratives, narrative therapy so understood might still have powerful tools at its disposal for resetting a person's future trajectory by opening up new, live possibilities for action for them to pursue.

Conclusion

This chapter has sought to motivate taking narrative practices seriously in mental health. Drawing on analyses advanced in McConnell (2016a, 2016b) and McConnell and Snoek (2018), it has shown the plausible role that narrative therapy could play in aiding recovery from addiction as a case in point. Yet it also revealed that the preferred philosophical take on the aims and methods of narrative therapy encounters a series of potentially crippling challenges. In a bid to answer these challenges it was proposed that narrative therapy might adopt a fictive stance only, and that in doing so it could thereby recast its stated aims and methods so as to defuse the challenges. Admittedly, to test whether these changes are viable in practice would require further work involving "practitioners willing and able to go deep philosophically [and] philosophers on the other hand . . . going deep practically" (Fulford et al., 2013, p. 3). But that, as they say, is another story for another day.

Notes

1. Narrative therapy "is an established therapeutic system with a body of trained practitioners" (McConnell & Snoek, 2018, p. 41). It is widely used for personal, family, and community interventions and treatments around the world. It is especially popular in its home Australia, having its main base in the Dulwich Centre, Adelaide. Other centers and institutes of narrative therapy have been established in other parts of the English-speaking world, Canada, the United Kingdom, and the United States.
2. To use their own words, McConnell and Snoek (2018) stress that "the self-narrative effects we have identified are likely to be particularly pervasive and influential in addiction and so should be given widespread consideration in treatment" (p. 32).
3. McConnell and Snoek (2018) are very clear that they have the "modest aim of illustrating the ways in which self-narratives influence the many small steps toward recovery" (p. 39). However, the importance of their analysis is brought home by the fact that, given the stakes, any improvement in treatment efficiency is a significant payoff.
4. Background adherence to essentialist assumptions about selfhood would explain why "the established self-narratives of addicted people are frequently fatalistic. Joshua

characterizes his ongoing drug use as something that happens to him rather than something he does" (McConnell & Snoek, 2018, p. 39).

5. Thus, the crucial narrative work required on the part of the agent is "to better integrate recovery-directed narrative threads with the existing self-narrative by developing a network of plausible narrative connections between them" (McConnell & Snoek, 2018, p. 38).

6. McConnell and Snoek (2018) give the following example: "Joshua could reinterpret his cycles of drug use as something that he did, rather than something that happened to him, for example" (p. 38).

7. The only way out would be to achieve a complete reduction of narrative explanations to causal explanations offered by the sciences. That will be the only other option so long as it is accepted that "science can't accept interpretation as providing knowledge of human affairs if it can't at least in principle be absorbed into, perhaps even reduced to, neuroscience" (Rosenberg, 2014, p. 41).

8. Rosenberg (2018) offers up reasons—though questionable ones—for thinking that "[t]he same science that reveals why we view the world through the lens of narrative also shows that the lens not only distorts what we see but is the source of illusions we can neither shake nor even correct for most of the time" (p. 3).

9. Loftus (1997) speculates that this belief may be instilled because "an act of imagination simply makes the event seem more familiar" (p. 75).

10. The sort of empirical investigation envisaged would dovetail with testing the Narrative Practice Hypothesis, which predicts that if cultures diverge in significant ways in their narrative practices then they will diverge in their folk psychologies (see Hutto, 2008, p. 188). To make progress on the latter research, Mills (2001) is correct that "[i]deally, the requirement is for strongly supported, comprehensive studies of folk psychologies, which display widespread major differences between the concepts of those folk psychologies and those of western folk psychology" (p. 505).

11. Morag (2016), too, has done some important spadework in clarifying the episodic nature of emotions that places emphasis on connective and synthetic imaginative processes that operate below the level of awareness.

References

Allen, J., Fonagy, P., & Bateman, A. (2008). *Mentalizing in clinical practice*. American Psychiatric Publishing.

Bouchard, M., Lecours, S., Tremblay, L.-M., Target, M., Fonagy, P., Schachter, A., & Stein, H. (2008). Mentalization in adult attachment narratives: Reflective functioning, mental states, and affect elaboration compared. *Psychoanalytic Psychology*, 25(1), 47–66.

Currie, G. 2010. *Narratives and narrators: A philosophy of stories*. Oxford University Press.

Denborough, D. 2014. *Retelling the stories of our lives*. W. W. Norton.

de Shazer, S., & Dolan, Y. 2007. *More than miracles: The state of the art of solution-focused brief therapy*. Haworth Press.

Fulford, K. W. M., Davies, M., Gipps, R. G. T., Graham, G., Sadler, J. Z., Stanghellini, G., & Thornton, T. (2013). Introduction. In K. W. M. Fulford, M. Davies, R. G. T. Gipps, G.

Graham, J. Z. Sadler, G. Stanghellini, & T. Thornton (Eds.), *Oxford handbook of philosophy and psychiatry* (pp. 15–17). Oxford University Press.

Gallagher, S. (2017). *Enactivist interventions.* Oxford University Press.

Gallagher, S. (2020). *Action and interaction.* Oxford University Press.

Gerrans, G. (2014). *The measure of madness.* MIT Press.

Goldie, P. (2012). *The mess inside.* Oxford: Oxford University Press.

Graham, G. (2010). *The disordered mind.* Routledge.

Gray, C., & Garand, J. (1993). Social stories: Improving responses of students with autism with accurate social information. *Focus on Autistic Behavior, 8*(1), 1–10.

Gwozdziewycz, N., & Mehl-Madrona, L. (2013). Meta-analysis of the use of narrative exposure therapy for the effects of trauma among refugee populations. *Permanente Journal, 17*(1), 70–76.

Hutto, D. D. (2008). *Folk psychological narratives.* MIT Press.

Hutto, D. D. (2015). Overly enactive imagination? Radically re-imagining imagining. *Southern Journal of Philosophy, 53,* 68–89.

Hutto, D. D. (2016a). Narrative self-shaping: A modest proposal. *Phenomenology and the Cognitive Sciences, 15*(1), 21–41.

Hutto, D. D. (2016b). Memory and narrativity. In S. Bernecker & K. Michaelian (Eds.), *Routledge handbook of philosophy of memory* (pp. 192–204). Routledge.

Hutto, D. D., & Gallagher, S. (2017). Re-authoring narrative therapy. *Philosophy, Psychiatry and Psychology, 24,* 157–67.

Hutto, D. D., & Myin, E. (2013). *Radicalizing enactivism.* MIT Press.

Hutto, D. D., & Myin, E. (2017). *Evolving enactivism.* MIT Press.

Klapproth, D. M. (2004). *Narrative as social practice: Anglo-Western and Australian Aboriginal oral traditions.* Mouton de Gruyter.

Launer J. (1999). Narrative based medicine: A narrative approach to mental health in general practice. *BMJ, 318*(7176), 117–119.

Loftus, E. (1979). *Eyewitness testimony.* Harvard University Press.

Loftus, E. (1997). Creating false memories. *Scientific American, 277*(3), 71–75.

Loftus, E., & Ketcham, K. (1994). *The myth of repressed memory: False memories and allegations of sexual abuse.* St. Martin's Press.

MacIntyre, A. C. (1984). *After virtue.* University of Notre Dame Press.

McConnell, D. (2016a). Narrative self-constitution and recovery from addiction. *American Philosophical Quarterly, 53,* 307–22.

McConnell, D. (2016b). Narrative self-constitution and vulnerability to co-authoring. *Theoretical Medicine and Bioethics, 37*(1), 29–43.

McConnell, D., & Snoek, A. (2018). The importance of self-narration in recovery from addiction. *Philosophy, Psychiatry and Psychology, 25*(3), 31–44.

Mills, S. (2001). The idea of different folk psychologies. *International Journal of Philosophical Studies, 9*(4), 501–519.

Morag, T. (2016). *Emotion, imagination, and the limits of reason.* Routledge.

Rosenberg, A. (2014). Disenchanted naturalism. In B. Bashour & H. D. Muller (Eds.), *Contemporary philosophical naturalism and its* implications (pp. 17–36). Routledge.

Rosenberg, A. (2018). *How history gets things wrong: The neuroscience of our addiction to stories.* MIT Press.

Rudd, A. (2012). *Self, value, and narrative.* Oxford University Press.

Sainsbury, R. M. (2010). *Fiction and fictionalism.* Routledge.

Schechtman, M. (1996). *The constitution of selves.* Cornell University Press.

Schechtman, M. (2007). Stories, lives, and basic survival. In D. D. Hutto (Ed.), *Narrative and understanding persons* (pp. 155–178). Cambridge University Press.

Schechtman, M. (2011). The narrative self. In S. Gallagher (Ed.), *Oxford handbook of the self* (pp. 394–416). Oxford University Press.

Singer, J. A. (2001). Living in the amber cloud: A life story analysis of a heroin addict. In P. McAdams, R. Josselson, & A. Lieblich (Eds.), *Turns in the road: Narrative studies of lives in transition* (pp. 253–277). American Psychological Association.

Strawson, G. (2004). Against narrativity. *Ratio, 17*(4), 428–542.

Strawson, G. (2020). On the use of the notion of narrative in ethics and psychology. In E. Nahmias, T. W. Polger, & W. Zhao (Eds.), *The natural method: Essays on mind, ethics, and self in honor of Owen Flanagan* (pp. 119–155). MIT Press.

White, M. (2004). Folk psychology and narrative practices. In L. E. Angus & J. McLeod (Eds.), *Handbook of narrative and psychotherapy* (pp. 15–51). Sage.

White, M., & Epston, D. (1990). *Narrative means to therapeutic ends.* W. W. Norton.

Wilker, S., Catani, C., Wittmann, J. et al. (2020). The efficacy of Narrative Exposure Therapy for Children (KIDNET) as a treatment for traumatized young refugees versus treatment as usual: Study protocol for a multi-center randomized controlled trial (YOURTREAT). *Trials, 21,* 185.

Wingard, B., Carolynanha J., & Drahm-Butler, T. (2015). *Aboriginal narrative practice.* Dulwich Centre.

PART II
CURRENT NARRATIVE PRACTICES IN PSYCHOLOGY AND PSYCHOTHERAPY

4

The Art of Teaching the Art of Listening

An Interview Study with University Teachers in Clinical Psychology and Social Work

Elisabeth Punzi and Malgorzata Erikson

When clients encounter practitioners in mental health care, a great deal of what goes on is centered on narratives. The client asks questions and describes difficulties, memories, and experiences. The practitioner asks questions and encourages the client to move toward understanding and increased ability to respond to life's many challenges (Seikkula, 2003; Snyder, 1994). Since the birth of mental health care as a discipline, it has been emphasized that practitioners should strive to make sense of their clients' narratives, situation, suffering, and experiences (Dessel, 2011; Frie, 2010; Lewis, 2011). Clients' narratives are, however, not straightforward. They involve explicit as well as implicit stories that practitioners need to perceive and present to the client (Guilfoyle, 2015). The explicit story might, for example, concern symptoms, whereas the implicit story concerns the meaning of symptoms, or traumatic experiences that are connected to the symptoms. Allen (2008) describes mental health care as an art and emphasizes that practitioners need to be creative. The practitioner needs to perceive nuances, "read between the lines" (Elkins, 2004), and strive for mutual understanding and meaning making (Dessel, 2011). Such an approach to clinical encounters is based in a dialogic perspective in which the other is recognized as a complex, unpredictable, and unique human being (Buber, 1923; Friedman, 2002). The encounter becomes a medium for change and development, precisely because it is unpredictable and complex (Lewis, 2011). A prerequisite is, however, that the practitioner approaches the client openly. Therefore, practicing psychologists, social workers, psychotherapists, and many others need to acquire the ability to engage in dialogues and listen to their clients. Such a skill is a form of practical wisdom that involves judgment (e.g., what parts of the narrative should be followed up, and what questions to pose), reflexivity

Elisabeth Punzi and Malgorzata Erikson, *The Art of Teaching the Art of Listening* In: *Narrative and Mental Health.* Edited by: Jarmila Mildorf, Elisabeth Punzi, and Christoph Singer, Oxford University Press. © Oxford University Press 2023. DOI: 10.1093/oso/9780197620540.003.0005 (e.g., the ability to perceive the complexity of unique situations and acknowledge one's own part of the situation), and ethical considerations (e.g., awareness of dilemmas, contextual factors that contribute to difficulties, and the need to evaluate conflicting ethical principles) (Hickson, 2011; Schön, 1983). In mental health care, such practical wisdom is fundamental (Snyder, 1994). Banerjee and Basu (2016), for example, found that clients perceive the practitioner's ability to listen and "contain" overwhelming experiences as curative. Wilhelmsson Göstas and co-workers (2012) likewise found that clients consider the practitioner's ability to listen and "hold the client" as curative.

In current mental health care, however, there is a tendency to focus on diagnoses, rating scales, and manualized methods. To "facilitate" the process, diagnostic criteria and results from questionnaires have to a considerable extent come to substitute for the narrative (Timimi, 2014). Practitioners are expected to inform clients about their "disorders" and how they should handle their symptoms, and thereby become providers of methods and information (Seikkula, 2003) rather than listeners.

The tendency to downplay the importance of narratives, and the practitioner's ability to listen, has however met with resistance. In the United Kingdom, the Power Threat Meaning Framework (Johnstone et al., 2018) was published. It is a method for conceptualizing the client's difficulties that recognizes the importance of narrative understanding as well as the client's life narrative. It is as an alternative to psychiatric classifications and the tendency to exclude contextual and narrative understanding. Moreover, the United Nations special rapporteur on the right to physical and mental health (Puras & Gooding, 2019) and an editorial in the medical scientific journal *The Lancet* (2021) have identified the weaknesses of mental health care that excludes contextual factors and have underlined the need to acknowledge social determinants and holistic perspectives.

Nevertheless, the tendency to prioritize classification, rating scales, and manualized methods has influenced higher education in clinical psychology and social work, disciplines in which dialogue and narratives traditionally have had a pivotal role. An education that prioritizes such methods is based on the idea that the situations the students will encounter are invariant, while they rather are unpredictable and varying (Schön, 1987, 1992). Therefore, the ability to encounter clients and listen to their narratives needs to be strengthened through an education that involves practice, interaction, and reflection (Werkmeister Rozas, 2004). In this process, students need guidance from experienced teachers. They also need a holding environment in which they might practice, reflect, and make mistakes. In this process, role-play might be important. Peterson (2014), for example, found that social work students improved their understanding of dialogues when engaging in video-recorded role-play. However, it needs to be acknowledged that students might be scared of "looking stupid," and therefore role-play should be used to empower students, not risking that they feel exposed (Kinney & Aspinwall-Roberts, 2010).

A research study investigating how Canadian social work teachers educate students about mental health showed that teachers strive to support their students' skills in active listening, asking open-ended questions, and reflection, which needs a holding environment (Kourgiantakis et al., 2021). Studies have also shown that psychology students request feedback that is personal and supportive so that they can improve (Ali et al., 2015; Erikson et al., 2016). It should also be noted that the ability to listen and reflect on the client's narratives requires teachers who are supported to create safe environments in which there is enough time for reflection (Marshall et al., 2021). Learning activities centered on self-reflection might support the ability to encounter clients in reflective and empathic ways (Punzi, 2015a), and it has been argued that practical wisdom should be central to clinical practice education (Keville et al., 2013; Schön, 1987; Sofronoff et al., 2011; Thompson & West, 2013). Nevertheless, relatively few studies have focused on how university teachers actually do so when they support students to develop their ability to encounter clients and listen to their narratives. We submit that teachers' experiences are important for understanding the prerequisites for teaching the skill of listening. Therefore, the purpose of this study was to investigate university teachers' experiences of teaching the ability to listen to clients' narratives, to students in clinical psychology and social work.

Methodology

Procedure and Participants

Psychology and social work are different disciplines, yet there is no discrete boundary between them. Psychologists engaged in the social work sector often encounter clients with complex psychosocial needs (Punzi, 2015b), and social workers engaged in mental health care organizations often encounter clients with psychological suffering (Probst, 2012). Moreover, both psychologists and social workers need to develop the generic skill of encountering clients, listening to their narratives, and understanding their unique situation and life history. Accordingly, teachers from both psychology and social work were included in this study.

The participants were teachers in the Department of Psychology or the Department of Social Work at Gothenburg University, Sweden. These departments belong to the Faculty of Social Science and co-arrange some courses. The psychology department manages education in individual psychotherapy; the social work department manages education in systemic psychotherapy. This means that our participants were involved in clinical psychology, social work, and psychotherapy education.

The participants were recruited through strategic sampling. Teachers who were involved in teaching nonstructured assessment and interviews were identified through examining the curriculums and through asking the directors of study at each department. Five teachers in the psychology department were identified and asked to participate. One of them could not participate due to a heavy workload. Six teachers in the social work department were identified and asked to participate. Three of them were unable to participate due to a heavy workload. Thus, seven teachers (two men and five women), four from the psychology department and three from the social work department, participated. Three participants from the psychology department were clinical psychologists and licensed psychotherapists; the fourth was a clinical psychologist and a doctoral student. The participants from the social work department were clinical social workers and licensed psychotherapists. All participants had clinical experience in working with adolescents, adults, and families. They had been involved in education from three to 25 years.

Interview and Analysis

During the interviews, the perspectives and experiences of the participants were the focus of attention (Larkin et al., 2006). Elisabeth Punzi conducted the interviews. The initial interview question was open-ended, and follow-up questions were formulated to support the participants to expand on the topics they discussed (Smith et al., 2009). The participants were initially asked to describe their experiences of teaching and to describe the courses in which they were involved. Thereafter the following topics were covered: (1) how the participants discussed clinical encounters, narratives, and nonverbal communication with their students, (2) complexities and paradoxes in clinical practice and in teaching/learning situations, and (3) difficulties and possibilities in teaching narrative practice and listening skills.

The interviewer strove to adopt a not-knowing mode of inquiry, thereby focusing on the experiences and understandings of the participants. The participants were continuously encouraged to describe their experiences and give concrete examples. Rich interview data can thereby be supported, and unpredictable aspects of the studied phenomenon might be illuminated (Ogden & Cornwell, 2010). Simultaneously, it needs to be acknowledged that the research process is influenced by the interviewer and his or her pre-understanding (Potter & Hepburn, 2005). The position of the interviewer will therefore be described under the subheading "Methodological and Ethical Considerations."

The interviews were conducted at the department of each participant, and they lasted between 40 and 60 minutes. Five individual interviews were conducted. At their request, two teachers from the social work department were interviewed together since they wished to learn from each other and use the interview to develop their own teaching. The audio-recorded interviews were transcribed by Malgorzata Erikson.

The transcripts were analyzed using Interpretative Phenomenological Analysis (IPA). In IPA, the aim is to understand how the participants understand the studied phenomenon (Smith et al., 2009). To permit an idiographic approach, each interview was analyzed individually. In the first step, both authors listened to each interview and then read the transcriptions in their entirety. In the next step, statements with relevance for the aim of the study were identified and labeled with provisional codes. To avoid foreclosure, relevance was understood as a broad concept. In the third step, codes that captured understandings shared by the participants were analyzed together, and individual codes were analyzed separately. In the fourth step, individual as well as shared codes were grouped together, thereby identifying the themes that are to be presented. In this step, the analysis reached a more abstract level. In the fifth step, the themes were compared to the interview transcripts to ensure that the participants' narratives had not been distorted during the analysis. The final step was to write the report and illustrate the findings with relevant quotes.

Methodological and Ethical Considerations

The interviewer is a researcher, lecturer, and licensed psychologist who has worked with clients in socially marginalized positions. She has experience in teaching nonstructured and semistructured methods in the same departments as the participants. She was familiar with some participants but had not carried out teaching or research together with them. It cannot be excluded that the participants adapted to the interviewer's perspective. Simultaneously, the familiarity might have encouraged them to express themselves to a listener who was sympathetic to their perspective. Moreover, the interviewer's familiarity might have contributed a sensitivity vis-à-vis the participants' narratives so that nuances and implicit themes could be perceived and explored. However, a false understanding might develop. The interviewer strove to counteract this by continuously asking for examples and lived experiences. During the interviews she continuously told the participants how she perceived what they had communicated and asked them to correct misunderstandings.

Since the interviews were co-analyzed, the risk of false understanding and self-confirmation was diminished. Malgorzata Erikson is a researcher, lecturer, and director of studies at the Department of Public Administration, Gothenburg University, which also belongs to the Faculty of Social Science. She is not connected to the education at the social work or psychology department.

The topic of this paper is not anxiety-provoking and the participants are not in a disadvantaged position vis-à-vis the authors. Nevertheless, it is important to approach the participants with ethical awareness. All participants expressed that they appreciated the interview and our interest in their experiences. They found it meaningful to support students and simultaneously they reflected on difficulties. Therefore, we want to protect their privacy. Quotes are not connected to any specific participant, and we will not present the participants' understandings as holistic narratives since this could permit identification.

Results

The participants' narratives concerned the following themes: (1) avoiding foreclosure, (2) balancing theory and practice, (3) providing supportive teaching/learning activities, and (4) resisting the temptation to "cure" clients.

Avoiding Foreclosure

Throughout the interviews, the participants emphasized the importance of patience when encountering clients and described how they strove to support their students to be open to the client's evolving narrative. According to our participants, an important clinical task is to avoid coming to a conclusion too soon, but to acknowledge that there probably is a lot one does not know about the client. They also wanted to communicate to their students that practitioners cannot control the process. Rather, one needs to listen to the client and use empathy and imagination to grasp explicit communication as well as silences and implicit themes. Together with the students, the participants reflected on case studies, recorded clinical sessions, role-play, and the students' experiences from clinical encounters, and discussed how understanding could be grasped.

The participants reflected on their own clinical work and integrated their clinical experience in their teaching. Time and patience, with clients as well as with students, were understood as prerequisites for building trust and sharing narratives. Our participants, however, described that the students could find it necessary to come to quick decisions. These tendencies were understood as connected to the current prevailing idea that diagnoses are more important than narrative understanding. The participants reflected on the current emphasis on diagnosis and manualized methods and how hard it might be for students to think beyond them. They also reflected on how such tendencies could be overcome.

One participant encouraged students to discuss how clients could be pathologized if they expressed themselves in ways that differed from the expected. This participant presented a "case" to the students and integrated questions about class, gender, and ethnicity, and together they reflected on the normative aspects of diagnostic entities and theoretical concepts. The students were asked to discuss implicit themes that showed the client's abilities. By doing so they could identify concern and compassion toward family members, and ability to handle frustration and carry on with duties despite difficult circumstances. This was described in the following quote:

> It's so powerful. The students . . . they discuss how we need to be careful . . . with our own prejudices and . . . that there's so much we don't know . . . and people might be nervous and therefore might sound aggressive or unreasonable. But that . . . there are so many more sides to a person.

Some participants also reflected on their own confidence in the students. Just as clients tend to develop, students also do so. One cannot expect them to practice the art of listening without support and practice. Some participants understood themselves as role models. Through being patient and confident, they could provide students with experiences of being trusted, which in turn could support students to be patient and confident themselves and to listen to clients' evolving narratives.

Balancing Theory and Practice

The participants also reflected on the interaction between theory and practice; through theory, the practical work was developed, and through practical work, the understanding of theory was developed. The participants from the psychology department tended to dwell more on theoretical topics. They could, for example, reflect on psychodynamic theoretical concepts and how these could be used to elucidate the importance of listening to implicit narrative themes. The participants from the social work department tended to emphasize that personal experience was fundamental for learning theories; theory became relevant, and possible to understand, when connected to personal experiences. It was, for example, described that if theoretical perspectives were overly emphasized early in the education, this could inhibit the students' trust in themselves:

> The students might sense that it's an enormous assignment to encounter a client. We shouldn't portray dialogues as extremely difficult . . . it makes the students . . . scared. Instead, we should encourage students to view everything that happens as encounters. It might be very important to watch TV together with clients at a treatment unit, for example. That's also an encounter . . . and a possibility for dialogue.

Regardless of method or theoretical perspective, the ability to listen to clients' narratives, including silences and nonverbal forms of communication, was seen as fundamental for the developing practitioner. Some participants, however, sensed that theoretical perspectives on narratives were needed in order to position narratives as central to education and clinical practice.

The participants also sensed that theory was needed in order to avoid an "anything goes" attitude among students. The students need to know what they are doing and why, and they need to understand the limitations of the perspectives they are working from. Theory should not be rigidly adhered to; rather, it should support reflection on the interaction between client and practitioner and the meaning of the client's narratives.

Providing Supportive Teaching/Learning Activities

Our participants also spoke about the various teaching/learning activities they used. One approach was to present their own clinical experiences to the students; another was to describe their own shortcomings that illustrate the complexity of clinical work and how difficult it might be to understand clients' narratives. Their own shortcomings could also mitigate stress among students.

The ability to listen to narratives and understand silences, complexities, and subtle topics was described as an art. Some participants used poetry, literature, art, or popular music in their teaching and could describe to students how their own experiences of fiction or theatrical plays had been illuminative for their theoretical understanding, clinical work, or teaching. It could be difficult for some students to understand the silences and the implicit messages in clients' narratives, and they could be overly concerned with the explicit material. The overestimation of explicit material could become a shield against the overwhelming emotions connected to the intense suffering experienced by clients. Some students could disconnect emotionally when sensitive topics such as suicidal thoughts or forms of self-destructive behavior were discussed. Such sensitive topics could, however, become less threatening if they were approached through art, literature, and popular music. Therefore, creative expressions were integrated in teaching/learning activities.

Those who were engaged in psychotherapy education described that some students could be difficult to reach since they had developed their own ways of working, or had their favorite theories or methods, which they sensed were sufficient:

> . . . students who sense that they are very competent and wise and have read a lot. And they lose the clients all the time . . . It's sensitive. It's easy to say to someone who is 22 that we all have to handle that we cannot accomplish everything. It's harder for someone who is 42 who has built the

identity on . . . it's harder to be in a crisis at 42. They might be very skeptical toward someone who presents an idea they don't identify with. And show it in a nonchalant, even rude, way.

In such situations, the participants strove to make difficulties explicit and thereby possible to handle. Most often, the psychotherapy students were thus able to reflect and handle the varying perspectives. In rare cases, students could endure in their worldview, and in such cases the curriculum became important. It was communicated that learning new theoretical and method-ological perspectives was necessary for examination, while opinions were welcomed in the course evaluation.

Another participant engaged in role-play with students and took the role of the client. The students interviewed "the client" and could thereby prac-tice in a safe environment. The participant communicated to the students that the task was not to conduct a "perfect" interview or dialogue—such do not exist—but the task was to interact, listen to the narrative, and reflect. Students thus gained experiences of encountering another human being in an unpredictable way. Moreover, the students experienced what it means to listen, understand, decide when to ask questions and when to remain silent, and permit the client's narrative to evolve.

Resisting the Temptation to "Cure" Clients

The participants underlined that in order to encounter clients and listen to their narratives, one needs to resist temptations to "know" what is best for the clients and "cure" them. The temptation to "cure" clients could be connected to desires to be efficient, which in turn could be connected to the current em-phasis on symptom reduction, or to a personal ideal of being competent. The ideal of being competent could make students preoccupied with themselves and thereby inattentive to the client. Moreover, it could be difficult to admit difficulties. According to our participants, the ability to handle uncertainty was fundamental for clinical practice. It could be difficult for some young students who came from privileged backgrounds to grasp the immense suf-fering and marginalization that some clients experience. In such cases the participants encouraged the students to reflect on their own needs to avoid suffering and whether striving to "do something" and "cure" the client ac-tually was their own desire. Together with the students, they also discussed how difficult it could be to perceive the complex suffering of others. Our participants did not underestimate that clients might need concrete help. However, they reflected on the fact that as practitioners we do not know everything, and we cannot control our clients' lives but rather need to listen and support clients to find their own meaning and solutions and make changes for the better. The participants also reflected on how difficult it might be to encounter traumatized clients and grasp how terrible their situation and suffering is. They acknowledged that it takes time for students to handle their own emotional reactions to trauma. Moreover, it might be overwhelming for students to realize that as human beings we might cause ourselves immense pain and we do not always do what is good for us.

According to our participants, resisting the temptation to "cure" clients is a matter of transition. Most students who early in their education sense that their task is to solve clients' difficulties later on realize that psychosocial difficulties are seldom possible to solve with a distinct intervention. Through practice and reflection, students come to understand that well-intentioned interventions or recommendations might be unsatisfactory; in fact, sometimes they might even provoke clients' anger or frustration. Students also learn from listening to each other. Our participants recognized that just as practitioners need to be patient, teachers need to be patient and learn that students need to learn; it is impossible to hurry narrative understanding and ability to listen.

Discussion

The purpose of this study was to investigate the experiences and practices of teachers who teach the skill of listening to clients' narratives to students in clinical psychology, social work, and psychotherapy education. Our participants strove to communicate to the students that it was important to avoid foreclosure and the temptation to "cure" clients. They also described a move back and forth between clinical material and theory, and a need to develop teaching/learning activities that support reflection. They strove to support students to learn how to endure insecurity and adapt a not-knowing approach to their clients, thereby fostering an ability for active listening. The ability to be open, to endure insecurity, to avoid absolute positions, and to strive to examine each situation in its own right is indeed fundamental for a reflective and responsible practice (Marshall et al., 2021).

Throughout the themes there was a common implicit thread: the importance of trusting the process. The process concerned the relationship between practitioner and client as well as the relation between teacher and student. As a practitioner, one cannot change clients' lives and "cure" them. As a teacher, one cannot do the learning for the students. Students' skills at encountering clients and listening to their narratives developed through reflecting on their own reactions and shortcomings, as well as through clinical practice and theoretical discussions. In other words, narrative understanding is a question of student transition in a safe environment. This approach is in accordance with prior research that has found that clinical education needs to be performed with ethical awareness and opportunities for students to reflect on themselves (Kinney & Aspinwall-Roberts, 2010; Punzi, 2015a).

There was a difference between participants from the two departments. The participants from the social work department underlined the connection between clinical practice and teaching more than those from the psychology department. Since its birth as a discipline, social work has had a close connection to clinical experience, justice, acknowledgment of clients' needs, and practical knowledge (Danto, 2009; Olsson, 1999). This is reflected in the interviews with the participants from the social work department. Likewise, Kourgiantakis and co-workers (2021) found that teachers in social work departments strive to balance established guidelines, biomedical approaches, and structured methods with a social justice framework. Psychology, on the other hand, has had a closer connection to theoretical concepts and variables, and methodology (Danziger, 1997; Schiff, 2017). The participants from the psychology department tended to underline theory more than the participants from the social work department. We therefore suggest that teachers in psychology and social work could inspire each other to develop teaching/learning activities that balance theory and practice. Moreover, they could develop a theoretical perspective on narratives and a methodology for integrating them in education. Thus, the position of clients' narratives could be strengthened in curriculums that currently tend to underline the importance of diagnosis and structured and manualized methods (Punzi, 2015a; Thompson & West, 2013).

Our participants underlined the need to be attentive to the client and reflect on one's own position and ideas about "cure." Their approach is in accordance with the importance of encountering clients with openness and engaging in a mutual dialogue in which the practitioner is touched and transformed as well (Freeman, 2015). This does not, however, mean that practitioners should overidentify with their clients. On the contrary, encounters require maintaining a distance between oneself and the other. In overidentification, there is no other to encounter. Distance does not mean objectification, but rather a genuine acknowledgment of the other as a complex, unpredictable, and uniquely experiencing human being (Buber, 1923, 1951). Practitioners need to deepen their ability for attentiveness so that the concern of the other is in focus (Freeman, 2015). To develop the ability to listen to the many-layered narratives of the clients, including nonverbal communication and silences, students need training and theoretical insight and they also need to approach clinical work as an art (Gadamer, 1996). Given the current emphasis on diagnoses, standardization, and time-limited interventions (Seikkula, 2003; Timimi, 2014), our participants' insistence on avoiding foreclosure and temptations to cure clients and on trusting the process might be seen as a form of resistance. The teachers we interviewed could have complied with the insistence on diagnosis and manualized interventions and focused their teaching on methodology and techniques rather than communicating that clinical practice should be perceived as a form of art. They framed their teaching in a narrative perspective, underlining practical knowledge, human uniqueness, the many levels of narratives, the importance of listening, and the need to trust the process. Their perspective is in line with results from studies that have found that, according to clients, the practitioner's abiity to listen and acknowledge complexity is fundamental for recovery (Banerjee & Basu, 2016; Topor & Matscheck, 2021; Wilhelmsson et al., 2012). This acknowledgment of narratives, listening, and meaning making is also central to narrative psychiatry (Lewis, 2011), narrative social work (Burack-Weiss et al., 2017), and the Power Threat Meaning Framework (Johnstone et al., 2018).

Prior studies have shown that students appreciate teaching/learning activities that support them to reflect and interact with clinical material as well as with each other and with teachers, and they perceive that such approaches support their learning (Binks et al., 2013; Erikson et al. 2016; Gardner, 2001). Therefore, we argue that teachers in psychology and social work should be supported to engage in teaching centered on reflection, narrative understanding, and listening rather than adapting to diagnostic procedures and manualized methods. This would support the students' understanding of the immense suffering and marginalization their future clients might experience as well as their ability to listen to their clients' narratives about their life situation and themselves. We would like to underline that teachers have important contributions to make when it comes to teaching/learning activities.

They find their own models and activities and, for example, involve artistic expression or take the role of the client in role-playing. We submit that such creativity should be encouraged and seen as a contribution.

Based on the results of this study, time and patience seem fundamental for learning/teaching activities that place narratives in the center of attention. Just as time and patience are fundamental for permitting the clients' narratives to evolve and be understood, teachers need to be patient and give their students time to develop the skill of listening to clients' narratives. The ability to listen to clients' narratives was described as an art. It seems as if teaching the art of listening also needs to be respected as a form of art.

Limitations

It should be noted that our study has several limitations. The results are, for example, not easily transferred to other departments, teachers, or countries. Hopefully, the results nevertheless provide insights about the prerequisites for teaching narratives and the art of listening. We also understand that the limited details provided about the participants hinder a holistic understanding of the results. Moreover, differences between varying courses and teaching/learning activities could not be acknowledged, which makes the study somewhat imprecise. Future studies could focus on specific disciplines or courses and thus provide more detailed knowledge. Hopefully, our study could give some inspiration.

References

Ali, N., Rose, S., & Ahmed, L. (2015). Psychology students' perception of and engagement with feedback as a function of year of study. *Assessment & Evaluation on Higher Education, 40*(4), 574–586.

Allen, J. G. (2008). Psychotherapy: The useful art of science. *Smith College Studies in Social Work, 78,* 159–187.

Banerjee, P., & Basu, J. (2016). Therapeutic relationship as a change agent in psychotherapy: An interpretative phenomenological analysis. *The Journal of Humanistic Psychology, 56,* 171–193.

Binks, C., Jones, F. W., & Knight, K. (2013). Facilitating reflective practice groups in clinical psychology training: A phenomenological study. *Reflective Practice, 14,* 305–318.

Buber, M. (1923). *Ich und Du* [I and Thou]. Insel Verlag.

Buber, M. (1951). *Urdistanz und Beziehung* [Distance and relation]. Lambert Schneider.

Burack-Weiss, A., Lawrence, L. S., & Mijangos, L. B. (2017). *Narrative in social work practice: The power and possibility of story.* Columbia University Press.

Danto, E. A. (2009). "A new sort of Salvation Army": Historical perspectives on the confluence of psychoanalysis and social work. *Clinical Social Work Journal, 37*(1), 67–76.

Danziger, K. (1997). *Naming the mind.* Sage.

Dessel, A. B. (2011). Dialogue and social change: An interdisciplinary and transformative history. *Smith College Studies in Social Work, 81,* 167–183.

Elkins, D. N. (2004). The deep poetic soul: An alternative vision of psychotherapy. *Humanistic Psychologist, 32,* 76–102. doi:10.1080/08873267.2004.9961746

Erikson, M., Erikson, M. G., & Punzi, E. (2016). Students' responses to a reflexive course evaluation. *Reflective Practice, 17*(6), 663–675.

Freeman, M. (2015). Beholding and being beheld: Simone Weil, Iris Murdoch, and the ethics of attention. *Humanistic Psychologist, 43,* 160–172. doi:10.1080/08873267.2014.990458

Frie, R. (2010). A hermeneutics of exploration: The interpretative turn from Binswanger to Gadamer. *Journal of Theoretical and Philosophical Psychology, 30,* 79–93.

Friedman, M. (2002). Martin Buber and dialogical psychotherapy. *Journal of Humanistic Psychology, 42,* 7–36. doi:10.1177/002216702237122

Gadamer, H.-G. (1996). *The enigma of health.* Stanford University Press.

Gardner, F. (2001). Social work students and awareness: How does it happen? *Reflective Practice, 2*(1), 27–40.

Guilfoyle, M. (2015). Listening in narrative therapy: Double listening and empathic positioning. *South African Journal of Psychology, 45*(1), 36–49. doi:10.1177/0081246314556711

Hickson, H. (2011). Critical reflection: Reflecting on learning to be reflective. *Reflective Practice, 12*(6), 829–839.

Johnstone, L., Boyle, M., Cromby, J., Dillon, J., Harper, D., Kinderman, P., Longden, E., Pilgrim, D., & Read, J. (2018). *The Power Threat Meaning Framework: Towards the identification of patterns in emotional distress, unusual experiences and troubled or troubling behaviour, as an alternative to functional psychiatric diagnosis.* British Psychological Society.

Keville, S., Siddaway, A. P., Rhodes, L., Horley, N., Brown, R., Dove, L., & White, L. (2013). Learning on the front line: Can personal development during problem-based learning facilitate professional development in trainee clinical psychologists? *Reflective Practice, 14,* 717–728.

Kinney, M., & Aspinwall-Roberts, E. (2010). The use of self and role play in social work education. *Journal of Mental Health Training, Education and Practice, 5,* 27–33. doi:10.5042/jmhtep.2010.0688

Kourgiantakis, T., Sewell, K., Ashcroft, R., & Lee, E. (2021). Canadian social work education in mental health and addictions: Understanding perspectives of faculty members. *Social Work Education.* doi:10.1080/02615479.2021.1985104

Larkin, M., Watts, S., & Clifton, E. (2006). Giving voice and making sense in interpretative phenomenological analysis. *Qualitative Research in Psychology, 3,* 102–120.

Lewis, B. (2011). *Narrative psychiatry: How stories can shape clinical practice.* John Hopkins University Press.

Marshall, T., Keville, S., Cain, A., & Adler, J. R. (2021). On being open-minded, wholehearted, and responsible: A review and synthesis exploring factors enabling practitioner development in reflective practice. *Reflective Practice, 22*(6), 860–876. doi:10.1080/14623943.2021.1976131

Ogden, J., & Cornwell, D. (2010). The role of topic, interviewee and question in predicting rich interview data in the field of health research. *Sociology of Health & Illness, 32*(7), 1059–1071. doi:10.1111/j.1467-9566.2010.01272.x

Olsson, S. (1999). *Kuratorn förr och nu: Sjukhuskuratorns arbete i ett historiskt perspektiv* [The almoner, then and now: Social work in hospitals from a historical perspective]. Doctoral dissertation, Department of Social Work, Gothenburg University.

Peterson, L. (2014). Using technology in peer role-play assignments to enhance competence in clinical dyadic treatment: A pilot study. *Journal of Technology in Human Service, 32*, 4–21. doi:10.1080/15228835.2014.885403

Potter, J., & Hepburn, A. (2005). Qualitative interviews in psychology: Problems and possibilities. *Qualitative Research in Psychology, 2*, 281–307.

Probst, B. (2012). Not quite colleagues: Issues of power and purview between social work and psychiatry. *Social Work in Mental Health, 10*, 367–383.

Punzi, E. (2015a). "These are the things I may never learn from books": Clinical psychology students' experiences of their development of practical wisdom. *Reflective Practice, 16*, 347–360. doi:10.1080/14623943.2015.1023280

Punzi, E. (2015b). Neuropsychological assessment in substance abuse treatment: Focusing on the effects of substances and on neuropsychological assessment as a collaborative process. *Smith College Studies in Social Work, 85*, 128–145. doi:10.1080/00377317.2015.1017357

Puras, D., & Gooding, P. (2019). Mental health and human rights in the 21st century. *World Psychiatry, 18*(1), 42–43.

Schiff, B. (2017). *A new narrative for psychology.* Oxford University Press.

Schön, D. (1983). *The reflective practitioner: How professionals think in action.* Maurice Temple Smith.

Schön, D. (1987). *Educating the reflective practitioner.* Jossey-Bass.

Schön, D. (1992). The crisis of professional knowledge and the pursuit of an epistemology of practice. *Journal of Interprofessional Care, 6*(1), 49–63.

Seikkula, J. (2003). Open dialogue integrates individual and systemic approaches on serious psychiatric crises. *Smith College Studies in Social Work, 73*(2), 227–245.

Smith, J. A., Flowers, P., & Larkin, M. (2009). *Interpretative phenomenological analysis: Theory, method and research.* Sage.

Snyder, M. (1994). The development of social intelligence in psychotherapy: Empathic and dialogic processes. *Journal of Humanistic Psychology, 34*, 84–108.

Sofronoff, K., Helmes, E., & Pachana, N. (2011). Fitness to practice in the profession of psychology: Should we assess this during clinical training? *Australian Psychologist, 46*, 126–132.

The Lancet. (2021). Brain health and its social determinants [editorial]. *Lancet, 398*, 1021.

Thompson, L. J., & West, D. (2013). Professional development in the contemporary educational context: Encouraging practice wisdom. *Social Work Education, 31*, 118–133.

Timimi, S. (2014). No more psychiatric labels: Why formal psychiatric systems should be abolished. *International Journal of Clinical and Health Psychology, 14*, 208–215. doi:10.1016/j.ijchp.2014.03.004

Topor, A., & Matscheck, D. (2021). Diversity, complexity and ordinality: Mental health services outside the institutions—service users' and professionals' experience-based practices and knowledges, and new public management. *International Journal of Environmental Research and Public Health, 18*(13), 7075.

Werkmeister Rozas, L. (2004). On translating ourselves: Understanding dialogue and its role in social work education. *Smith College Studies in Social Work, 74*(2), 229–242.

Wilhelmsson Göstas, M., Wiberg, B., Neander, K., & Kjellin, L. (2012). "Hard work" in a new context: Clients' experiences of psychotherapy. *Qualitative Social Work, 12*, 340–357. doi:10.1177/1473325011431649

5

The Aftermath of Silencing the Trauma

A Narrative Case Study

Soly Erlandsson and Nicolas Dauman

In an open society in which gender equality and ethical principles are regarded as valued, we would expect women's narratives about sexual violence to be heard and respected. As many as one in five women over the course of their lifetime will be sexually assaulted. According to Armstadter and co-workers (2011), epidemiological investigations indicate that the rate of rape among women across a lifetime in the United States is between 12.6% and 16.1%. Most sexual crimes are not reported, however, and the percentage of reports worldwide is approximately 11% (Turquet et al., 2012). Rape and sexual assault against women are not only an act of violence but foremost a way to harm some of the victims for the rest of their lives (e.g., make them powerless and silent). Whether the worldwide "MeToo" movement will lead to changes regarding women's rights to be heard and trustfully met after sexual violence in our societies remains to be seen. Young women in a subordinate position who are sexually assaulted might keep silent about the assault due to fear of losing their job or being neglected by superiors in their field. This is a scenario narrated by women in Sweden who came forward and disclosed their experiences of sexual harassment and assaults that took place during several decades in association with an esteemed cultural scene in Stockholm (Gustavsson, 2019). Gustavsson, who collected the women's narratives, describes her astonishment about the fact that men who seem to understand the problem of sexual assault still lack deeper theoretical knowledge and have no access to the narratives of these victims, as if the women's hostile experiences belong to a parallel or underworld. This is even the case when the men share the streets and the offices with some of the offended women. In other words, we can start out from the presumption that women in general know more about men's lives and world than men know about the world of women. Bourdieu (1998) suggests in his thesis *La domination*

Soly Erlandsson and Nicolas Dauman, *The Aftermath of Silencing the Trauma* In: *Narrative and Mental Health.* Edited by: Jarmila Mildorf, Elisabeth Punzi, and Christoph Singer, Oxford University Press. © Oxford University Press 2023. DOI: 10.1093/oso/9780197620540.003.0006 *masculine* that the androcentric worldview was probably constructed as far back as an archaic era in the history of our societies. Hence, the historical unconscious, which cannot be characterized as biological or psychological in nature, should not be explained by differences between the sexes, as is claimed by psychoanalysis; instead, it must, in Bourdieu's view (1998), be understood as historical constructional work.

Rape Victims, Silence, and Culture

In other parts of our world, sexual violence in its most extreme form (e.g., rape and torture of innocent women and children) is a strategy used to destroy the enemy in armed conflicts. Nadia Murad, one of two persons (together with Dr. Denis Mukwege) to receive the Nobel Peace Prize of 2018, was recognized and honored for her brave narration about what she experienced after being captured and sexually abused in a slave-like way by Islamic State (IS) men in Iraq. The acts of cruelty that she and other female war prisoners were exposed to are of such a magnitude that it is hard to believe anyone can survive, physically and mentally. Nadia Murad decided not to keep silent about what she went through during the time she was captivated by IS, although she knew that she would risk being regarded as a "persona non grata" by people in her village. Many women (and men) keep silent because the consequences of speaking out are not always met with empathy, as reported by Ahrens (2006). In Ahrens's investigation, eight women, all rape victims, were interviewed about their experiences of having disclosed the assault either to a person close to them, to a police officer, or to an informal support giver. The women included in the study had all been traumatized by negative social reactions, which made them keep silent about the trauma. It is likely, according to the author, that the association between silence and powerlessness is one reason behind rape victims' decision to remain silent about the assault (Ahrens, 2006). It is, however, rather common for rape victims to disclose the assault to at least one person (Ullman & Filipas, 2001). However, victims who are blamed for their own inappropriate behavior and thus almost accused of having caused the assault might feel that they are being raped a second time; they experience what one may call "secondary victimization."

Research has shown that rape by a stranger is viewed as a stereotypical form of sexual assault and deviates from rape by an acquaintance; in the latter, victim blaming is greater (Grubb & Harrower, 2008). Myths about rape stating that women are themselves responsible in some way or another have been around for a very long time; for example, questioning women's behaviors and how they dress, believing that women enjoy sexual domination, or thinking that only promiscuous women are rape victims. Those rape myths and their ideological grounds can have an impact on how society and institutions fail to acknowledge the event and assist and support the victims (Lebowitz, 1985; quoted by Roth & Lebowitz, 1988). Hill and Marshall (2018) studied beliefs about sexual assault in two different cultures by asking 112 Indian and 117 British adults about their views on rape myths. A greater acceptance of myths was found in the Indian sample; according to the authors, this points to more traditional gender roles and hostile sexism in the Indian culture compared to an egalitarian culture such as Britain. Findings that culture has a role to play in terms of how rape myths are spread and kept alive underline the importance of preventive actions to raise awareness about how patriarchal societies may influence women's lives and health. Gravelin and co-workers (2019) investigated in two different cohorts (Study 1 and 2) the impact of power and powerlessness on blaming and denying feelings of rape victims and found some interesting results when they compared the attitudes of female and male study participants. In Study 1, who were primarily Caucasians (N = 139) were recruited via a mechanical company in the United States. They were randomly assigned to three different power conditions (high, low, and neutral power). Results showed that women in high-power conditions adhered to the perspective of victims to a larger extent (lower ratings of blame) than women in neutral and low-power conditions. Almost the opposite was true for the male participants: Men feeling powerless adopted the perspective of the assaulted individual more often than men in high-power and neutral conditions. The authors' suggestion for future research is to study possible links between powerlessness in men and their perspective taking associated with emotional state and empathy (Gravelin et al., 2019).

Women who have been raped have a significantly higher risk for poor health compared to women without a history of assault. The percentage of victims of sexual violence in the United States who are diagnosed with depression or anxiety disorders is reported to be 55% compared to 17% in a sample of non-victimized individuals (Choudharry et al., 2012). A history of sexual assault was found to be associated with a higher prevalence of post-traumatic stress disorder (PTSD) in comparison with other forms of traumatic events (Armstadter et al., 2011). PTSD symptoms have been reported by an estimated 33% to 45% of rape survivors (Campbell et al., 2008). Rape victims, who most often are traumatized, face a wide array of negative experiences as a consequence of the violence. Affective responses found among rape victims are terror, rage, loss, guilt, shame, and betrayal (see Roth & Lebowitz, 1988). Being victimized can influence a person's basic assumptions about the framework of life—for example, that you live in a meaningful, orderly world with people who are mostly fair, and that you experience yourself as a worthy person (Janoff-Bulman, 1985).

Epstein (1986; quoted by Roth & Lebowitz, 1988) suggested that losing important basic assumptions of the world can make the rape victims feel that life is unmanageable and paradoxical, leading them to either reconstruct their vision of a previously experienced safe place or to change their view of themselves. Judith Alpert (2015) recounts memories from her childhood and a mother who was afraid of almost everything, and somehow the mother's fears were passed on to her daughter, Judith. In her youth, the mother had, for unknown reasons, suddenly become withdrawn, frightened, and silent. At a later point in life Alpert realized how transgenerational history had bearings on her mother's silence, but also on a family that was silent. She refers back to both the mother's trauma and to the history of her grandmother's life in one of many pogroms in Russia. Before her death at age 87, Alpert's mother finally told her daughter about a trauma that had severe consequences in life for both mother and child: "I was raped by the dress shop owner when I was 15" (Alpert, 2015, p. 299). The author describes how silence after an unresolved trauma can pass from one generation to the next, and thus silence becomes the screen on which fear and suffering are projected (Alpert, 2015). The French child psychoanalyst Françoise Dolto defines the small child as an independent person with his or her own subject position and with desires from birth. She also considers how the structure of the child originates from the collective speech of the family. Painful and repressed experiences that parents are carrying can be imprinted in the family's communication and expressed in an unrecognizable form through the child's symptoms (Dolto, 1971/1997).

In a psychodynamic approach to an individual's suffering, the term *trauma* refers to a specific kind of adverse event. Not only does trauma induce stress and strain upon the individual body, but it basically also constitutes a disruption in the life course of the traumatized person. As Mills noted (2008, p. 382): "The present becomes merged with the past in temporal diffusion and post-traumatic stress subsequently becomes the symptomatic outcome." Unlike a stressful event, a traumatic event cannot be integrated into a previous pattern of ego experiences (which would suit such a statement such as "this happened to me"). It cannot be clustered to individual memories of the past because it is incommensurate with one's lived social interactions and shared emotions. If a trauma was to be compared to a painting, it should be seen as an empty frame—that is, with no form or shape to narrate a story about what happened there. A trauma is a shortcut in the ongoing meaning-making process of representing oneself in relation to others, and others in relation to oneself. What happened to a traumatized individual has been subjected to a specific defensive process, which relies on an altered sense of time. As was wisely observed by the British psychoanalyst and pediatrician Donald W. Winnicott, the traumatic event is not remembered as a past event; rather, it is anticipated with fear as a disaster to come. This "fear of breakdown," as Winnicott called it (1963), focuses the individual's attention on details from the material reality that he or she is searching for with a sense of an imminent threat. The individual's tense experience might be accompanied by a change in self-perception and perception of the world. Hallucinations, for instance, can trigger odd feelings about what is happening around the individual. This altered relationship to one's external reality results from a threat to the organization of the ego—that is, a fragmentation of the individual's inner experience.

The Narrative-Psychological Approach in Research

The *narrative method* is an umbrella term for several narrative approaches in psychology that use personal stories to help interpret and understand how people struggle to create meaning from their life experiences. This meaning-making process is natural and important for one's well-being and mental health. Researchers using the narrative method assume that we have an inner drive to create meaning and that we recreate our view of ourselves concomitantly with life changes. In this way, narration can contribute to a sense of coherence, and it can also inspire one to initiate changes and to adapt to new conditions (McMahon et al., 2012). Personal narratives are shaped by social and psychological forces both conscious and unconscious. Although a narrative is focused on one individual, it is possible to also interpret the socio-cultural norms and values that the person holds. In social science, it is not unusual to view identity as determined by the prevailing discourse in society, built on how we understand our position in the world and the social context (McMahon et al., 2012). A narrative psychological approach has developed as a way to understand the psychology of trauma and how people adhere and respond to traumatizing events (Crossley, 2000). The ability to create an integrated narrative about life can be difficult for a person with a history of severe trauma, for example, due to disassociation. Through storytelling, a person can find a way to create order out of chaos by linking their past story to the present time. Narrative can also facilitate the search for a genuine self and identity. This search raises existential questions, which can help people to formulate for themselves how they would prefer to live their lives. A narrative is never static: Its meaning can be seen through an alternative discourse in which social phenomena are reinterpreted.

We now turn to our case study, where we pull the various strands of our previous discussion together. At the heart of this trauma narrative is the case of Lucie, a 70-year-old female patient, and what she disclosed during psychotherapy.

Lucie's Narrative of a Hidden Trauma

Lucie consulted a tinnitus clinic for a severe and annoying tinnitus that she, from a psychological viewpoint, experienced as a life-threatening symptom. Following the consultation, she was referred to a psychotherapist for treatment (Dauman & Erlandsson, 2012). At the end of the psychotherapy sessions, Lucie gave informed consent to publish parts of the notes on how tinnitus interfered with her present and past experiences of discomfort and agony. Ethical permission was given by the Ethical Committee CPP du Sud-Ouest et Outre-mer III (People Protection Committee). Reviewing and reanalyzing the therapy notes provided some new perspectives on the story of her life and trauma that were worth recognizing.

In Lucie's narrative, time seems to be of subordinate significance for the memory of a traumatic event that took place half a century earlier. Memories of her trauma were well stored but continued to dwell under the surface until she was prepared to share the experience with someone she trusted, her psychotherapist. Lucie could not afford to travel to the psychotherapy sessions at the hospital, so when the clinician suggested continuing the therapy over the phone, she agreed to do so. The opportunity to be in regular contact over the phone with the psychotherapist gave Lucie a break from her isolation.

Tinnitus is usually described as the perception of sound that results exclusively from activity within the nervous system without any corresponding mechanical, vibratory activity within the cochlea; it is not related to external stimulation of any kind (Jastreboff & Hazell, 2004). The definition of tinnitus as a sound can be somewhat misleading, however, as the experience is often too complex to be characterized as a sound. Hence, by focusing on an outside source (sound), the subjective experience of an inner phenomenon may become objectified and devalued (Erlandsson & Dauman, 2013). Dauman and co-workers (2017) showed in a qualitative grounded theory study that an underestimated part of tinnitus-induced disability is related to frustration. The authors stress that the frustration hypothesis in disabling tinnitus may contribute to a more comprehensive understanding of the patient's experienced distress. Based on the study results, significant tinnitus-related health issues can be raised and incorporated in a clinical dialogue with the patient.

A long-term disability such as tinnitus can have harmful effects on an individual's life, sense of identity, and social relationships, as was illustrated by the narratives of the participants in a study by Erlandsson and colleagues (2020). The single most widely used approach in research discovering the difficulties patients experienced in connection with tinnitus is the quantitative approach, which involves measuring scales and questionnaires. Considering their limited knowledge of an inside personal perspective on the annoyance people may experience with tinnitus, the researchers decided to use a narrative-psychological approach to investigate the condition's impact on quality of life and demands for one's future life. The study demonstrated the complexity of the problem as well as the severe consequences it had on the participants' personal resources, which foregrounds the importance of listening to the individual patient's unique story (Erlandsson et al., 2020). The onset of tinnitus can in certain cases follow a strong, emotion-driven experience, as described by Erlandsson (1998) in an article focusing on counseling in medical settings. Sometimes tinnitus is perceived as the cause behind both bodily and mental splitting and fear of being overwhelmed by the sound. A condition that restricts someone from having a "normal life" without the presence of a serious physical illness conveys an important psychological message. Cognitive distortions and impaired information processing can lead to an unproportionally aggravated attention to tinnitus, which in severe cases can be compared with a form of sensory deprivation (Erlandsson,

2000a). Severe tinnitus may exacerbate symptoms that are related to mental health problems, and research has demonstrated a link between personality disorders and severe tinnitus suffering (Erlandsson & Persson, 2006).

Lucie had a history of mental health problems and had been hospitalized a number of times. She recalled being very anxious prior to the onset of tinnitus and used to walk at nights in the streets near her apartment. Lucie was afraid of the noises that she thought came from the apartment above hers. She asked for help from one of her neighbors but did not receive any support from this person. During one psychotherapy session, Lucie described her alarming reactions with vivid, yet elusive words: "I had an anxiety attack . . . started to panic! I could not stay at home . . . was too scared. All that noise they were making. I walked out of my apartment during the night; I couldn't manage to bear it anymore." Tinnitus first occurred when Lucie returned home after admission to a psychiatric hospital for treatment. At first, she thought that the new noise she heard came from a fan, an explanation that Lucie's daughter doubted. She told her mother not to pay attention to the noise and so did the consulting psychiatrist, who advised her to keep busy with daily routines. People's attitudes toward her suffering evoked sadness and resentment in Lucie: "They told me that it was all in my head . . . that I invented the tinnitus." Some time later, Lucie recalled that tinnitus occurred after the installation of a third radio relay near her apartment. As she remembered, the installation took place during school holidays, an observation that made sense to her: "There might be much more traffic on the radio relay then, because family members call each other more frequently." Lucie felt the Hertzian waves of the radio relay to be intrusive but had nobody to share her frustration with: "No one believed me about the waves of the radio relay . . . .but yourself, do you believe me?" she asked the psychotherapist. Another of Lucie's suspicions was that the medication she had taken at the hospital contributed to damaging her ears. Back home she consulted her family physician about tinnitus, but his answer did not reassure her: "You have tinnitus, Madam . . . It is your ears, they are worn out."

The confrontation with irresistible noises scared Lucie to the point that she began to think about suicide and ending her life by jumping from a viaduct close to her home. The reason why she did not follow through with suicide was her concern for her grandson. A couple of months earlier, her grandson had told his grandmother that he no longer wanted to be in contact with her and hung up the phone. Before he walked out on her, she had hosted him in her apartment, giving him money and encouraging him to find a job so that he could have a life with dignity. She worried about her grandson's acquaintances, whom she feared could have a bad influence on him. She expressed her fears: "I am always afraid that something will happen to him with the police force." When Lucie heard police sirens in the street or saw the arrest of young people on TV, she thought about her grandson. She felt that she had a close relationship with him: "He is everything for me—I recognize myself in him." Several months after the start of the psychotherapy, Lucie was still bothered by intrusive tinnitus, and still had no news from her grandson. A proposal by her psychotherapist to visit her in the apartment was accepted. While talking over a cup of tea, Lucie seemed withdrawn and absorbed in her thoughts. She questioned the reason behind the frightening events in her life, when the only wish she had was to "be happy," and said: "Something happened inside me that I did not understand. What is it that has made me fall over like this? [...] Something in me betrayed me. My body ... it must be something that has triggered all of this."

Lucie had her own reason to think about betrayal and to worry about her grandson being involved in fishy business. During the last session of psychotherapy, in her home, Lucie told the therapist about a gruesome event that had happened to her at the age of 22, about the same age as her grandson and her psychotherapist. At the time, Lucie was searching for a job, and a man who informed her about job vacancies made an appointment with her. She remembered walking downstairs to a room, empty with the exception of a bed and a mirror. In this room the man violated her sexually. She did not report the rape and kept silent about her trauma, because, as she said, "no one took notice about those events back then." Who would believe a young woman with no position accusing a man of rape 50 years ago? Lucie remembers where the assault took place (the frame), but she cannot recall the memory of her as a victim (the content) or the aftermath of the trauma. Lucie perceives the present suffering as deeper compared to how she felt at the time when the rape happened. She has no words to describe her suffering other than as a reason to be depressed and contrasts her past and present mood in the following way: "I can remember the frame (where it happened), but what happened there I can't ... but that is nothing compared to what I am suffering now ... That is the reason why I was depressed."

Lucie's experiences and unresolved trauma from almost 50 years earlier seem to have a link to her upsetting thoughts about what she believes are the "Hertzian waves of the radio relay" above her apartment. As back then, she keeps silent because she feels that no one wants to know about her story.

With the psychotherapist Lucie shared her observation of three men who entered an apartment upstairs and made noises related to fishy business:

> They were trafficking upstairs, making false credit cards and cheque books with their machine. I heard them . . . [then Lucie made some moves, clutching her fists as if she was mimicking a fight] They were struggling upstairs . . . I remember one day, when I was shopping, and the cashier asked me if I lived in town when I paid with my credit card. I thought to myself that the policemen searched for the traffickers and they asked for checking every credit card owner . . . The police came eventually, and the men upstairs were arrested, and the noises stopped.

Tinnitus occurred in the wake of what Lucie called the "arrest" of the three men upstairs. Her feelings of being intruded upon by the upstairs noise stopped after the intervention of the police. This did not, however, lead to relief from her hallucinatory resolution, and she still feared that her grandson could be arrested for drug trafficking. Tinnitus continued to plague her, although she seemed relieved from having shared her trauma with her psychotherapist.

During a final contact over the phone Lucie wanted to share "something extraordinary" with the therapist. A few days before, she awoke with a strange feeling "that something was missing." She realized that the tinnitus was gone: "They left me, eventually." In the evening on the same day, her tinnitus reappeared, but she found it to be softer and more tolerable. Lucie's last, meaningful words were: "I found someone I could talk to about what happened to me. I will never forget that."

The Metaphorization of Suffering Through Narrative

More than 100 years ago Pierre Janet explained what he believed to be the forces behind dissociation. Janet was, however, not the first psychiatrist to observe and describe dissociation in patients suffering from hysteria (Van der Hart & Horst, 1989). Janet argued that traumatic experiences are relived unconsciously as highly vivid memories through sensory fragments like images or sounds, or through compulsive ruminations or reenactments of the trauma. Janet's disassociation theory should be of special value for researchers and clinicians with a focus on trauma-induced tinnitus. Van der

Hart and Horst (1989) reported that Janet tried to analyze and describe in psychological terms the poorly understood multidimensional regulating system. According to Kaminer (2006), more recent evidence has shown that emotionally charged memories are not stored as a unified and integrated whole, but rather as sensory fragments and without coherent verbal element. The memory of the trauma is in itself the feared stimulus as it has a strong connection to danger (Kaminer, 2006). In the context of a trustworthy psychotherapeutic relationship, however, an explanatory narrative can be developed. Through the exploration of the unconscious processes that influence emotions, thoughts, and behavior, psychotherapy may help the patient to fill out the "plot" of her story (Crossley, 2000). As Spence (1982) suggested, the elaboration of self-narratives in psychotherapy contributes to the exploration of a sense of oneself in relation to time and past events. Accordingly, the discovery of the unconscious and its meaning can help the clients to understand the causal link between present and past events in their life. The present case study illustrates the complex relationship between sensory fragments (i.e., hallucinations and tinnitus) and the disclosure of a hidden trauma that occurred half a century earlier.

In his pioneering work, the Hungarian psychoanalyst Ferenczi (1934) emphasized that the setting of psychotherapy offers the sufferer a context of careful listening that does not contest the fact that the trauma is incommensurate with the patient's daily routines. In accordance with this, building a trustful therapeutic alliance is essential for restoring a patient's sense of belonging to a reality that can be shared with someone else. Ferenczi also made several clear statements about the non-technical presence of the therapist by the patient's side. This form of presence can be seen as the therapist's affordability as a human being, including a flexible attitude and tolerance to the confusion that the sufferer displays (Ferenczi, 1932). Within the therapeutic encounter, Lucie feels confident and safe enough to approach what is hidden and forgotten. A second feature of the psychotherapeutic approach to trauma concerns the alteration of the sense of oneself in the sufferer. Notably, ego fragmentation also brings the patient's inner experience closer to dream processes. In his famous study on dreams, Freud (1900) made a major contribution to the understanding of the unconscious by elaborating on the processes of translation of the seemingly disorganized images and speeches of dreams into a coherent narrative about the dreamer's concerns and wishes. Every detail from the dream stands for a myriad of thoughts and associations that are intertwined with each other through the poetry of language. As we shall consider below, an approach to ego fragmentation as a process of translation of unconscious thoughts offers the royal road to the integration of the sufferer's fragmented memories and disorientation.

The word *traffic* in Lucie's narrative is illustrative of the overdetermination Freud found essential to the dream thought. Many associations of thoughts that surround the word *traffic* are pervasive in the way Lucie presented her anguish for the psychotherapist. These individual associations of thoughts appear to be intertwined with the historical meaning of the word. In French (Lucie's mother tongue) as in English, the word *traffic* initially referred to some hidden business associated with illegal or immoral benefits (in the fourteenth century, see Rey-Debove & Rey, 2000; Stevenson, 2007). As noted above, Lucie used the word *traffic* when she talked about her grandson, whom she identified with ("He is everything for me" . . . "I recognize myself in him"). She was afraid that her grandson would fall into drug trafficking, not being able to resist the influence of bad acquaintances forcing him to do things against his will. Later, the word *traffic* came to refer to a hidden influence associated with power and lobbies (Rey-Debove & Rey, 2000). In the mid-nineteenth century, the word was connected to the rise of industrial life and the halo of mystery that surrounded the technology of trains. Lucie's intuition regarding her feeling of being overwhelmed by the Hertzian waves from the radio relay, when tinnitus occurred, testifies to the meaning of the following words: "There might be much more traffic on the radio relay then," she said, "because family members call each other more frequently." Talking about the traffic of the Hertzian waves, Lucie unconsciously tried to figure out some mysterious technological influence that could explain what she was going through. She also used the word *trafficking* when mentioning the noises that the three mysterious men above her apartment were making. The word *trafficking* later came to stand for manipulation of something through the use of a secret means, or with the purpose to fool someone, and it became synonymous with falsification. The men upstairs who frightened Lucie were making "false credit cards and cheque books" and the neighbor next to her apartment had been "arrested" by the police for a similar crime.

The disclosure of Lucie's sexual trauma resonates as an underlying motif for the repetition of the numerous meanings of the word *traffic*. The assault was an act of power, illegal and immoral, that remained hidden and a secret between Lucie and her aggressor for half a century. By referring to her bodily experience and tinnitus, Lucie expressed her bewilderment by using words that pointed to her aggressor: "Something in me betrayed me. My body . . ."

In truth, she was betrayed by the man whom she encountered in the hope of finding a job (see Roth & Lebowitz, 1988, about betrayal as a response to rape). Essential to Lucie's worries, prior to her hospitalization, was her fear that the grandson would not find a job and live with dignity. As was disclosed in the psychotherapy, her fear about a coming threat toward her grandson had already happened, but to herself (Winnicott, 1963). Unconsciously, the fragmented intuitions and perceptions Lucie tried to communicate contained a piece of historical truth (Freud, 1911).

In her book *Metaphor and Meaning in Psychotherapy*, the American psychoanalyst Ellen Siegelman (1990) contrasted bodily symptoms with metaphors. She pointed out the bodily matrix of self-knowledge in relation to others' attitudes, and how self-narratives are built up from the primacy of body experience. In this perspective, Siegelman considered symptoms as unfinished metaphors, which conceal dilemmas and conflicts that sufferers are confronted with in their relationships to other people. Symptoms indicate a history of events that remain unnamable to the sufferer, and also unarticulated to her self-perception. Unconsciously, the person shows an attitude of fear and turning away from threatening past events. In contrast, the metaphors acknowledge and articulate the threats patients experience from others. Metaphors also reveal the insights that a patient gains from paying attention to bodily experiences and true desires. The healing process of psychotherapy, advocated by Siegelman, can be described as the creation of metaphors originating from the symptoms. Lucie's perceptions of threats that surrounded her remained merely as abnormal symptoms to herself, as well as to her entourage. In the dialogue with the therapist, credence was given to her intuitions, allowing for an elaboration of self-knowledge from an initially confused bodily experience (i.e., hallucinations, delusions, and intuitions). It was a relief to Lucie to be able to share her tragedy, the sexual trauma, with her psychotherapist—a life experience that she might have wished to also share with her grandson. As we pointed out above, according to Alpert the transmission of the unresolved trauma can be characterized as transgenerational—a trauma that is passed on to the next generation through unconscious fantasies, stemming from events that the child had not even experienced (Alpert, 2015). The fact that Lucie has given consent to publish her narrative is proof of her courage to integrate her trauma into her life story, but also passing on her narrative to others to read and learn from.

At the time of the rape, Lucie felt that recognition and support would not be there for her. For the same and for other reasons, many sexually assaulted women come to the same conclusion as Lucie that reporting the crime is useless. The assault becomes disassociated and repressed as the victims try to go on with their lives. But silence has a price and implies that the victimized person is violated a second time, detached from her own narrative and memories of what happened. In her testimony, Lucie explains that she feels betrayed, but not by someone else. Instead, she feels that her own body has betrayed her and, unconsciously, she touches upon a fragmented memory that has been denied materialization. The body does not lie to her; it makes her realize that something is wrong. In a broader, narrative sense, Lucie's past trauma scene is explored through her body scene in the form of sounds, both inner (tinnitus) and outer (the noise she hears above the apartment). In the process of keeping disturbing thoughts and feelings underneath, focusing on tinnitus helps her to survive mentally. The child psychoanalyst Melanie Klein (1975) suggested that elementary, mental formations of anxiety and depression are part of the normal child's as well as of the adult's mental life. She described anxiety during the child's first three months as a fear of being destroyed and exterminated by an attack from inner objects—a condition imprinted by life or death, which Klein called the paranoid-schizoid position. A more mature state, according to the model, is the depressive position, which is established during the first year of life and is characterized by guilt, reparation, and the development of ambivalence. Klein proposed that an individual who is struggling with an exceptionally frustrating situation might fall back into the paranoid-schizoid position. Considering Klein's developmental model, some of the defensive reactions found in patients with chronic, severe tinnitus might be perceived as characteristic expressions of the paranoid-schizoid position, implying that the noise will pursue, attack, and/or destroy the person from inside (Erlandsson, 2000b). Like other sufferers, Lucie personified the presence of tinnitus in her ear as the materialization of some kind of intention, saying, for instance, "*They* are awakened now" or "*They* left me, eventually."

Epilogue

Psychodynamic psychotherapy relies on the assumption that personal and existential issues will arise from, and during, the course of therapy. Even though neither the patient nor the therapist can know in advance when and how a disclosure will occur, both believe that telling the story of the patient's suffering can help him or her go through unbearable experiences (whatever they are). Enabling the patient to experience limitations and hardships instead of repressing those experiences (i.e., protecting oneself from them) is the underlying theme of the psychodynamic process (Bion, 1964; Winnicott, 1971). To deal with the anxiety of being alive, and to repeatedly negotiate their desires with those of others, is an issue waiting for patients to deal with at the end of the process. One can expect patients to be more confident as they dare to live as persons with sorrows and renewed desires. We also like to underscore the importance of acknowledging the psychotherapist's own horizon of experience to be used as a guide to the inner life of the patient. This implies bringing ourselves in harmony with the other's experience of the world (Olsson, 2016). At the end of therapy, Lucie told her psychotherapist about an intersubjective experience of this kind: "I found someone I could talk to about what happened to me. I will never forget that."

Narrative psychology is concerned with subjectivity and the lived experience of the person, in contrast to social constructivist approaches in which there is a tendency to "lose the subject" (Crossley, 2000). As clinical researchers and practitioners, we are responsible for helping to illuminate our patients' narrative about their suffering and contributing to a story that is true to them. The clinical setting may offer the patient, for the first time after the trauma, the right not to be contested by another about the suffering (Ferenczi, 1934). A confidential therapeutic alliance is necessary for a sustained integration of fragmented experiences of the trauma into a personal history, as we saw in the case of Lucie. Social factors such as emotional support, compassion, and the quality of the encounters with professionals and caregivers are of considerable importance as well. To recognize the psychological aspect of tinnitus means also acknowledging the clients' narratives about their own experiences and relationships to a social network (Tyler & Erlandsson, 2002). A prevailing aim in all psychotherapeutic work is to create a "fuller plot," which can lead to a more dynamic plot—perhaps, we could say, to a more coherent life story (Polkinghorne, 1988).

Women's opportunities to narrate what sexual abuse does to their self-confidence and psychological health need to be facilitated and encouraged in society. Their impact can be twofold: (1) increase awareness about and insight (among men) into the fact that women's rights include legal rights to be protected from sexual violence and (2) contribute to a positive influence on women's physical and mental health as their story can be told and heard by a respectful listener. Not only the victim but also the perpetrators and those who are witnesses are affected by the trauma. Alpert (2015) draws our attention to the perpetrators' children, who might be traumatized by inheriting "the damage and the ghosts from the past, because they are deprived of their memory" (p. 309). The author takes as an example children and grandchildren of Germans who had been involved in the Holocaust. Dr. Denis Mukwege, gynecologist and activist, has for many years helped women to heal physically and mentally after they have been sexually abused and tortured in wars in Kongo-Kinshasa. In an interview in October 2018, following the announcement of the Nobel Peace Prize Dr. Mukwege gave his vision of how to deal with sexual violence: "This is not a women's issue; it is an issue for humanity and men must take responsibility for ending these assaults."

Acknowledgments

The authors are most grateful to Lucie for her willingness to allow publication of her narrative. Most quotations that belong to Lucie's story originate from the article by Dauman and Erlandsson (2012), which was published in the *International Journal of Qualitative Studies on Health and Well-Being* (IJQHW). We are thankful to Associate Professor Henrika Jormfeld, Chief Editor of the IJQHW, for giving us permission to use and reinterpret the original material.

References

Ahrens, C. E. (2006). Being silenced: The impact of negative social reactions on the disclosure of rape. *American Journal of Community Psychology, 38*, 263–274.

Alpert, J. L. (2015). Enduring mothers, enduring knowledge: On rape and history. *Contemporary Psychoanalysis, 51*(2), 296–311. doi:10.1080/00107530.2015.1037236

Armstadter, A. B., McCauley, J. L., Ruggiero, K. J., Resnick, H. S., & Kilpatrick, D. G. (2011). Self-rated health in relation to rape and mental health disorders in a national sample of women. *American Journal of Orthopsychiatry, 81*(2), 202–210.

Bion, W. R. (1963/2005). *Elements of psychoanalysis*. Karnac Books Ltd.

Bourdieu, P. (1998). *La domination masculine*. Éditions du Seuil.

Campbell, R., Greeson, M. R., Bybee, D., & Raja, S. (2008). The co-occurrence of childhood sexual abuse, adult sexual assault, intimate partner violence, and sexual harassment: A meditational model of post-traumatic stress disorder and physical health outcomes. *Journal of Consulting and Clinical Psychology, 76*, 194–207. http://dx.doi.org/10.1037/0022-006X.76.2.194

Choudharry, E., Smith, M., & Bossarte, R. M. (2012). Depression, anxiety, and symptom profiles among female and male victims of sexual violence. *American Journal of Men's Health, 6*, 28–36. http://dx.doi.org/10.1177/1557988311414045.

Crossley, M. L. (2000). *Introducing narrative psychology: Self, trauma and the construction of meaning.* Open University Press.

Dauman, N., & Erlandsson, S. I. (2012). Learning from tinnitus patients' narratives—a case study in the psychodynamic approach. *International Journal of Qualitative Studies on Health and Well-Being, 2*, 33–44.

Dauman, N., Erlandsson, S. I., Albarracin, D., & Dauman, R. (2017). Exploring tinnitus-induced disablement by persistent frustration in aging individuals: A grounded theory study. *Frontiers in Aging Neuroscience.* doi:10.3389/fnagi.2017.00272

Dolto, F. (1971/1997). *Le cas Dominique.* Éditions du Seuil. *Fallet Dominique*, Swedish translation by G. Hallerstedt & M. Fatton. Rabén Prisma.

Epstein, S. (1986). *The self-concept, the traumatic neurosis, and the structure of personality.* Unpublished manuscript.

Erlandsson, S. I. (1998). Psychological counselling in the medical setting—some clinical examples given by patients with tinnitus and Ménière's disease. *International Journal for the Advancement of Counselling, 20*, 265–276.

Erlandsson, S. I. (2000a). Psychological profiles of tinnitus patients. In R. D. Tyler (Ed.), *Handbook on tinnitus* (pp. 25–58). Singular Publishing Co.

Erlandsson, S. I. (2000b). Tinnitus: ljud som bärare av psykisk smärta—empiriska och teoretiska perspektiv [Tinnitus: Sounds as carrier of psychological pain—empirical and theoretical perspectives]. In S. G. Carlsson, E. Hjelmqvist, & I. Lundberg (Eds.), *Hälsa och handikapp ur ett psykologiskt perspektiv* (pp. 105–125). Boréa Bokförlag.

Erlandsson, S. I., & Dauman, N. (2013). Categorization of tinnitus in view of history and medical discourse [editorial]. *International Journal of Qualitative Studies on Health and Well-Being, 8*, 23530. http://dx.doi.org/10.3402/qhw.v8i0.23530

Erlandsson, S. I., Lundin, L., & Dauman, N. (2020). The experience of tinnitus and its interaction with unique life histories—life events, trauma and inner resources narrated by patients with tinnitus. *Frontiers in Psychiatry, 11*, 136. doi:10.3389/fpsyt.2020.00136

Erlandsson, S. I., & Persson, M.-L. (2006). A longitudinal study investigating the contribution of mental illness in chronic tinnitus patients. *Audiological Medicine, 4*, 124–133.

Ferenczi, S. (1932/1994). Confusion of tongues between adults and children: The language of tenderness and passion. In M. Balint (Ed.), *Final contributions to the problems and methods in psychoanalysis.* Karnac Books Ltd, 156–167.

Ferenczi, S. (1934). Gedanken über das Trauma [Some thoughts about trauma]. *Internationale Zeitschrift für Psychoanalyse, 20*(1): 5–12.

Freud, S. (1900/2008). *The interpretation of dreams.* Oxford University Press.

Freud, S. (1911/2002). *The Schreber case: Psychoanalytic remarks on an autobiographically described case of paranoia (Dementia Paranoides).* Penguin Group.

Gravelin, C. R., Biernat, M., & Baldwin, M. (2019). The impact of power and powerlessness on blaming the victim of sexual assault. *Group Processes & Intergroup Relations, 22*(1), 98–115.

Grubb, A., & Harrower, J. (2008). Attribution of blame in cases of rape: An analysis of participant gender, type of rape and perceived similarity to the victim. *Aggression and Violent Behavior, 13*(5), 396–405. https://doi.org/10.1016/j.avb.2008.06.006

Gustavsson, M. (2019). *Klubben. En undersökning [The club. An investigation].* Albert Bonniers Förlag.

Hill, S., & Marshall, T. C. (2018). Beliefs about sexual assaults in India and Britain are explained by attitudes toward women and hostile sexism. *Sex Roles, 79*, 421–430. https://doi.org/10.1007/s11199-017-0880-6

Janoff-Bulman, R. (1985). The aftermath of victimization: Rebuilding shattered assumptions. In C. R. Figley (Ed.), *Trauma and its wake: The study and treatment of post-traumatic stress disorder* (pp. 15–35). Brunner/Mazel.

Jastreboff, P. J., & Hazell, J. W. P. (2004). *Tinnitus retraining therapy: Implementing the neurophysiological model.* Cambridge University Press.

Kaminer, D. (2006). Healing processes in trauma narratives: A review. *South African Journal of Psychology, 33*(6), 481–499.

Klein, M. (1975). *The writings of Melanie Klein*, volume III. *Envy and gratitude and other works (1946–1963).* Free Press.

Lebowitz, L. (1985). *The cultural context of rape.* Unpublished manuscript.

McMahon, L., Murray, C., & Simpson, J. (2012). The potential benefits of applying a narrative analytic approach for understanding the experience of fibromyalgia: A review. *Disability and Rehabilitation, 34*, 1121–1130.

Mills, J. (2008). Attachment deficits, personality structure, and PTSD. *Psychoanalytic Psychology, 25*(2), 380–385.

Olsson, G. (2016). *Det svåra samtalet [The difficult dialogue]. Psykoterapi,* 2016, No. 4.

Polkinghorne, D. P. (1988). *Narrative knowing and the human sciences.* SUNY Press.

Rey-Debove, J., & Rey, A. (2000). *Le nouveau Petit Robert.* Dictionnaires Le Robert.

Roth, S., & Lebowitz, L. (1988). The experience of sexual trauma. *Journal of Traumatic Stress, 1*(1), 79–107.

Siegelman, E. (1990). *Metaphor and meaning in psychotherapy.* Guilford Press.

Spence, D. (1982). *Narrative truth and historical truth.* Norton.

Stevenson, A. (2007). *Harrap's unabridged dictionary.* Chambers Harrap Publishers.

Turquet, L., Seck, P., Azcona, G., Menon, R., Boyce, C., Pierron, N., & Harbour, E. (2012). *Progress of the world's women, 2011–2012: In pursuit of justice.* UN Women. https://www.unwomen.org/sites/default/files/Headquarters/Attachments/Sections/Library/Publications/2011/ProgressOfTheWorldsWomen-2011-en.pdf.

Tyler, R. S., & Erlandsson, S. I. (2002). Management of the tinnitus patient. In L. M. Luxon, J. M. Furman, A. Martini, & D. Stephens (Eds.), *Textbook of audiological medicine* (pp. 571–578). Isis Publications.

Ullman, S. E., & Filipas, H. H. (2001). Correlates of formal and informal support seeking in sexual assaults victims. *Journal of Interpersonal Violence, 16*(10), 1028–1047.

Van der Hart, O., & Horst, R. (1989). The disassociation theory of Pierre Janet. *Journal of Traumatic Stress, 2*(4), 1–11.

Winnicott, D. W. (1963/2010). Fear of breakdown. In C. Winnicott, R. Sheperd, & M. Davis (Eds.), *Psycho-analytic explorations* (pp. 87–95). Karnac Books.

Winnicott, D. W. (1971/2005). *Playing and reality.* Routledge Classics.

6

Writing as Narrative Resource in Therapeutic Settings

Diaries, Sketches, Notes

Jarmila Mildorf and Daniel Ketteler

Introduction

This chapter[1] is a joint endeavor by a clinical psychiatrist with an interest in studying and writing literature, and an English studies scholar with expertise in sociolinguistics and literary studies, especially narratology. The chapter aims at reflecting on a hitherto under-researched method in psychotherapy: the use of patient diaries (cf. Bolger et al., 2003; Le et al., 2006; Wheeler & Reis, 1991). We want to have a closer look at possible functions of literary sketches and diary entries in the context of psychotherapeutic processes. We discuss the benefits of this qualitative method for the therapeutic context as it offers clients means of creative self-expression and therapists an alternative way of accessing emotional states and of discussing illnesses with their clients. We analyze the example of a diary kept by a graphic designer who suffered from depression, drawing on narrative discourse analysis as a methodological framework, as well as more "literary" examples, most prominently among them Roland Barthes's *Mourning Diary*. The approach we take here connects questions and methods from our two disciplinary backgrounds: psychiatry on the one hand and philology on the other. Perhaps surprisingly, the psychiatrist is responsible for the discussion of most of the literary examples, while the philologist largely undertook the analysis of the psychiatric case study. Each part was commented upon and complemented by the other author. In that regard, this chapter is interdisciplinary in the best sense of the word, and we believe that such interdisciplinarity is the way forward when it comes to tackling issues such as mental health.

Jarmila Mildorf and Daniel Ketteler, *Writing as Narrative Resource in Therapeutic Settings* In: *Narrative and Mental Health*. Edited by: Jarmila Mildorf, Elisabeth Punzi, and Christoph Singer, Oxford University Press. © Oxford University Press 2023. DOI: 10.1093/oso/9780197620540.003.0007

Diaries, notes, and similar text forms prove to be very helpful aids, especially for clients with an interest in creative activities. These text types allow for self-reflection and may thus support psychotherapeutic strategies and interventions. By picking up a pen (or typing on a PC), clients literally take their own life courses into hand again; they have the possibility to integrate their traumas, failures, and conflicts into the plot trajectory of their life narratives. In writing down their own personal life "novel," in using narrative strategies such as describing circumstances and "characters" or oscillating between different perspectives, they may eventually be in a better position to endure ambivalences and difficulties in their lives. However, one needs to be careful not to impose a normative value on "narrative," especially if this term is associated with notions of coherence, structure, and order. The good thing about diaries is that there are not a priori any hard-and-fast rules for how to write down one's experiences, even though certain conventions may have been established over time in actual practice (e.g., to note the date for a certain event). So, diaries in principle offer room even for nonnarrative or, as in our example, nonverbal material—all of which may be relevant for the ongoing therapy.

The structure of our argument is as follows. First, we will survey some of the literature on uses of diaries in various settings and look at some examples of literary diaries. Then, we will discuss one specific case study: One of the psychiatrist's clients, a graphic designer, used a diary as an additional resource in the course of his psychotherapeutic treatment. He took notes, wrote short narrative and nonnarrative[2] texts on his experiences, and drew sketches and icons that expressed his emotional states. These textual and pictorial materials delineate and attest to the client's development from having mental health problems (he suffered from a severe episode of depression) to an eventual improvement of his condition. We are grateful to the client for consenting to making his diary available for this research. We approach the materials using a qualitative analysis including thematic and narrative-discourse-linguistic perspectives, focusing not only on *what* the client wrote but how he *worded* his experiences. We also assess the therapeutic effects the use of this diary had on the client. Indeed, the therapy proved successful in that the client started to feel better—due to clinical intervention and guidance on the one hand but also and especially because of his own creative engagement with and reflections on his situation by means of the diary. The client regarded his diary as a "co-therapeutic you" that replaced or reinforced the effects of the therapy even in the absence of the actual therapist; it thus assumed the function of an intra-individual, abstract-dialectical communication process. The client's speedy remission was surprising given the severity of his initial depression. In the early stages of the therapy, his diary entries were used during therapy sessions to draw up mood protocols and to analyze his behavior. The written protocols were used to identify and analyze concrete situations and behaviors with regard to how they influenced the client's mood and aspects of cognition, specifically if they did so in a negative way. At present, the client deliberately and independently continues to use his diary and notebook, even though his therapy has ended.

Diaries in Research and Practice: A Brief Overview

Diary entries offer a broad spectrum of possibilities to come closer to one's inner self on the verbal level. They typically combine the retelling of everyday experiences with moments of self-reflection, a pause in the narrative that allows one to take stock and evaluate what one has experienced. What exactly one writes about will of course very much depend on the actual purpose one has assigned to the diary, and also on one's specific interests and agendas. The famous diaries of Samuel Pepys, Member of Parliament and Secretary to the Admiralty in seventeenth-century England, for example, serve as sociohistorical documents because the author wrote in them about current political affairs as well as about the Great Fire of London in 1666 and the theater plays he attended. At the same time, one can read about Pepys's problems with dyspepsia, which he describes in painstaking detail. Travel diaries document one's experiences during a journey; reading diaries capture the impressions one has formed while reading books. In sociology, diaries are used as a research method to find out more about how participants in a study relate to a particular issue or how they deal with it on a daily basis. The topic may be, for example, illness (Broom et al., 2015) or relational dynamics in the diarists' families (Haldar & Wærdahl, 2009), or how people spend their time more generally (Sullivan & Gershuny, 2018).

From sociolinguistic and psychological perspectives, diaries constitute an interesting research object insofar as they not only contain personal experiences but also demonstrate how these experiences are verbalized and, indeed, narrativized. This narrativization signals the imposition of a certain logic—or a lack thereof—that is given to lived experience with hindsight (Freeman, 2010; Herman, 2002). As a rule, diaries—unlike published autobiographies—do not presuppose an audience to which the diary is addressed or a larger institutional frame within which it is written. For this reason, autobiography scholar Philippe Lejeune (2007) considers what is written in diaries as potentially more authentic. However, this view perhaps needs to be modified in that even a personal diary is still written for oneself— an audience of one, as it were. It stands to reason that this quasi-dialogical set-up may also lead to textual strategies that bear witness to the difficulties some diarists may have in facing their own predicaments, emotions, and motivations.

In psychotherapy, the diary is used as an instrument for self-reflection. However, it is only in recent years that its benefits have also been acknowledged in the research literature—albeit by no means widely, given clinical psychology's and psychiatry's preoccupation with evidence-based, quantitative methods. For example, a recent study conducted in Jena, Germany, by Suhr and colleagues (2017) found that a group of 44 clients who had received treatment for depression experienced a stabilizing effect through writing a diary in the post-therapy phase. Alexander and co-workers (2016) deplore the fact that the potential resources that creative or "literary" applications of diaries have to offer remain untapped and are not sufficiently explored for mental health research and practice. Empirical psychology seems to shy away from this rather subjective and nonquantifiable method of "self-therapy." There is a constant push for quantification, even where methods similar to diary writing are employed. Thus, notes are used in the context of pain treatment to document the severity of the pain experienced by clients (whereby pain is measured in various degrees). Similarly, mood protocols are employed in the treatment of depression. Here, too, quantification is still the main purpose. In the context of cognitive-behavioral therapy, for example, such notes and protocols are used to quantify clients' experience of pain or the intensity of their mood swings, which they are asked to assess themselves. In cases of depression, the SORC scheme is used to analyze clients' behavior. The scheme seeks to identify how stimuli (S) affect an organism (O) (i.e., people) and lead to physical, cognitive, and emotional reactions (R), which in turn have certain consequences (C) (Goldfried & Sprafkin, 1976; Nelson-Gray & Farmer, 1999). The aim is to raise awareness about the complexity of one's emotions and emotional responses and to change those responses accordingly. After all, these responses are also influenced by the thoughts that clients have in phases of depression, for example, and the idea is that such thoughts can in turn be influenced if duly identified. The purpose of the abovementioned notes and protocols, then, is to document and quantify a client's thoughts and emotions throughout a day and to correlate them with specific events or experiences (Beck, 2013).

Protocols are also used when people experienced panic attacks, somatic illness, bulimia, and alcohol abuse (Seiffge-Krenke et al., 1997). Why, then, are clinicians still skeptical about using the open form of a (literary) diary in their practice? One answer could be that they mistrust the "truth-value" of what clients write about their experiences (see also Hutto, Chapter 3 in this volume). Seiffge-Krenke and colleagues (1997) point out in their overview of the diary method in research and therapy that Sigmund Freud himself wrote diaries for many years, but then destroyed them only to later retrieve his notes from memory, thus documenting them again retrospectively (p. 47). They link this to the fact that Freud also had severe doubts about the truthfulness of some of the incidents his clients reported during psychoanalysis (p. 36). Indeed, truthfulness is a question that is central to all therapy forms in psychology. What is interesting about Freud's diaries is the ambivalence with which he—and, by implication, early psychology—already reacted to his own, possibly more honest, notes. The "half-baked" truths that literary or personal writing may harbor seem to be perceived as a threat because they are perhaps revelatory of some deeper meaning after all and therefore must be "filtered" through scientific processes before they can be allowed to appear on the surface of what is deemed publishable. By drawing clear demarcation lines, psychology has from the start kept the potential reputation of coming suspiciously close to literary production at arm's length from its own "science." More provocatively, one could say that the analyst Freud mistrusts not only the ill person and his or her impulsive-emotional sense of judgment, but in fact himself as someone who writes a diary. A recent study about the role of reading and writing as tools in psychology seems to confirm that psychologists are reluctant to admit to using such qualitative methods because they are afraid of coming across as "non-scientific" (Bergqvist & Punzi, 2020). The question arises—and we want to posit this question here, too—whether there is any better source of information for psychotherapists than the spontaneous and unmonitored (to a degree) output of clients and whether it is not precisely the subjective reality of clients that ought to be the starting point for every therapy.

Furthermore, is artistic-literary production—and perhaps the distinction between artistic and non-artistic writing is a matter of degree rather than of kind—not a much better source of knowledge about one's own psychological disposition precisely because it constitutes a more ambivalent, and therefore more authentic, source than the claims and assertions made by clients in psychotherapy that may follow expectable and rehearsed social scripts? Psychiatrist and founder of existential psychotherapy Irvin D. Yalom repeatedly points out in his book *Becoming Myself: A Psychiatrist's Memoir* (2017) that he considers literary authors and philosophers as the better psychologists because they discuss things that matter to humans in general and to his clients—aging, loss, death, life decisions such as taking a job or choosing a partner, and so on—much more adequately than his own colleagues did. In the 1970s, Integrative Therapy already employed open diary forms for analysis and therapeutic purposes. Hilarion Petzold, who published a three-volume book on Integrative Therapy (1991–1993), for example, used diaries because, in his view, they chronicled his clients' lives, offered instances of remembering, and helped reduce mechanisms of repression.[3] Relapse rates after psychotherapy are particularly high for socially less privileged clients. Perhaps using creative methods such as (diary) writing, which empower clients to engage with their predicament more independently, may open vistas onto new methods that are less quantitative and more holistic in nature and thus more effective in the long term.

Literary Diaries

The diary as a medium has long been used by writers as a literary-therapeutic resource in times of grief, disruption, or sadness, or simply to document the multifaceted nature of lived experience and at times even the tediousness of one's life. Roland Barthes's *Mourning Diary* is a case in point. He wrote it between 1977 and 1979 to try and come to terms with the death of his beloved mother. It is a good example for the potential self-reflexivity and the language-philosophical dimensions inherent in the diary as a narrative medium. It also illustrates the paradox, expressed succinctly by Antoine Compagnon (2017), that "mourning rejects literature, but there is no greater literature than that of mourning" (p. 7). While Barthes was mourning the death of his mother, he had to write his inaugural lecture, fully aware of the fact that his mother's seat would remain empty in the auditorium. In his diary, he reflects on his emotions, his difficulties to let go. With reference to psychoanalyst Winnicott, who studied the bonds between mother and child, Barthes comments on his anxiety in view of a catastrophe that has in fact already happened (Barthes, 2010, p. 214). The symbiosis between mother and child has been disrupted; the "inner child" is alone now and has to face his fears on his own. Barthes realizes the pettiness of everyday concerns in the face of loss and grief and in this connection reflects on the significance and value of a true and intensive bond such as that with his mother, which he compares to a love relationship (Barthes, 2010, p. 49). To finally realize what really matters in life is perhaps a clichéd outcome of and experience in moments when one faces bereavement, illness, birth, and death, yet it is an experience that people in such situations have and also often verbalize. Barthes's reflections can ultimately be regarded as not only a dialogue with himself through his diary, but in fact a dialogue with his deceased mother. As Ottmar Ette (2011, p. 32) succinctly puts it, Barthes's diary represents a crying out or scream expressive of the author's fear (*Aufschrei der Angst*). Fittingly, the French language allows for a pun: One could say that the scream (*cri*) is in fact an intrinsic part of the writing (*écriture*). This pun opens the door to the philosophical and psychological dimensions of writing: For Barthes, literature, language philosophy, and life were inseparable, and he practiced a special form of literary studies by drawing on literary techniques in his writings (*Literaturwissenschaft im Modus der Literatur*) (Ette, 2011, p. 32). In the *Mourning Diary*, Barthes mentions not only the breaking up of the "love relationship" but also his difficulty talking about this incisive event (Barthes, 2010, p. 50)—a difficulty that can be traced in dashes marking the path to what cannot be said. Barthes is concerned with overpowering emotions that remain hard to verbalize. He consequently ponders on—and explores in quasi-literary form—the limits of language itself, a language that has partially left him in this time of distress. An existentialist awareness of the futility of life and language alternates with his attempts at reclaiming life, with assertions of a will to live and to have courage (p. 51). The diary thus encompasses a movement from despair to hope, and in the separate entries one can notice a dialogical engagement with a therapeutic "you" that enables the author to use writing as a means of self-healing. Human experience is condensed into the literary shape of the diary; the speechlessness attending his life crisis and the very crisis itself are integrated into a life story that unfolds in the diary's narrative. What Barthes's example shows is that the "inner talk" that diaries make possible can become a universal resource for people in times of psychological crisis, whether it is the experience of grief, pain, anger, sadness, or trauma.

Many other examples of literary diaries can be mentioned here. For example, German author Helmut Krausser (2006) engaged in a diary project spanning 13 years, in each of which (with the exception of the year 2000) he published a diary covering one month of the year (starting in May until he reached the month of April in his final diary). These diaries, like *Mourning Diary*, offer unmitigated insight into the heights and depths of an author's life. Diary and blog thus become instruments for navel gazing, which in itself can be considered narcissistic to a certain degree, but perhaps as a "healthy" form of narcissism that is needed to engage with oneself honestly. There are obviously differences between private or even secret diaries that one writes only for oneself and those that are intended for publication. One has to be quite egocentric to believe that other people might be interested in what one writes down about one's life and inner states. Blogger and author Alban Nikolai Herbst writes about the exposure of one's life in diaries: "Some reactions to my opened inner life are painful. To endure this pain is definitely part of a public diary. In fact, this is where the genre's very own strength lies" (Herbst, 2011, p. 75; our translation).[4] A radical, perhaps the most radical, form was chosen by Wolfgang Herrndorf, author of the bestselling German novel *Tschick*, who ironically became successful only when he was also diagnosed with a terminal brain tumor, a glioblastoma. In his blog (2010–2013), he documents the development and consequences of his tumor and what effects this had on his life until he committed suicide in 2013. He reflects on his situation, describes moments of psychosis, exposes his innermost ambivalences that reach the limits of what can be considered human, and gives expression to his anxiety, his struggle with his impending death and his decay. Authors like Gerhard Henschel (2018) in Germany and Karl Ove Knausgård (2013) in Norway are further examples for writers who, sometimes using a fictionalized alter ego, presented their lives in great detail—occasionally almost painfully so—and in sublimated literary form.

One could ask more critically: Does the sheer amount of examples of such self-exposure point to more general exhibitionist trends in our modern-day society that increasingly acts in narcissist ways? A study by Vater and colleagues (2018) seems to point in this direction as it finds more narcissism (as measured by means of the Narcissistic Personality Inventory [NPI] and the Pathological Narcissism Inventory [PNI]) among young adults today. Another study by Hunt and colleagues (2018) even suggests that the use of social media like Facebook, Twitter, and Instagram can lead to depression, perhaps precisely because, unlike a private diary, they are intended for a wide public audience and foster an expectation of (positive) responses in users. We suggest that we need to distinguish between such open-space "diary" forms and the more intimate space that traditional diaries offer. In the latter, engagement with oneself seems to be more salutary as it does not lead to the same frustrations of feeling rejected, for example, and thus can even strengthen one's sense of self-worth. The following case study illustrates these points.

The Diary in Psychotherapeutic Practice: A Case Study

Writing a diary proved especially useful in Daniel Ketteler's therapeutic work, especially with clients who already worked in creative jobs and thus had a propensity for creative methods. These clients used the diary as a kind of "self-monitoring" instrument, and this impressively improved the outcomes of the therapy sessions by reinforcing synergistic effects. There was also an added level of meta-reflection in that the clients felt encouraged to ponder upon the progress they had made. One case, which is at the center of the present study, was a graphic designer who experienced the onset of a major depression. In the course of a separation, he had suffered from anxiety attacks and symptoms of unrest. To this day, he has used his diary actively to engage with his emotional life. As he wrote to Ketteler: "This system of structure allows space for the daily writings: expression, resolving issues, self-psychoanalysis etc, and a focus on things that are coming up: purpose = meaning = good." For us to be able to illustrate in short excerpts how this client went about writing his diary, the client kindly agreed to contribute to this study by allowing us to use examples from his diary entries and thus to make them available for a broader audience. He gave written consent for the written material presented here. The diary also contains a lot of pictorial material, little sketches that capture the client's emotional state or his perception of his current situation. In the following analysis, we draw mainly on transcriptions of various diary entries and only in passing on his sketches, which all illustrate how the client creatively-artistically (both verbally and graphically) engaged with himself. We refrain from printing the original autographs or sketches to ensure anonymity, and also because including pictures would have raised further ethical and copyright issues. The transcripts reproduce the text as it was written by the client. Amendments and corrections as well as anonymizations of names are inserted in square brackets for better readability.

Reflection, Implied Audience, and Daily Life in the Diary of Client S.

As already discussed above, diaries can be used to complement therapies as a further instrument to foster self-reflection. With the client's consent, diaries can also be made available to the therapist for further analysis, and they can be used in psychotherapy sessions as starting points for discussing the client's current situation. In the present case study, the client's relationship to what he writes is further complicated because there is a concrete reader, the psychotherapist or psychiatrist, that one has to bear in mind and a larger institutional context in which the writing is situated: the psychotherapy. The diarist no longer writes merely for himself but is aware of the larger context in which his texts are received.

In the excerpts from Client S.'s diary that we discuss here, the author's orientation toward an audience can be seen in the occasional direct *you*-address in phrases like "I tell ya" (entry Wed[nesday] 31). This could be a form of self-address, whereby S. communicates with himself through his diary, or he could be addressing his therapist, knowing that he was going to read the diary. At any rate, such phrases create a communicative situation, and they even simulate an oral speech situation through linguistic features that are typical for an oral style: for example, the colloquial contracted form of the second-person pronoun ("ya") or expletives such as "fuckin" (entry FRI[DAY] 2), where the deletion of the final consonant "g" also marks a typical phonetic feature of spoken English. Spelling mistakes and a kind of telegram style, where the subject is left out in many sentences, also point to the spontaneity of what is written down: "Went back to sleep at 6:09 am. Woke up at 11:30 am. Swept through facebook + instagram for a[n] hour. Now listening to Jordan Peterson whi[l]st tidying the apartment" (entry SAT[URDAY] 3). This example furthermore shows how diarists, this one included, often document rather mundane daily routines in their diaries: Falling asleep, waking up, using social media are activities that belong to most people's lives today. In the context of a diary, such activities suggest "normality" and form the backdrop to potentially more exciting or disruptive experiences. Activities that are less to be expected stand out. In this case, the fact that the client listened to an audiobook by Canadian psychologist Jordan Peterson while tidying up his flat becomes noteworthy. S.'s marked interest in psychological topics and psychological literature can already be seen at the beginning of the same entry, where he made a note about a book by another psychologist,

Eric Neuman. On the one hand, S.'s interest in psychology shows his readiness to engage meta-reflexively with his own situation. On the other hand, from the vantage point of the therapeutic process, these entries suggest that the client engages at least indirectly with the results of the preceding therapy session, where the focus was on mindful living, on paying attention to even small things and regular routines in order not to become paralyzed by a kind of thinking that centers on success and achievement and that may lead to a sense of inner emptiness. The point was to focus less on the big achievements in life than on those little moments where something can be enjoyed very intensely and to strengthen the feeling that one can treasure such moments. These recent psychotherapeutic concepts are borrowed and adapted, among others, from Buddhist theories.

Work and Relationships

In the selected excerpts, two thematic clusters stand out: the client's professional life and, in connection with that, his financial situation, as well as his relationships to other people. At the beginning of his entry on "WED[NESDAY] 31," S. writes in a tone that suggests he was somewhat put out: "It must be over 2 weeks without having any real money to play with." The phrasal verb "play with" is conspicuous here since it does not commonly collocate with the noun "money," as verbs like "have," "spend," "earn," or "waste" do. To "play with" money suggests rather careless spending of money for things that are not necessarily needed. On the other hand, "play" also implies a sense of enjoyment and gratification when spending money. S.'s comment suggests that he was temporarily deprived of this sense of enjoyment, one of the reasons being that he did not receive the full amount he had been promised for services offered to an acquaintance ("to look after [name]") as he explains in the same entry: "[name] gave me 50 instead of 60 €." The client also debates whether he should now confront this other person about this: "Was I really going to pull him up on this?" He writes that he has not done so yet: "Well, I didn't, or rather—I haven't yet." The change in tense from the preterite or simple past to perfect tense indicates a change in the speaker's/writer's attitude toward the situation he depicts. While "I didn't" simply indicates that the confrontation has not yet taken place, "I haven't yet" suggests that the matter is by no means resolved and that S. still intends to confront his acquaintance about the money. Here, one can see a moment of hesitation and the client's ambivalence about a relationship that also entails a "business" component.

The same entry refers to another, similarly ambivalent relationship the client has with a female friend: He expressly mentions that he does not find her attractive ("I don't fancy her" and "I generally don't find her that attractive") because apparently she talks like a robot and appears to be like a wild cat ("od[d]ly ferral [*sic*]"); at the same time, he admits that he enjoys spending time with her: "BUT—I do enjoy hanging out with her." The discourse marker "but," which is here even emphasized by being written in capital letters, suggests a point contrary or opposite to what has just been said and thus a (perhaps unexpected) turn. Together with the *do*-periphrasis in the following sentence, which confers special emphasis on the verb "enjoy," "but" introduces an explanation for the client's ambivalent relationship to this woman: Even though he does not find her attractive, he feels well when he is with her. In the text that follows, S. then ascribes to this woman a role that is still possible in this seemingly paradoxical relationship: "She could become an awesom[e] friend" but not his lover. In this connection, the modal verb "could" signals potentiality, but also a degree of uncertainty about whether this friendship can actually be realized in the end.

Friendships play a major role fort the client's sense of well-being, as his diary entries show. Thus, for example, he describes a moment of crisis in the following terms (entry "13/01 FRI[DAY]": "Semi turbulent couple of days. Inner turbulence, speaking with [name] really helped center myself. I feel it had that effect on both of us. Communication. Sharing con[s]ciously what is going on for us. Can I help? Yes, sometimes I can." The "inner turbulence" the client experienced could only be alleviated in and through conversation with a good friend. The metaphor of "centering" that the client uses is quite telling because it inversely points to a feeling of being "decentered" during emotional-psychological crises. Interpersonal communication, which is here depicted as a conscious and deliberate mutual exchange about one's innermost feelings, plays a vital role for overcoming such emotional turmoil and psychological crises, according to S. What seems to be particularly important for the client is that, through talking, he can also contribute something to his various friendships. The question "Can I help?" suggests a degree of uncertainty about whether and to what extent he himself can be of help to others. In this excerpt, he answers this question in the positive, albeit in slightly mitigated form, as can be seen in the restrictive temporal adverbial "sometimes." This thought could be used as a fruitful starting point for further reflections on the meaning and relevance of dialogue between human beings more generally and between therapist and client in particular (see also Punzi & Erikson, Chapter 4 in this volume). The main function of conversation, S. suggests, does not seem to be that one verbalizes one's own problems in the sense of a "talking cure," but that one's sense of self-worth is heightened because one also listens carefully to what the other person has to say and thus offers a "service" in friendship. At another point in his notes, the client regrets that there is so little intimacy in his life, a feeling he apparently experiences quite strongly on some days (entry SAT[URDAY] 3). Again, one can see here how the client oscillates between loneliness and experiencing strong friendships.

Another topic to emerge from the notes is the client's sense of inclusion or exclusion, of belonging and not belonging. In the same entry in which the client describes the helpful talk with his friend, he also mentions that he changed his medication, which, in this case, luckily did not lead to "strange brain zaps." Quite on the contrary, the client takes the opportunity of being in relative emotional equilibrium to go out and have fun at the night club West Germany: "A chance to get a little silly at WEST GERMANY this [eve]." Significantly, this form of entertainment is understood as "getting" or "being silly"—that is, it basically constitutes a "minor" form of entertainment where you behave in a way that is not utterly appropriate. Despite this slightly derogatory assessment, the client continues to write how important it is to occasionally behave this way: "It's good to be silly once per ever so often"—not least because it allows one to belong, at least temporarily, to a community: "Be part of the silliness." In what follows, the client then half-jokingly anticipates the negative consequences of a pleasant night out: "I can already feel my poor lungs, smell the temptation of Kebab meet [sic] wafting into my crusty nostrils triggering a premature urge to consume." What is linguistically noteworthy here is the juxtaposition of trivial experiences—such as perceiving the tempting smells of kebab meat—with an elevated style in his vocabulary and grammar as, for instance, in the complex noun phrase "premature urge to consume." This kind of discrepancy is very typical for an ironic mode of writing. The empty space in the text, which is then followed by four words—"Home. Soup. Love. Meditation."—does not make it sufficiently clear for the reader whether the client really went to the nightclub, and this final line captures what happened when he came back home, or whether these four words depict what he did or imagined he would do instead of going out.

This entry also offers another hint to the client's therapy. Apart from getting himself to adopt a more mindful and less egocentric perspective on things, another aim of the client's cognitive-behavioral therapy was to restructure his previous thought patterns—for example, away from a black-and-white dichotomy in judgment to a more differentiated view of smaller details. The aim generally was to encourage a less global and generalized evaluation, which, in a state of depression, leads to quick devaluation, and instead to allow for a more multifaceted perspective on things and thus a richer emotional response.

Orientation Toward the Future

This example shows a special feature of diaries: They offer room not only for remembering and writing down the experiences one has had during the day, but also for verbalizing future plans and expectations. Thus, the client's diary also contains pages where he simply made lists of things to do. In the entry "6 May," for example, S. jotted down his "plan" for the day by listing various activities preceded by dashes. Another list, where the same activities have been placed inside boxes, shows in retrospect which of these activities have actually been completed. For example, the client did not manage to register with a fitness studio as he had intended to do or to have tea in a coffeeshop. An emoji with a frowning face right beside this entry suggests a generally negative feeling on that day. It does not become entirely clear, however, whether this feeling (of sadness or disappointment) is caused by the fact that the client did not manage to accomplish certain activities or whether, conversely, he did not accomplish them because he was not in the mood for them.

Hints to anticipated or planned actions are of particular importance with clients suffering from depression since depression leads to a lack of motivation and future orientation. In the context of the therapy, taking stock at the end of the day is a key element. Apart from a general assessment of the day that is measured in different numbers, the therapist also encourages the client to note down three positive experiences or moments. Thus, the client's perspective is shifted away from a purely negative evaluation, and even a "bad" day can be reassessed more positively by recognizing that one's mood evidently swings and that bad days are followed by better days. A depressed person tends to think in absolutes and therefore often overlooks these connections, thus turning bad situations apodictically into catastrophes.

Orienting toward the future can also be seen as an attempt to motivate oneself. Thus, for example, S. takes the decision in his diary entry "SAT[URDAY] 3" to go running in the afternoon even if it rains. In the entry "Wed[ne]s[day] 31," he comments on the positive structure that his work gave him on that day, and he hopes to be able to replicate the same structure the next day: "Let[']s try again tomorrow." As an afterthought, the client adds the remark that he was in fact much more productive because he did not work in cafés. Two days later, in his entry "FRI[DAY] 2," he has to make more of an effort to motivate himself for work: "Let[']s get to work," and even stronger than that: "Let[']s fuckin DO IT." The underlined and capitalized letters in the verb phrase "do it" convey a sense of the urgency the client felt about his task, and perhaps of the difficulty he had getting himself to do it on that day.

Quasi-philosophical Introspection

Apart from allowing S. to note down these daily activities and chores and the problems he occasionally has with them, his diary also offers him space for more abstract reflections, for moments of thought and insight. A good example is his entry "14/01 SAT[URDAY]," in which the client thinks about his loneliness. A feeling of emptiness is expressed in words like "emptiness," "void"—which, significantly, is written twice in capital letters—and "darkness." These terms are common expressions, if not even clichés in (literary) texts about psychological illness (see also Iakushevich, Chapter 11 in this volume). The client reflects on what people typically try to do to avoid having to face this emptiness. Thus, he writes: "It's easy to react to this by quickly filling up that space with things: people, tasks, appointments—anything that offers us reassurance." He suggests that basically everyone is running away from this emptiness—in other words, that this state of mind is by no means pathological. This kind of reasoning reminds one of the writings of Søren Kierkegaard (1975), who was one of the predecessors of existentialist philosophy and who also described how we try to escape into a life of (aesthetic) pleasure to avoid the truth.

S. likewise interprets people's taking refuge in meeting others, in taking on tasks and appointments as a "reaction" to our inner state that keeps us "running. Sweating. Fretting." The progressive verb forms suggest dynamism and movement—features that also correspond to S.'s image of the "treadmill." The client sketches here the idea of a stimulus-and-response reaction to which human beings willingly subject themselves in order to avoid facing the emptiness in their lives. In his view, it would be better for us to familiarize ourselves with this emptiness, to experience its color, shape, and size, and thus "to become intimate with this part of ourselves." Only by doing this, he continues to write, can one reach a state of "awar[e]ness, balance, stability, contentment, peace." The term "inner emptiness" was thematized during therapy because it plays a role in depressions marked by narcissism; the aim of discussing this was to show the client ways for experiencing closeness and more intensive relationships with others and to foster more empathetic feelings for others in his social environment. The client managed to adopt these ideas very quickly and thus to leave the narcissist cul-de-sac of self-pity, isolation, and low self-esteem.

Another term, "lighter" in the noun phrase "lighter life," was interestingly crossed out again, probably in recognition of the fact that a life as he envisaged it—being fully conscious of the void—can never be a "lighter" life. The expression "to make peace with this VOID" is potentially ambiguous as it may also point to the possibility of suicide. This possibility is to be discarded here, however, since the following reflections point toward ways of living *with* this void, rather than escaping it. A sense of emptiness and futility is precisely what people suffering from depression know all too well. We can see in the diary entries how the client uses his writing to engage with his own life experience and perhaps to look at it from a distance through abstract reflection.

Conclusion

What this example shows is once again the malleability of the textual genre of the diary. As we indicated above, the client also included drawings—some of them quite disturbing—to give expression to his current mood or to reflect on his life in this other medium. As we saw, many of the entries are not even narrative in nature, strictly speaking, but contain plans or to-do lists, or general reflections that have a philosophical quality. Lasse Gammelgaard quite rightly argues in Chapter 13 in this volume that it is not only narrative forms that can have healing effects when it comes to the expression of suffering. The diary, sketches, or other forms of notetaking are useful because they give this freedom to writers to include whatever they deem fit and necessary at any given moment. In that sense, the diary and, to an extent, its more recent equivalent, the (literary) blog, thus perhaps constitute some of the most honest genres that allow for an authentic relationship with the world—often in literary form. One could of course object that any kind of self-writing may involve a degree of posturing and thus insincerity. However, as scholars in autobiography studies have time and again argued, the very choice of one's posture may be even more telling about who one is. Any autobiography in that sense contains an "autobiographical truth" (Smith & Watson, 2010, p. 15). It is the search for one's own truth that diary writing and other forms of creative expression can support. As already pointed out above, creatively minded clients in particular may benefit immensely from using such an outlet. Since all people, and not just those working in creative sectors, can potentially engage in a variety of creative activities, such activities may prove useful across a wide range of contexts and offer clients the possibility to express themselves and find meaning. And we may ultimately learn from our clients.

Notes

1. This chapter is a revised and extended version of a contribution published in German in *Jahrbuch Literatur und Medizin* (*Yearbook of Literature and Medicine*; 2019). The translation was done by one of the authors, Jarmila Mildorf. We thank the chief editor, Florian Steger, and the publishing house Universitätsverlag Winter for allowing us to reprint this modified version in English.
2. One of the minimal definitions of narrative in narratology is that it should capture a sequence of two related events over time and thus mark a change or disruption in the story world. To distinguish narratives from mere reports, one can include further criteria such as the quality that the narrative text should give readers an idea of how the presented events were experienced by the characters involved (the question of "qualia") (Herman, 2009).
3. In 1974 Petzold, together with Johanna Sieper and Hildegund Heinl, founded the German *Fritz Perls Institut für Integrative Therapie, Gestalttherapie und Kreativitätsförderung*, and in this context introduced the latest creative methods in psychotherapy, which had already been tested in the United States (see Pennebaker, 2004), into German psychology.
4. The original reads: "*Manche Reaktionen auf geöffnetes Inneres sind schmerzhaft. Das auszuhalten, gehört zu einem öffentlichen Tagebuch unbedingt hinzu. Darin liegt sogar seine ureigene Kraft.*"

References

Alexander, J., Mcallister, M., & Brien, D. L. (2016). Exploring the diary as a recovery-oriented therapeutic tool. *International Journal of Mental Health Nursing, 25*, 19–26.

Barthes, R. (2010). *Tagebuch der Trauer* (transl. H. Brühmann). Carl Hanser.

Beck, J. (2013). *Praxis der kognitiven Verhaltenstherapie* (2nd ed.). Beltz.

Bergqvist, P., & Punzi, E. (2020). Living poets society—a qualitative study of how Swedish psychologists incorporate reading and writing in clinical work. *Journal of Poetry Therapy, 33*(3), 152–163. https://doi.org/10.1080/08893675.2020.1776963

Bolger, N., Davis, A., & Rafaeli, E. (2003). Diary methods: Capturing life as it is lived. *Annual Review of Psychology, 54*, 579–616.

Broom, A. F., Kirby, E. R., Adams, J., & Refshauge, K. M. (2015). On illegitimacy, suffering and recognition: A diary study of women living with chronic pain. *Sociology, 49*, 712–731.

Compagnon, A. (2017). Writing mourning (transl. S. Ferguson). In N. Badmington (Ed.), *Deliberations: The journals of Roland Barthes* (pp. 5–15). Routledge.

Ette, O. (2011). *Roland Barthes zur Einführung.* Junius.

Freeman, M. (2010). *Hindsight: The promise and peril of looking backward.* Oxford University Press.

Goldfried, M. R., & Sprafkin, J. N. (1976). Behavioral personality assessment. In J. Spence, R. Carson, & J. Thibaut (Eds.), *Behavioral approaches to therapy* (pp. 295–321). General Learning Press.

Haldar, M., & Wærdahl, R (2009). Teddy diaries: A method for studying the display of family life. *Sociology, 43*, 1141–1150.

Henschel, G. (2018). *Erfolgsroman.* Hoffmann und Campe.

Herbst, A. N. (2011). *Kleine Theorie des Literarischen Bloggens: Erste Lieferung.* Edition Taberna Kritika.

Herman, D. (2002). *Story logic: Problems and possibilities of narrative.* University of Nebraska Press.

Herman, D. (2009). *Basic elements of narrative.* Wiley-Blackwell.

Herrndorf, W. (2010–2013). *Arbeit und Struktur* [Blog]. http://www.wolfgang-herrndorf.de/2010/04/daemmerung/

Hunt, M., Marx, R., Lipson, C., & Young, J. (2018). No more FOMO: Limiting social media decreases loneliness and depression. *Journal of Social and Clinical Psychology, 37*, 751–768.

Kierkegaard, S. (1975). *Entweder—oder: Teil I und II* (ed. H. Diem & W. Rest; transl. H. Fauteck). Deutscher Taschenbuch Verlag.

Knausgård, K. O. (2013). *Sterben* (transl. P. Berf). Luchterhand.

Krausser, H. (2006) *März, April: Tagebuch des März 2003, Tagebuch des April 2004.* Rowohlt.

Le, B., Choi, H. N., & Beal, D. J. (2006). Pocket-sized psychology studies: Exploring daily diary software for Palm Pilots. *Behavior Research Methods, 38*(2), 325–332.

Lejeune, P. (2007). Le journal comme "antifiction." *Poétique, 149*, 3–14.

Nelson-Gray, R. O., & Farmer, R. F. (1999). Behavioral assessment of personality disorders. *Behaviour Research and Therapy, 37*, 347–368.

Pennebaker, J. (2004). *Writing to heal: A guided journal for recovering from trauma & emotional upheaval.* New Harbinger.

Petzold, H. (1991–1993). *Integrative Therapie: Modelle, Theorien und Methoden für eine schulenübergreifende Psychotherapie* (3 vols.). Junfermann.

Seiffge-Krenke,   I.,   Scherbaum,   S.,   &   Aengenheister,   N.   (1997).   Das "Tagebuch": Ein Überblick über die Anwendung der Tagebuchmethode in Forschung und Therapiepraxis. In G. Wilz & E. Brähler (Eds.), *Tagebücher in Therapie und Forschung: Ein anwendungsorientierter Leitfaden* (pp. 34–60). Hogrefe.

Smith, S., & Watson, J. (2010). *Reading autobiography: A guide for interpreting life narratives* (2nd ed.). University of Minnesota Press.

Suhr, M., Risch, A. K., & Wilz, G. (2017). Maintaining mental health through positive writing: Effects of a resource diary on depression and emotion regulation. *Journal of Clinical Psychology, 73,* 1586–1598.

Sullivan, O., & Gershuny, J. (2018). Speed-up society? Evidence from the UK 2000 and 2015 time use diary surveys. *Sociology, 52,* 20–38.

Vater, A., Moritz, S., & Roepke, S. (2018). Does a narcissism epidemic exist in modern western societies? Comparing subclinical narcissism, pathological narcissism, and self-esteem in East and West Germany. *PLoS One, 13*(5), e0198386. https://doi.org/10.1371/journal.pone.0188287

Wheeler, L., & Reis, H. T. (1991). Self-recording of everyday life events: Origins, types, and uses. *Journal of Personality, 59,* 339–354.

Yalom, I. D. (2017). *Becoming myself: A psychiatrist's memoir.* Basic Books.

7

What Constitutes Mad Behavior?

Changes in the Grand Narrative of Disorder Delineated in Psychiatric Diagnoses Between 1832 and 1980

Malin Hildebrand Karlén

What behavior is always mad and what is only mad sometimes? In this chapter, the stability and change that has characterized the grand narrative (Lyotard, 1979/1984) of mental disorder is described from the perspective of overarching paradigms outlined through psychiatric diagnoses. Before psychiatry's establishment as a distinct clinical and scientific discipline in the beginning of the nineteenth century, madness was a comparatively more homogenous concept. Later, towards the end of the twentieth century, "madness" was divided into several hundred psychiatric diagnoses. With their distinct names, these psychiatric diagnoses give the impression of capturing underlying, qualitatively different, categories of concrete disease entities (here: disorder). But how did the narrative of madness change from "being outside one's own mind" into a plethora of different mental disorders? And within this grand narrative, which social behaviors have always been considered mad and therefore enduring parts of the grand narrative of human problems for the psychiatric profession to define, and which have only been considered mad during some periods of time and therefore must be considered in parentheses in this grand narrative? The purpose of the present chapter is to nuance the present image of mental disorder by describing changes in grand narratives of mental disorder through analyzing historical changes regarding inclusion (and exclusion) of certain types of social behavior within psychiatric diagnoses. What characterizes these stable versus unstable disordered social behaviors? If unstable, why are they only included within psychiatric diagnoses at certain points in time and not others? If stable, what is "mad" about them?

Malin Hildebrand Karlén, *What Constitutes Mad Behavior?* In: *Narrative and Mental Health*. Edited by: Jarmila Mildorf, Elisabeth Punzi, and Christoph Singer, Oxford University Press. © Oxford University Press 2023.
DOI: 10.1093/oso/9780197620540.003.0008

From God to Nature: The Medical Narrative
of Psychiatric Diagnoses

Until the eighteenth century, the grand narrative of madness—as influenced by Judeo-Christian and Greek/Hellenistic ideologies—entailed primarily two images of the mad person: the religious fool, possessed by demons or angels, and the medical fool, suffering from brain and nerve sickness and a disturbed physical and mental balance (Johannisson, 2002). The medical fool can also be divided into two types, and both are relevant to the establishment of psychiatry as a medical discipline during the Enlightenment: the Hippocratic and the Platonic perspectives (Qvarsell, 1982). These perspectives gained in explanatory value during the Enlightenment since new humanistic ideals spread across Europe and thus also the notion that humans had a capacity for change. Madness was reconceptualized as a disease, which made medical treatment an option and increased the relevance of more nuanced diagnoses of psychological states, to more closely study its behavioral expressions and physiology. Hence, around the time of the Enlightenment, the divine perspective on madness successively lost its explanatory value. Madness was no longer considered as being due to a divine inspiration, a divine punishment for sins, or demonic possession, where prayer was the only course of action. The person's mad behavior was instead an expression of one of many forms of mental disorders. This change from a religious/moral perspective into a medical/moral perspective in the early nineteenth century contributed to theoretical assumptions that something could actively be done instead of hoping for divine redemption.

From Hippocrates and Plato to Hippocrates Versus Plato

The Enlightenment's emphasis on reason and empirical investigations required reason to be clearly defined. Even though many psychiatrists at the time avoided polarized views of the origins of madness, this created discord between psychiatrists who emphasized somatic aspects (advocated by Hippocrates) and psychic aspects (advocated by Plato), although in their original form, these two perspectives both emphasize imbalance. According to Qvarsell, the eighteenth-century psychic school emphasized the platonic thoughts of psychic disharmony—where a person's thoughts are disturbed by sinful living—and for some thinkers also divine intervention. Propagating this school was Johann Christian August Heinroth (1773–1843), who advocated deeply moralizing ideas that only weak, immoral persons, not strong enough to withstand their animal passions and environmental temptations, were afflicted by mental illness. This conceptualization implies that social or psychological treatment methods (e.g., moral treatment) were needed to cure the ailment. The somatic school, here represented by Johannes Baptista Friedrich (1796–1832), instead emphasized the Hippocratic explanation that madness was caused by a disruption of the essential balance between somatic fluids (i.e., by physical injuries and illness) and argued that its treatment therefore needed to be physical. Despite these differences in perceived causes of madness, the two perspectives had a common goal of establishing psychiatry as a unitary discipline, which was more or less reached toward the early nineteenth century. This created a psychiatric discipline in which diagnoses and treatments were based on both perspectives regarding causes for madness, and in the beginning of the nineteenth century, Sweden (following other European countries such as France) established central hospitals to administer treatments based on psychiatric diagnoses.

Grand Narratives and Paradigm Shifts: 1832 Versus 1980

Erklären Versus Verstehen (Explain vs. Understand)

When the contraposition between priests and medical doctors regarding the responsibility of caring for "mad" persons was at least temporarily solved in the beginning of the nineteenth century, an internal conflict within the nascent psychiatric discipline concerning causes of madness blossomed instead. This conflict is still actively debated and marks a dividing line between the biological and psychological perspectives within psychiatry today. The conflict can be traced to the concepts of *erklären* versus *verstehen*, between biologically/objectively explaining a mental state and psychologically/subjectively understanding a person (Ghaemi, 2003, pp. 78–80).

Biology, Psychology, and Sociology

The ontological positioning of psychiatry today is a complex affair and its vague ontological foundation has created confusion regarding where the discipline's boundaries really are (see analysis in Ghaemi, 2003). Considerable attempts to solve this theoretical schism between mainly biology and psychology have been made and the biopsychosocial (BPS) model and the pluralistic approach by existential psychiatrist Karl Jaspers (1959/1997) are prime examples of this. Ghaemi argues that the BPS model encompasses psychiatry's key perspectives, but that praxis has become too eclectic and has led to an arbitrary use of theoretical perspectives based on individual preferences. Ghaemi instead argues for the virtues of the pluralistic approach, where the use of each basic perspective is founded on quantitative and qualitative empirical research (pp. 7–13).

To Cure an Ailment or to Remedy a Deviation from a Norm?

Two functional approaches are currently used within psychiatry according to Ghaemi (2003, pp. 241–242). The generally dominant approach, generally framed since the 1980s by the third edition of the *Diagnostic and Statistical Manual of Mental Disorders* (DSM-III, APA, 1980), is founded on a biomedical model where the disease is assumed to change or break down the body so that a medical treatment is needed to reinstate the physical function. The "enhancement approach" is instead based on the assumption that the mental disorder is a deviation from a statistical norm and from an expected emotional state, perception of the world, or behavior. From the end of the 1990s (e.g., Henriques, 2002; Wakefield, 1992; see also DSM-IV-TR and DSM-5), the enhancement approach has increased as an explanatory value (e.g., if the individual cannot function in areas important for sustaining a healthy and fulfilling life in his or her environment). Therefore, changes in how diagnoses are construed can mirror variations over time in the emphasis placed within psychiatric praxis on (1) how a disorder causes biomedical decline and (2) how different kinds of behaviors deviate from a societal norm.[1] Examples of such use of psychological norms within the diagnostic process involve the contrasting of behaviors inherent in symptoms, such as "excessive vigilance," "hypersensitivity to rejection," "eccentricities of behavior," and "odd speech" (examples of symptoms taken from several DSM-III-disorders; see American Psychological Association, 1980). The societal norm can be defined as the authorities' notion of how persons in society should behave, mirrored in laws regulating rights and responsibilities, and legal decisions regulating the psychiatric discipline. Psychiatric praxis in Sweden between 1832 and 1980 was centrally organized and financed, and its diagnoses were tied to other governmental authorities that can reimburse and support citizens with certain diagnoses. Hence, diagnoses have for a long time been influenced by attitudes held by the government at the time, as well as society at large, about what should be considered sane or sick.

According to Kuhn (1962), the establishment of a paradigm (i.e., what is perceived at the time as "normal" science) is preceded by a pre-paradigmatic situation where the problems the research tries to solve cannot be satisfactorily answered. In this situation, as was the case during the decades preceding the 1980s, psychoanalytical research was perceived as unsystematic from a positivist medical perspective and lacked the universal definitions needed to base research on (Ghaemi, 2003). Systematic explanations and reliably operationalized definitions were instead a strong aspect of biological medicine's theories. With its basis in human physiology, nomothetic lines of enquiry within psychiatry were encouraged, and based on this ontological positioning and on metaphysical assumptions, they formed solutions for psychiatry's problems with its lack of systematic research. With the publication of DSM-III in 1980, the use of diagnosis within higher education in psychiatry and psychology has exploded, and thus also teaching criteria and norms for acceptable diagnoses. Through these contributions, which fulfill several of Kuhn's criteria for a paradigm, a biomedical/empirical paradigm shift can be said to have occurred within psychiatry.

Diagnostic Expressions of the Grand Narrative and Perspectives on Mental Disorder

As the preceding argument indicates, the grand narratives within psychiatry are infused by norms, principally the norms of psychiatric health (here defined as physical balance) and societal functionality, and also by three perspectives: biology, psychology, and sociology. The theoretical implication of accepting a changed emphasis over time between these two norms and the three perspectives is that diagnoses are culturally influenced and capture different kinds or aspects of human behavior to a varying extent in different societal contexts.

In the present chapter, in an attempt to nuance the present image of psychiatric disorder, the perspective of social interaction is used to create an overview of the changes in which social behaviors were incorporated within the diagnoses used in Swedish psychiatry in 1832 (based on the diagnostic system devised by Georg Engström) and 1980 (the diagnostic system as reflected in the DSM-III), respectively (see also Hildebrand Karlén, 2013, and below). When studying grand narratives in mental disorders, critical discourse analysis (Achugar, 2017) and Michel Foucault's concept of genealogical archaeology (Foucault, 1961/2010; Foucault 1969/2011) are useful. Through these methods, the groupings and characteristics of diagnoses at different points in time can be used to understand how and which social behaviors were described within these concepts, and thus, if possible, to get an understanding of why these were singled out. Hence, following Foucault's genealogical archeology used in his *History of Madness* (1961/2010), I selected social behaviors on the basis of a thematic analysis of diagnoses, and discussed the changes in prevalence of these themes in relation to the changing grand narrative of mental disorder. This was done on the assumption that some social behaviors have always been included in descriptions of "mad functioning," while some behaviors have slinked in and out of this concept, crossing the boundaries between healthy and disordered states. Although ideal types are not portraits of reality and tend to emphasize differences between the types, an ideal type analysis based on social behaviors is utilized here since it can also highlight and systematize developments over time and thus constitute a basis for comparisons. The chosen diagnostic system from 1832 was created by Georg Engström, psychiatrist at one of Sweden's first governmentally directed central hospitals, Vadstena Central Hospital.[2] It was one of the first psychiatric diagnostic systems used in Sweden and was also heavily influenced by a German diagnostic system by Johan Christian Reil (1759–1813). The other, the DSM-III, was chosen since it was the first version that had a primarily biological frame of reference rather than a psychodynamic one (Mayes & Horwitz, 2005, p. 258) and has had a major impact internationally on psychiatric praxis and research. The thematic analysis (presented in Table 7.1) showed similarities over time in why a social behavior was considered disordered (left column) and resulted in four themes, here termed *social behavioral categories* (right column), that are used in the present chapter to discuss changes in the grand narrative of psychiatric disorder.

1832: Engström's Diagnoses

Georg Engström was the psychiatrist at Vadstena Central Hospital from 1826 to 1846. At the time, psychiatrists' education included a holistic view

Table 7.1. Social Behavior Categories Used for Comparison

The notion that mental disorders change by changing societal behavioral norms is based on the following:	*The social behavior categories used for the comparison were the following:*
• Cause the person suffering • Are socially maladaptive • Are considered irrational by his or her environment • Are unpredictable and the person does not seem to be in control of them • Are unusual and unconventional • Cause others distress or discomfort • Violate norms and rules in social contexts and in society as a whole	*Melancholy/mania:* Depression, passivity, internalized anxiety with self-destructive traits, a feverish hyperactivity that at times may generate euphoria *Psychosis:* A: Hallucinations B: Paranoia, eccentricity with externalized anxiety or frustration turned into nervous agitated and/or aggressive outbursts *Withdrawal:* Apathy, solitary behavior, and insensitivity in the face of one's own or others' pain *Specific extreme behaviors:* Defined behaviors that deviate from the norm in a person who, in other regards, has a relatively socially well-adjusted personality, such as sexual interests deviating from the adult heterosexual norm, strong fear of specific things or places, memory problems, and other specific acts that are either disliked or considered disturbing or offensive by the person or his or her environment

Adapted from Hildebrand Karlén, 2013.

of patients, both theoretical (concerning mental disorders' causes) and practical (concerning aspects of lifestyle). During the 1820s through 1840s, many physicians were also educated in the spirit of natural science and were therefore also open to Hippocrates' physiological perspective, including biological, psychological, and social causes, even though Engström emphasized the psychological perspective that was based on a perceived imbalance between psychic functions. In line with this education, treatment at Vadstena was partly based on the medicinal effects of substances and partly on safe and wholesome physical, psychological, and social environments (Qvarsell, 1982, p. 176). Engström was the first psychiatrist in Sweden who, through his diagnostic system, characterized and classified mental disorder based on clinical observation, and in this he was influenced by two European pathbreakers of psychiatry, Philippe Pinel (1745–1816) and Johan Christian Reil (1759–1813). This influence made Engström's diagnostic views and constructed systems highly similar to those of Pinel and Reil, who both worked empirically to map the phenomenon of madness/mental disorder using a nosological (symptomatic) classification (Qvarsell, 1982, p. 33). However, their perceptions of causes and cures were still heavily influenced by moral notions of mental disorder. This can be seen in ideas that immoral habits and a bad social and physiological environment created and maintained psychic illness, as well as in the notion that psychically ill persons were confused and needed a strong father figure (i.e., the doctor) to show them the right way (pp. 32–33; see also Johannisson, 2013, pp. 54–55). Psychic disorder was considered to be caused by the disturbance of psychic energy between different parts of one's consciousness, which in turn emanated from strong emotions and a bad milieu. The physiological balance of Hippocrates was another, but not as often cited, cause of mental disorder for Engström. Disturbed menstruation, obstructed sweating, or having colds were possible somatic causes of a disrupted somatic balance. Even though both Plato and Hippocrates were represented in Engström's ideas regarding diagnoses and causes, strong emotions and passions disturbing psychological balance (i.e., Plato) became more important as explanations of mental disorders in his framework. The "moral depravation" that was central to his arguments for environmental causes of mental disorders (e.g., bad heritable traits or upbringing, masturbation, poverty, or substance abuse) were a considerable part of both the somatic and psychological perspective on causes for developing mental disorder. One can see here that the ancestors of the biological, psychological, and social perspectives coexisted within Swedish psychiatry at the time, and often a combination of causes was found for patients' distress. The diagnostic classification from 1832 used by Engström included four groups of diagnoses for mental disorder. In total, these categories contained 13 diagnoses (see Table 7.2).

Engström's diagnoses were captured by only three social behavioral categories, with *Psychosis* being most frequently represented (75% of the diagnoses), but almost all included at least some trait from this behavioral category. Diagnoses dominated by *Withdrawal* were less frequent (approximately 20%), and only one diagnosis was dominated by *Melancholy/mania*, which was characterized by the oscillation between passivity and hyperactivity. Manic behaviors (e.g., strong emotional engagement and hyperactivity) were also included in some of Engström's diagnoses, together with several behaviors included in *Psychosis*, so that the manic activity was perceived as aggressive rather than just intense. *Specific extreme behaviors* were not represented by any diagnosis, and all persons diagnosed by Engström had

Table 7.2. Engström's Diagnostic Categories and Their Causes and Diagnoses

Stupidity (too low energy): Three diagnoses	Stupidity had three grades (i.e., diagnoses): *imbecillitas* (low impairment), *fatuitas* (moderate), and *stupiditas/idiotismus* (high). Stupidity was a well-defined diagnostic category and other diagnoses were seldom used to specify the diagnostic state. The states today termed intellectual disability were the main part of the diagnostic category. The category's diagnoses were primarily considered to have somatic causes, a disturbed balance in somatic fluids. Stupidity was often considered to be innate, characterized by a weak and insufficient energy. Within *fatuitas* and *stupiditas*, the person was considered to have impaired cognitive capacities and "dulled faculties of body and soul," illustrated by being calm and seeming to understand only simple concepts such as everyday objects and events (pp. 121–126, 139, 179).
Fury/mania (too high energy): Three diagnoses	Caused by a strong psychic energy, in turn caused by a neglected childhood where the child's passions had been given an unbridled outlet together with other disadvantageous environmental factors (pp. 121, 127, 179), the category contained four diagnoses: nymphomania, "simple mania" (i.e., only manic in periods), and two complex forms of mania where the rage either could be combined with confusion (third diagnosis) or lethargy (fourth diagnosis). Persons with rage had too strong psychic energy that could not be controlled, resulting in violent behavior. Persons with a raging/manic diagnosis had periodic outbursts that could result in increased physical tension (e.g., forced speech, darting eyes) but also exaggerated or violent actions.
Derangement: Four diagnoses	An imbalance within the patient's psychic life where fantasy had taken over and lacking logical ability. It was a vague diagnostic category often used with other specifying diagnoses from other categories that described the nature of the derangement. The category included many disorders incorporating general anxiety or confusion. It could have a somatic, psychological, or moral/environmental cause, but the common factor for the diagnostic group was that some part of one's psychic life had an overly controlling role (pp. 121, 128, 139, 179). A subheading within this diagnostic category was *Melancholy*; in later versions of Engström's system, this developed into a diagnostic category in its own right including distress and persecutory ideas (p. 132).
Fixed insanity: Three diagnoses	Caused primarily by strong feelings (p. 139), *fixed madness* consisted of a strong feeling of a general impending threat where the person was fixated on a single thing (pp. 121, 179). The diagnostic category was divided into diagnoses such as "religious madness" and "demonomania," as well as other examples of fixed ideas that were given a specific diagnostic name (varying over Engström's diagnostic classifications) (p. 133).

considerable psychic problems encompassing traits from several behavioral categories. Even though extreme behaviors were found among Engström's diagnoses, they are included in more severe mental disorders with disrupted perception, cognition, motivation, and communication.

1980: DSM-III and the Diagnostic Description of Mental Disorder

The background to the development of the DSM system was Emil Kraepelin's system, established in 1893. In developing DSM-III, a descriptive biological perspective was used instead of a psychodynamic perspective, as it had been in DSM-I and DSM-II. After the launch of DSM-III in 1980, the DSM became one of the principal diagnostic systems used by clinical and research psychiatrists, and it used essentially overt (and biologically explained) symptoms in diagnosis. The structure of DSM-III is complex, consisting of three structural levels: main categories, sub-categories, and diagnoses (265 diagnoses in total, 191 diagnoses included in the present analysis). Four main categories of DSM-III were excluded from the diagnostic comparison in the present analysis, since its diagnoses were only applicable to children and youths or their symptomatology was physical rather than psychological. Hence, the inclusion of these two aspects, child diagnoses and diagnoses manifesting mainly physical symptoms, differed from how Engström had conceptualized mental disorder.

In total, 29 of the DSM-III diagnoses are incorporated in *Melancholy/ mania*—primarily affective disorders, different forms of acute intoxication (causing manic behaviors like, for example, elatedness, grandiosity, hyperactivity, irritability, drowsiness, and worry), and certain psychoses related to dementia and originating from organic damage. *Psychosis* was the next most frequent behavioral category in DSM-III diagnoses (characterized by lack of reality orientation, hallucination, and delirium), consisting primarily of personality disorder, dementia, and drug-related diagnoses. Characteristics were egocentricity, perceptual and cognitive distortions according to one's own focus, which could lead to delusions, impaired communication capacity, fear and altered cognition. Within this mental state, the person's manner of perceiveing and processing information do not follow the same association and symbols as others', making the person's train of thought very hard to follow or relate to by others. Examples of diagnoses were anxiety disorders, dissociative disorders, paranoid schizophrenia, and impulse control disorders.

Only eight diagnoses were characterized under the behavioral category *Withdrawal* (i.e., apathy, being solitary, decreased cognitive ability, lack of exhibited emotions, and perceived as insensitive to the pain of oneself or others). Examples for such diagnoses were hebephrenic and catatonic schizophrenia, adjustment disorder with social isolation, schizoid personality disorder, and different forms of dementia (i.e., generally low cognitive and social function, including unwillingness/inability to interact with others), but no other specific behaviors were mentioned (e.g., depression, delirium, or delusion).

The social behavioral category *Specific extreme behaviors* was the most frequently represented in DSM-III, consisting of 99 diagnoses and characterized by symptoms of specific extreme behaviors in an otherwise socially well-adjusted (or at least not diagnosed) personality. Examples of such specific behaviors were drug use, sexual interests deviating from the adult heterosexual norm, specific memory problems (e.g., amnestic syndrome and fugue), and circumscribed impulse control disorders (e.g., a strong urge to steal or set fire). Within all these diagnoses, the symptoms only affect specific aspects of the person—even with these symptoms the person could be considered to function relatively well socially—or certain aspects of the person's thinking totally blocked meaningful reflection. Drug abuse was the numerically largest diagnostic category among *Specific extreme behaviors* and the largest diagnostic category in the entire DSM-III (76 diagnoses). All diagnoses describe a type of drug use that was considered excessive (i.e., polarized against socially accepted alcohol use), and the diagnoses *only* focus on the person's drug habits. Psychosexual disorders were the next largest category in *Specific extreme behaviors* (13 diagnoses), only describing sexuality as disordered (Table 7.3).

Changes Within Behavioral Categories Between Diagnoses 1832 and 1980

The largest difference between Engström's diagnoses and DSM-III is that while the behavioral category *Specific extreme behaviors* does not exist in Engström's diagnoses, it is represented by the majority of the diagnoses (52%) in the 1980s, while the dominant behavioral category in 1832 was *Psychosis*

Table 7.3. Diagnoses Distributed over Behavioral Categories, 1832 and 1980

Behavioral categories	1832	1980
Melancholy/mania	8%	15% (29 diagnoses)
Psychosis (total)	69%	29% (55 diagnoses)
A	–	6% (12 diagnoses)
B	–	19% (37 diagnoses)
A + B, mixed	–	3% (6 diagnoses)
Withdrawal	23%	4% (8 diagnoses)
Specific extreme behaviors	–	52% (99 diagnoses)

(69%). The proportion of diagnoses containing behaviors from *Melancholy/mania* (15%) was higher in the 1980s, while *Withdrawal* had substantially decreased in DSM-III, in part due to the removal of intellectual disability from adult diagnoses to childhood diagnoses (but since it only consisted of four diagnoses, the effect was not considerable).

Changes in the Grand Narrative of Mental Disorder Between 1832 and 1980

Our relationship to an organism is different than our relationship to a person . . . One acts differently towards an organism than towards a person. (Laing, 1968, p. 17)

In general, the change regarding diagnoses described here shows that an increasingly nuanced mapping of certain aspects of human life (primarily addiction and sexuality) has developed since the start of psychiatry in Sweden (and in other Western countries), which has changed the narrative of mental disorder as well as narrowed the sphere of "normal behavior." More specifically, the outlined changes show that (1) singling out addiction and certain sexual behaviors as psychiatric pathology in specific and nuanced diagnoses is a relatively new phenomenon and (2) hallucinations, delusions, and severe mood swings from depression to mania are stable in their position as perceived pathological behaviors over these 150 years.

When Engström created his diagnostic system in 1832, the cause of mental disorder was first and foremost considered to be strong feelings or passions and an inability to handle and balance such emotions, which could be due to ill-breeding, bad morals, or lifestyle. In DSM-III, the aim was instead to replace vague diagnostic concepts and to find general patterns of observable symptoms that preferably had a biological basis. What preceded this shift in the grand narrative of mental disorder from the psychological imbalance observed by Plato, which was also used by Engström in 1832—strong emotion and immorality as causes of mental distress and curing the patient by retuning his or her psychological balance—to the somatic imbalance discussed by Hippocrates as it resurfaces in contemporary psychiatric practice, including an unbalanced humoral mix or physiological damage as perceived causes and the administration of substances or purging fluids to reinstate physiological balance?[3] How did this narrative shift concerning causes and cures affect the diagnostic delineation of mental disorder?

The BPS Model: A Paradigm Shift from "P" to "B" in Cause and Cure

A stable aspect of the grand narrative of mental disorders between 1832 and 1980 was the acknowledgment of the biological, psychological, and social perspectives regarding the causes and cures of mental disorders. However, the unstable aspect within this grand narrative is a shift in emphasis among these three perspectives, and with DSM-III, a biological emphasis became predominant. The BPS model of mental disorder introduced in 1977 (Engel, 1977) is the predominant solution to this ontological conflict in psychiatry today, but it has been criticized for having slid into arbitrary eclecticism (Ghaemi, 2003, pp. 11–12). Instead, the pluralistic model of Karl Jaspers (1959/1997) has been suggested as a better guide for how to apply clinical research and knowledge to the individual case. The purpose of the BPS model was to use a multi-perspective approach when defining and treating mental disorder, but the psychodynamic emphasis on psychology in DSM-I and DSM-II was instead exchanged for a biomedical emphasis on biology in DSM-III. Engström considered causes and cures from these three perspectives, although also with a different internal emphasis on psychology, but the perspectives themselves were for Engström more intertwined (or, put differently, not divided by the same demarcating lines as in the 1980s) and also more explicitly mixed with moral connotations—a kind of multiple-cause/multiple-cure BPS model. Examples of this are bad hereditary traits and somatic disease and damage during upbringing, masturbation, unhappy love, insatiable sexual pleasures, poverty, or substance abuse, and such moral decay was a strand of causal explanations often cited in Engström's journals, together with other causes, at admission to the hospital.

Regarding the paradigm shift in psychiatry from a psychological to biological emphasis with DSM-III against the four components of Thomas Kuhn, the lack of criteria and norms among psychodynamic theorists during the decades leading up to 1980 was at the time argued to be important for remedy. Such a lack of common, easy-to-use criteria and norms in higher education teaching was at the time considered a flaw within the discipline, opening up the discourse for further emphasis on the biological perspective since this aspect was perceived as one of psychiatry's strengths. Due to research from around the 1950s and onwards, the biological perspective had developed medical treatments based on perceived biological markers for psychosis and depression resulting in, for example, the dopamine hypothesis of psychosis and the serotonin hypothesis for depression. To be able to cite empirical biological findings regarding causes of mental disorder was a major, if not crucial, factor for the developers of DSM-III when using the diagnostic model of Emil Kraepelin to change the theoretical course of the DSM, and with that incorporating a biological ontology for mental disorders as a basis for their diagnoses. This shift, however, changed the balance among the biological, psychological, and social perspectives in the ontology and diagnoses of mental disorder from a predominantly psychological to a biological model, profoundly affecting how clinicians, researchers, and society nowadays are led to think about the nature and boundaries of mental disorder as a phenomenon.

Narrative Shifts in Cause and Cure

In line with Francois Lyotard's view on grand narratives, one could say that the natural "disorder" in the area of mental disorder had from the beginning of the nineteenth century been placed within the physician's domain, and was in the course of the 20th century organized in accordance with a narrative where the basic tenet of medicine explains and defines pathology as the presence of a damaged or disordered physiological state and thus can be measured by the traditional quantitative and representational methods of natural scientific empiricism. Based on such premises, the use of the BPS model becomes unbalanced, since it is "B" that forms the background against which definitions made within "P" and "S" need to accommodate their focus of investigation and choice of method and produce results that will be accepted in this narrative. According to how Jaspers (1959/1997) conceptualized empiricism and dynamism (Figure 7.1), psychiatry's use of the BPS model in such an ideological milieu always risks becoming too rigid in its explanatory emphasis, and hence loses its clinical functionality since a diagnosis must be malleable to a certain extent and also be adaptable to an understanding of the patient's problem that emerges in the clinical meeting with the person. In this meeting, meaningful connections between the emergence of disorder and the dissonance between how the person experiences the world and his or her hopes and wishes need to be made—connections that cannot be measured and are only accessible through empathy and understanding. Ideologically, Jaspers (1959/1997) argues, drawing on Wilhelm Dilthey's (1833–1911) work, that the development of psychiatry is under constant tension between explaining and understanding a person's psychic state, which is also in line with Kuhn's idea of paradigm shifts.

Jaspers proposes that pluralism, where the premise of a mental disorder as biologically observable (at least in theory) is not the only defining perspective available, is the best way to gain the most complete knowledge of a phenomenon possible. By using several different perspectives and their respective methods in research to illuminate a certain phenomenon (here, an aspect of mental disorder), an understanding of how to most correctly and reliably identify this phenomenon is outlined. As research progresses, this process leads to a constant refinement of the standard for how to alleviate this aspect of mental disorder in the afflicted, if perspectives from both the explanatory (e.g., biomedical/"from without") and the understanding pole (e.g., patient's own self-report/"from within") of the dimension are considered.

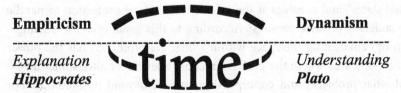

Empiricism   **Dynamism**

Explanation   **time**   *Understanding*
Hippocrates   *Plato*

Figure 7.1. The pendulum between dominance of empiricism and dynamism.

Development of Treatment and Its Effect on Diagnosis

> In fact, the most defensible justification of the steady increase in the number of officially recognized mental disorders that has occurred over the last 50 years is the development of an increasing range of at least partly effective therapies. (Rounsaville et al., 2002, p. 4)

When defining a disorder, not only the choice of perspective and wording matter. Another important aspect for the grand narrative of mental disorder is what we think we can remedy and are more prone to perceive as a problem (Carlberg, 2008, p. 101; Courtwright, 2005; Rounsaville et al., 2002). How did this biological emphasis in diagnosis change the ontology in the grand narrative in psychiatry regarding what should constitute a mental disorder and therefore be treated?

A major cause for the shift in psychiatric ontology from psychology to biology can be related to the development of psychiatric pharmaceuticals during the second half of the twentieth century. An example of how treatability becomes a central question when including problems among "what medical professionals treat" is alcoholism. Physicians Thomas Trotter (1760–1832) and Benjamin Rush (1746–1813) had for a long time argued that alcoholism should be perceived as an illness, but it was not until the 1940s, when the medication Antabuse was released, that the American Medical Association decided that alcoholism should be considered a disease since the medicine showed positive treatment effects.

And If No Physical Basis Has Been Found?

The Swedish psychiatrist Johan Cullberg (1988, cited in Carlberg, 2008) argues that if there are states of mental disorder that do not require medical assessment, have a non-biological cause, and should be treated with non-biological means, would it really be consistent to call these states "diseased states" and consider it the role of the medical profession to handle the suffering of these persons? According to this assumption, it is a question of demarcating the space within which the profession has the power to act—the area where the profession could alleviate or alter something—and what problems and conceptualizations lie beyond its methods. For psychiatry, this demarcation line was drawn between different areas over time: between priests and physicians in 1832, and between different ontological explanations (i.e., biology and psychology) in 1980. When it came to diagnosing a disorder in 1832, instead of identifying demonic possession as had previously been common, the physician was considered the right person to treat the disorder, rather than a priest (if the cause was not perceived as demonic possession, why pray for divine help?). At the time when DSM-III was published, diagnoses were still to a considerable extent outlined to safeguard the physician's right to define and treat mental disorder, despite the fact that the psychiatrists' leading position in defining this was no longer threatened by other professions. Instead, there was now an internal debate about causes between modern heirs to Engström's "psychics" (i.e., psychology) and "somatics" (i.e., biology) that divided psychiatry (Mayes & Horwitz, 2005, pp. 250, 269–270).

In my outline of narratives of mental disorder, the relative lack of focus on validity compared to reliability in the scientific discussion of diagnoses says something about the current biological paradigm's flaw—that the current ontological explanation is not enough. The lack of decisive empirical evidence for causes and treatments for mental disorders between Engström's system and DSM-III is important when considering psychiatry's grand narrative and shows the complex and individual etiology as well as processes of recovering from mental disorder. Cullberg (1988, numbers 32 and 33; cited in Carlberg, 2008, p. 148) argues in his clinical notes, in line with Jaspers (1959/1997), that the manner of talking to the patient—posing questions about the person's actual situation and relationships—is strongly affected if the psychiatrist's task is to diagnose a biological disturbance compared to considering symptoms as markers of the person's present state and seeking meaningful relationships behind them. A compromise suggested by Jaspers (1959/1997) between natural science's *Erklären* and the human science's *Verstehen* is that the psychiatrist has the role to understand the link between a scientific explanation and the individual's own interpretation of symptoms and his or her free will. This has actually been emphasized more recently through the broader implementation of person-focused care in Sweden, acknowledging the importance of patients' own narratives and understanding of their symptoms.

Healthy Morals and Disordered Immorality
in Psychiatric Diagnoses

Not only causes and cures but also the grand narrative of the prevention of mental disorder encompassed all three BPS perspectives: If the person was considered to have good hereditary traits and upbringing, managed well economically, did not drink too much, and lived quietly without strong emotions, the risk of developing a mental disorder was said to decrease considerably. This stability in assessing mental health factors over approximately 150 years is remarkable, and all of the BPS model's components are still considered salutary in psychiatric research and praxis today. This stability within what psychiatry considers that you yourself could do to avoid developing a psychiatric disturbance could be considered from various perspectives. It could mark the fact that some behavioral ideals in society are indeed stable for some reason (for example, are relatively universal or common in certain cultures, such as societal values in European thought), or perhaps that certain behaviors have been identified as universally beneficial for humans.

The considerable increase in the number of diagnoses capturing specific extreme behaviors in the 1980s can be related to Foucault's *History of Sexuality (1976/2004)*, where he describes an increasing normalization and medicalization of certain kinds of sexual behavior at the end of the nineteenth century (see also Johannisson, 2002, 2009). The societal context around this time is described by Johannisson (2013) as similar to that at the beginning of the twenty-first century: a state of anomia, where physical and psychological exertion is highly prevalent in the population due to a sharp increase in collective stress and uncertainty. Johannisson argued that such states increase societal pressure for absolute truths, which at the times in question increase the prevalence of medical explanations of these psychic states, since the medical discipline enjoyed a considerable "truth capital," was considered a reliable science, and could generate truths that were not based in theology. As a consequence, the uncertainty society felt was given a medical interpretation and a psychiatric or somatic diagnosis. This tendency to too quickly medicalize uncertainty, vague states of worry, stress, and melancholia and their varying behavioral expressions is an important factor to be wary of in times of increased societal uncertainty (Johannisson, 2002).[4] A similarly fast-changing societal context and increased uncertainty about previous societal values were present in the United States during the two decades predating DSM-III, which primarily became linked to a youth culture that included new avenues of sexual behavior and new types of drugs. Such a social tradition, to morally condemn intemperate pleasure and pathologizing it in the 1980s, is mirrored in the debate at the beginning of the twentieth century in Sweden, when youths' smoking habits and women's coffee-drinking were heavily criticized within the public debate (Lindgren, 1993).

Substance Abuse Diagnoses

The morally tainted term "intemperance," which was used previously to denote one cause of drug abuse, was exchanged in 1980 for "impaired impulse control,"[5] a term based on the notion that there was a biological deviation that, for a variety of reasons, decreased frontal lobe function.[6] This is an example of how a social and moral tradition, to condemn the use of a certain drug, is anchored scientifically in medical terminology, and as research continues, the less empirically founded moral aspects of the mental disorder (here, addiction diagnoses) fall away when the grand narrative changes (here, from psychologically and sociologically grounded explanatory models into biological ones). Consider that during the first decades of the twenty-first century, a whole debate has erupted surrounding possible addictions that do not include substances but only activate similar brain structures as seen (among many other states) in drug abuse. A diagnostic example of this kind of development can be seen in DSM-5 (published in 2013), where the first solely behavioral diagnosis—gambling disorder—was included in the addiction diagnoses. Since the reward system is a highly "general" brain system, activated by so much in our surroundings, the sole use of this kind of vague argument for the inclusion of behaviors among addiction diagnoses will most assuredly create problems in the future for psychiatry, especially regarding the danger of pathologizing certain kinds of behaviors solely on moral grounds—that the behavior in question is not functional in society and, since it is not functional, creates suffering for the person.

Sexuality

Johannisson (2002) describes the medicalization of sexuality in psychiatric diagnoses as follows: "From the end of the 18th century up to our century they slip through society's cracks, persecuted but not always by the law, often incarcerated, but not always in prison, perhaps sick but scandalous, dangerous victims, victims to a strange sickness that also carries the name of vice and sometimes crime" (p. 62). The medical view of nonreproductive sexuality (e.g., masturbation) in the nineteenth century built on the ancient assumption that sexual activity (and particularly its pleasure) led to a loss of energy/powerlessness, and at the end of the nineteenth century, it was assumed that this state could cause mental disorder, exhaustion, and ennui, which could result in suicide. Even in 1903, an excess of masturbation was seen as one cause of intellectual disability (Grünewald, 2009, p. 286). This traditional view of sexuality was combined, in psychiatry, with a moral stance regarding nonreproductive sexuality as immoral and as resulting from a lack of impulse control. Finally, the combination of these ideas was given medical terms, which sanctioned the concepts scientifically (Johannisson, 2013, pp. 116, 126). Even though DSM-III did not include the notion of sexuality as unhealthy and masturbation as an unnatural sexual practice, homosexuality was just barely exempted from diagnosis (it had been included in previous DSM versions), and other forms of sexuality that deviated from an adult heterosexual norm were still included in the diagnoses. Michel Foucault describes the end of the nineteenth century as the creation of a *scientia sexualis* in Europe,[7] when a discourse of the nature of sexuality and its many forms outside the adult heterosexual norm exploded in the halls of science, resulting in the shaping of a "world of perversities" separate from the old libertines, albeit still related to them (Foucault, 1976/2004, pp. 60–71). According to Johannisson (2013, p. 138), when doctors during the last decades of the nineteenth century broke down nonreproductive sexuality into different forms of "deviations," the thought that some individuals were "born homosexuals" was accepted, but they were considered to be pathological beings. Deviance from the adult heterosexual norm became pathologized from a biological perspective, with its assumptions based in genetics, and from then on sexuality became a matter for the physician, not for the priest or judge. At this time, the Victorian ideal included morality and temperance (Birch, 2007), and the threat presented in the grand narrative at the time was, as for Engström, that, while keeping to these behaviors protected the individual from mental disorder, their breach would result in somatic degeneration and the spreading of disease and in the long run in a "degenerated offspring" that would destroy human society. Hence, only submission to medical advice related to these ideals could hinder this threatening doom (Johannisson, 2013, pp. 116, 140–142, 148).

Addiction and Sexuality: Intemperance and Morality in Diagnoses Today

Regarding the grand narrative of morality in psychiatric diagnoses, especially surrounding substance abuse and sexuality, the moral heritage that psychiatry carries surfaces in Engström's diagnoses. However, a considerable mistake is made if it is presumed that basing diagnoses on observable symptoms rather than underlying causes removes the risk of formulating diagnoses with strong moral influences: A clinician's gaze when looking for symptoms is directed by the perspective that has formed the basis for choosing these particular diagnostic symptoms. The difficulty of separating a moral perspective from a care perspective is evident in several diagnoses both in 1832 and 1980, an example previously mentioned being the clearly moral term of intemperance, which had been changed to the more biologically oriented "impaired impulse control"—a term still used in several of the frequently used psychiatric diagnoses today (e.g., substance use disorder and attention-deficit/hyperactivity disorder). Especially interesting is the fact that with the publication of DSM-5, the narrative surrounding substance abuse and addiction has not only evolved to include pure behavior addiction but has also led to a discussion centering on other chemicals (i.e., sugar) and other pure behavioral addictions (e.g., computer gaming, sex addiction). In this narrative, the similarity of these states to drug addiction is based on their similarly compulsive use of a stimulus and an activation of the same neurological system that substance abuse activates. The alteration of this neurological system is the defining cause of all sorts of addicted states. In discussions about the cause of addiction as well as perceived difficulties connected to sexuality, the search during the 1960s for a genetic predisposition for drug abuse as well as deviations from an adult heterosexual norm has continued (Johannison, 2002). Should homosexuality be considered a medical deviation from a norm or a natural aspect of human variation with a biopsychosocial basis? Questions like these were not only part of the narrative surrounding mental disorder in 1832 and in the 1980s; they are still debated today. In the light of psychiatry's historical experiences, today's debates in psychiatry, with their increased emphasis on the individual's own responsibility, should not rest on the assumption that a nosological structure protects one against moral prejudice. There is therefore an often unnoticed and increased risk of giving moral answers to medical and psychological questions.

The Blind Spots: Problems with the Classic Medical Model of Diagnosis in Psychiatric Praxis

Since the establishment of the psychiatric discipline in Europe, its narrative has been influenced by the classic method of natural science: categorization and the isolation and analysis of singular variables' effects on outcomes.

This makes us much less likely to identify when the whole is more than the parts—such as identifying disorder processes developing over time, especially disorders that take different forms throughout such a process, and interaction effects between variables that in themselves have a weak relationship to disorder but in synergy may be a strong cause for disorder. Hence, meaningful connections of understanding may contribute greatly to develop cures.

A cornerstone in medical science and practice builds on the knowledge of a physiological cause of the disease, its course, and which treatments are available. This causes serious problems with psychiatric diagnoses. To categorize "madness" and to view its varying expressions from a classical disease perspective is more problematic than it is for many somatic diseases. A strong contributing factor is that the purpose of diagnoses used within psychiatry today is to identify pathological *states* and their nonfunctional behaviors rather than to illuminate processes within the person's context (e.g., intrapsychic patterns, patterns of social interaction, and historical and/or present stressors) that have created and/or maintain the suffering and the symptoms. Hence, one of the major questions when considering psychiatry's grand narrative is whether mental disorder should be perceived as a biomedical imbalance (which, at least in theory, is objectively measurable by methods traditionally used in natural science) or in psychosocial terms (more relative and related to subjective suffering and a normative comparison). Wakefield (1992) tried to assimilate the two perspectives by focusing on the decreased functionality of a certain physiological function. However, since psychiatric diagnoses are said to be BPS-based and psychiatry also is a behavioral science, the central questions for a narrative surrounding mental disorder—regarding its validity and reliability—are still problematic. Regarding validity, which phenomenon, defined by which theoretical framework, should the diagnosis try to capture? Regarding reliability, for whom should the diagnosis be reliable—for the physician (e.g., emphasizing the symptomatic similarity so that two physicians always state the same diagnosis), the patient (e.g., taking potential fluctuations in the disorder into consideration to always ascertain that the same diagnosis is made), or society (e.g., that the same diagnosis is made for all the persons with the same disorder despite interpersonal differences so that everyone deserving it receives the same assistance)? Considering the change in diagnoses, the narrative has shifted from *understanding* intemperance and normatively deviant behavior through a theoretical perspective to a descriptive symptom *explanation* in DSM-III. If the clinician only uses this explanation of the disorder by matching superficial symptoms to a diagnosis list of "markers," diagnoses become reliable but not valid and are therefore better suited for population-oriented and mean-value research (Mayes & Horwitz, 2005, pp. 251–252), while the individual patient's risk to suffer increases greatly. For example, despite similarities in symptoms generating the same psychiatric diagnosis, two persons can have very different levels of needs regarding societal assistance or the kind of psychotherapeutic treatment to be given. While one person may need both kinds of interventions, the other might need neither because of differences in person-oriented factors such as level and diversity of coping skills and the presence of other protective or mitigating factors that lessen the consequences or alter the experience of the symptoms.

How Can This Historical Account Inform Clinical Diagnoses Today?

According to Allen Frances (2014), new diagnoses can be as dangerous as new medicines since they affect how millions of people are treated without there being enough knowledge about whether that treatment is well founded. Despite this, Frances asserts that psychiatric diagnoses will be one of the most important tools for many decades to come since they are our best alternative today when it comes to defining and communicating the phenomenon of psychic disorder. In addition to the above-mentioned roles of diagnoses, the perspective that is allowed to define mental disorder does not only guide psychiatry's narrative by shaping its diagnoses and treatment. It also impacts society as a whole and often influences how much societal support—economically or socially—the afflicted person receives from society. By ignoring causes per se in diagnoses, by focusing on easily generalizable symptoms, or by trying to ignore other causes than those biologically observable, the psychiatric narrative delineates the accepted vocabulary and hence draws boundaries against what cannot be verbalized or considered an accepted argument in this narrative. According to a pluralistic view, as well as the original BPS standpoint, this effectively hinders the discipline's scientific development and its ability to develop clinically useful diagnoses whose application is based on multi-perspective research (Ghaemi, 2003; Lewis, 2012).

Another risk to consider with the trend to specifically outline more and more aspects of psychic life in diagnoses, psychiatry risks making itself unreliable because it remains unclear whether psychiatry describes "true" disorder, something relevant regarding the person. If this should happen, psychiatry may make itself irrelevant as a discipline by losing its legitimacy as a relevant narrative of causes and cures of mental disorder. The social role created by the diagnostic outline also creates expectations surrounding behavior that stems from the person's social context as well as from the person's own self-image, which makes it harder to distance oneself from such self-conceptualizations. It is likely that the more static the basic premise on which disorder is defined becomes, the harder it is to cast off the sick role. One perilous aspect of this line of reasoning is that the more static (i.e., biologically determined) a disorder is conceived to be, the more helpless the person would feel to remedy it. This would take away people's agency and, if the narrative is biological, create a tendency to turn to psychopharmaceuticals. The lesson learned by the rise of eugenics should make us extremely watchful of using broad theories of biological differences, even though the biological matter at hand can be measured in detail. If the basic conceptualization is entirely invalid, it does not matter how well the matter is measured. New theories, especially theories of biological differences as a cause or marker for a mental disorder, have a way of making psychiatry as a whole get too excited too soon—ascribing causes and administering cures far too generally on too scarce or too narrow a research. This kind of narrative about biological dissimilarities among groups in society easily feeds into humans' xenophobia, and with the appalling historical evidence in view, this should make us wary about using biological models to explain mental disorder.

Conclusion

> The original question: are there only stages and variants of one unitary psychosis or is there a series of disease-entities which we can delineate, now finds its answer: there are neither. (Jaspers, 1959/1997)

Psychiatry needs some way of structuring its knowledge in a purposeful manner, since without some kind of organization based on predefined or exploratory ideal types, we could not perform certain important kinds of research. However, humans' innate proclivity to reify abstract concepts, like the ideal type diagnoses of the DSM system mistaking them for something that actually exists as well-defined entities, has influenced social service systems and society in profound ways. Diagnoses as a clinical tool for structuring knowledge have today become perceived as a collection of real entities—things to be localized in the patient—and used to categorically separate those who need society's help from those who do not.

DSM-III's creators argued that it lacked a "theoretical orientation" and that its diagnoses therefore were neutral, also implying that they would be neutral in a moral sense. However, the nosological character of DSM-III separates a disordered state from a normal state, separating them with a certain number of symptoms over which a disorder emerges. A moral implication is always present when the notion of how the majority behaves is the point of comparison, which can be seen in several of the DSM-III diagnoses. That "normal" within the psychiatric discipline is something positive is taken for granted since "normal" implies "healthy." However, whether abnormal is deemed to be negative or not depends to a considerable degree on which form the abnormal behavior takes and in which social and societal context it is expressed. The "sometimes diagnosed" extreme behaviors regarding certain kinds of drug use and sexuality outlined in the present chapter were at some point in time considered as vices (but not disorders) and at other times as disorders (although still far from free from its simultaneous position in the contemporary narrative of "vices"). Social tradition, moral condemnation, and scientifically based diagnosis seemed in these cases often to coexist in a diagnostic system that lacked theory and did not take moral notions into account. In the case of the two diagnoses of drug abuse and sexuality, research findings on genes and brain structures have often been used to argue for a biological cause of these intemperate and normatively deviant behaviors—a tendency that has already had comprehensive and risky consequences (e.g., the use of eugenics and the argument surrounding biological differences as a narrative for rationalizing genocide). This is not to say that biology should not be a part of the construct of mental disorder, only that its emphasis in the current grand narrative may incline us to more uncritically accept new and unproven theories from the biological perspective compared to theories from other core perspectives of mental disorder, the psychological and the social. Through continued multi-perspective research, and awareness of our biological bias when we use psychiatric diagnoses, hopefully a more balanced pluralistic use of the biological, psychological, and social perspective on mental disorder can be developed in the future and as a result create a more balanced narrative of mental disorder.

Notes

1. Note that certain behaviors also can be left out of diagnoses, not because they are considered healthy, but since they are not considered to deviate from the statistical norm enough to merit inclusion in the mental disorder construct.
2. This system was also the first and last system of Swedish psychiatric diagnoses that contained a religious diagnosis, *demonomania*.
3. That Hippocrates represents a biological focus is of course a simplification, since the division between body and soul as we have known it since Descartes was not applicable back then. The balance between the body's fluids affected the psyche and vice versa. The Hippocratic/Platonic distinction is used here to illustrate the difference between a focus on reinstating a physiological balance of bodily fluids and a focus on reinstating a psychological balance between different aspects of the psyche (see Hippocrates, *On the Sacred Disease*).
4. For example, from being considered extremely rare at the time of DSM-III, a sharp increase in prevalence of the diagnosis "social phobia" (i.e., a strong anxiety when being at the center of attention, which often results in withdrawal and panic attacks) at the beginning of the twenty-first century indicates a medicalization of anxiety when every eighth Swedish person was considered to suffer from this condition, which was discussed as one of the greatest endemic diseases (Carlberg, 2008, p. 246ff).
5. Persons with substance use disorder are also often diagnosed with attention-deficit/hyperactivity disorder, where impaired impulse control is a core symptom.
6. The biological foundation for the deviation of impaired impulse control is broadly that the brain structure the striatum is flooded with dopamine, resulting in problems with maintaining focus when other impressions are perceived. One's focus is shifted, and it is more likely that one acts on one's impulses. What *causes* the striatum to be excessively flooded for certain persons is more unclear and debated among biological, psychological, and social perspectives.
7. Variants of sexual expressions in psychiatric diagnoses emerged at the end of the nineteenth century alongside their perceived characteristics such as transvestitism, zoophilia, and pedophilia, which were still represented in the 1980 DSM-III. Engström, by contrast, had not yet differentiated sexuality in this nuanced manner.

References

Achugar, M. (2017). Critical discourse analysis and history. In: J. Flowerdew & J. E. Richardson (Eds.), *The Routledge Handbook of Critical Discourse Studies*.

APA (1980). *Diagnostic and statistical manual of mental disorders (3rd Edition) (DSM-III)*. American Psychiatric Association, Washington DC.

Birch, D. (2007). *Our Victorian education*. Wiley-Blackwell.

Carlberg, I. (2008). *Pillret: en berättelse om depressioner och doktorer, forskare och Freud, människor och marknader*. Nordstedts förlag.

Courtwright, D. T. (2005). *Drogernas historia [Forces of habit]*. Historiska media.

Engel, G. L. (1977). The need for a new medical model: A challenge for biomedicine. *Science, 196*, 129–136.

Foucault, M. (1961/2001). *Vansinnets historia under den klassiska epoken [Madness and Civilization: A History of Insanity in the Age of Reason]*. Arkiv.

Foucault, M. (1969/2011). *Vetandets arkeologi [Archaeology of knowledge]*. Arkiv.

Foucault, M. (1976/2004). *Sexualitetens historia Band 1: viljan att veta. [The history of sexuality I: the will to knowledge]*. Daidalos.

Frances, A. (2014). *Saving normal: An insider's revolt against out-of-control psychiatric diagnosis, DSM-5, Big pharma and the medicalization of ordinary life*. Harper Collins.

Grünewald, K. (2009). *Från idiot till medborgare [From idiot to citizen]*. Gothia Förlag.

Henriques, G. R. (2002). The harmful dysfunction analysis and the differentiation between mental disorder and disease. *Scientific Review of Mental Health Practice, 1*(2), 157–173.

Hildebrand Karlén, M. (2013). *Vansinnets diagnoser: Om klassiska och möjliga perspektiv i svensk psykiatri*. Carlssons Bokförlag.

Hippocrates. On the sacred disease. Downloaded 2022-12-31 from: http://classics.mit. edu/Hippocrates/sacred.1b.txt

Jaspers, K. (1959/1997). *General psychopathology* (vol. I and II). John Hopkins University Press.

Johannisson, K. (1990/2013). *Medicinens öga: sjukdom, medicin och samhälle—historiska erfarenheter*. Nordstedts förlag.

Johannisson, K. (2002). Kroppen i den moderna medicinen: Ett historiskt perspektiv på moderniteten. *Slagmark, 35*, 39–68.

Johannisson, K. (2009). *Melankoliska rum: Om ångest, leda och sårbarhet i förfluten tid och nutid*. Albert Bonniers förlag.

Kuhn, T. S. (1962). *The structure of scientific revolutions*. University of Chicago Press: Chicago.

Laing, R. (1968). *Det kluvna jaget [The Divided Self: An Existential Study in Sanity and Madness]*. Aldus/Bonniers.

Lewis, B. (2012). *Narrative psychiatry: How stories can shape clinical practice*. Johns Hopkins University Press.

Lindgren, S.-Å. (1993). *Den hotfulla njutningen: Att etablera drogbruk som ett samhällsproblem 1890–1970*. Symposion graduale.

Lyotard, J. (1979/1984). *The postmodern condition: A report on knowledge*. Manchester University Press.

Mayes, R., & Horwitz, A. V. (2005). DSM-III and the revolution in classification of mental illness. *Journal of the History of the Behavioural Sciences, 41*, 249–267.

Ghaemi, S. N. (2003). *The concepts of psychiatry*. John Hopkins University Press.

Qvarsell, R. (1982). *Ordning och Behandling*. Göteborgs offsettryckeri.

Rounsaville, B. J., Alarcón, R. D., Andrews, G., Jackson, J. S., Kendell, R. E., & Kendler, K. (2002). Basic nomenclature issues for DSM-V. In D. J. Kupfer, M. B. First, & D. A. Regier (Eds.), *A research agenda for DSM-V* (pp. 1–29). American Psychiatric Association.

Wakefield, J. (1992). The concept of mental disorder: On the boundary between biological facts and social values. *American Psychologist, 47*, 373–88.

PART III

NARRATIVES OF AGING, DEMENTIA, AND DEPRESSION

8

How to Narrate a Healthy Life

Life Stories and Mental Health in Interviews with the Elderly Aged 90+

Mari Hatavara

Narrative studies today expand to such fields as narrative gerontology, introducing humanities methodology to the study of aging. From early on, a humanities perspective on gerontology has been understood as pivotal to understanding the experiential side of human life (Van Tassel, 1979), and recent studies have emphasized that narrative gerontology should shift its focus more on the act and context of storytelling instead of the content of what is told (Blix, 2016) as well as to understanding narratives as a use of symbols to understand the self (de Medeiros, 2014, pp. 2–4). This chapter suggests an interdisciplinary combination of narratology originating in literary studies and psychology as a methodology to study the ways of narrating lives in interviews with the elderly. The aim is to combine discourse-narratological methodology for the analysis of the narrating self with narrative positioning theory on the various levels of positioning in the interview. Discourse narratology targets the use of language as a symbolic system, and positioning theory examines the contextual act of storytelling in relation to story contents and cultural expectations. Previous studies have indicated that richness and flexibility in the process of narration correlate with mental health (see Westerhof & Bohlmeijer, 2012). With a methodological combination geared towards the analysis of the situated act of narrating and its linguistic form, this chapter proposes a possible model for analysis in narrative gerontology. The ways of narrating studied include the narrator's discursive and evaluative relation to their former self and how these relate to the levels of story, interaction, and identity in positioning.

Mari Hatavara, *How to Narrate a Healthy Life* In: *Narrative and Mental Health*. Edited by: Jarmila Mildorf, Elisabeth Punzi, and Christoph Singer, Oxford University Press. © Oxford University Press 2023.
DOI: 10.1093/oso/9780197620540.003.0009

Narrative Discourse Modes and Positioning in the Analyses of Life Storying

At least since the famous statement by Roland Barthes about narrative being pervasive, "simply there, like life itself" (1977, p. 79), narratives have been regarded as crucial to understanding and engaging with others as well as for shaping our identities. In the social sciences, for example, the whole life of a person has been equated with a narrative that would display life from birth until the moment of remembering—a view also criticized for its lack of nuance and ignorance towards the empirical difficulty to identify such complete narratives outside of a researcher's projection (see Hyvärinen, 2008, p. 261; Hyvärinen & Watanabe, 2017, pp. 337–337). Psychologist Jerome Bruner (2004/1987, pp. 691–693) also argues that autobiographical narratives consist of procedures for life making. For him, telling about one's own life is an interpretative act, which is necessarily reflexive as the narrator and protagonist are the same. As interpretative and situated acts, narratives are at least as much about the discursive ways of narrating as the contents of a story unfolding.

Narrative as a sense-making operation is highlighted in one of the recent definitions of narrative as "a basic human strategy for coming to terms with time, process, and change" (Herman et al., 2005). Besides this cognitive definition of narrative, at least two other main definitions can be identified: one with the emphasis on the rhetorical act of the situated telling of a story for a purpose, and one with the emphasis on the semiotic articulation of a story as a narrative, be it oral, written, or visual. Together with another literary scholar I have suggested that these strands of narrative research with their different definitions of narrative need to be brought together in order to study narratives as both sense-making operations and as discursive resources in communication and social action (Hatavara & Toikkanen, 2019). Therefore, it is crucial to maintain the distinction between story level, the content of what is told, and discourse level, the means of telling, in the analysis of narratives (cf. Björninen et al., 2020). This chapter brings together the study of narrative discourse modes developed in literary studies and positioning theory developed in the social sciences. The former enables one to undertake linguistically based analysis of the discourse features as well as the narrating I's relation to their former self, and the latter allows for the study of how story and discourse levels relate to identity. This combined methodology is used to explore how narration is linked with mental health in two interviews with elderly people in Finland.

Philosopher Daniel D. Hutto exposed the core assumptions of narrative medicine and narrative therapy, the two most prominent approaches that use narrative to improve (mental) health. Together with his colleagues Nicolle Marissa Brancazio and Jarrah Aubourg, Hutto reaffirms the link between narrative skills and quality of life: "[h]ow we narrate can shape who we are and what we do" (Hutto et al., 2017, p. 314). With philosophical scrutiny, the authors demonstrate that narrative is one of the most important ways of understanding and making sense of self and others, and they indicate that better narrative skills correspond with improved mental health (Hutto et al., 2017, pp. 310–312 and *passim*). Based on an empirical study, the importance of the ways of storytelling for an individual's mental health has been indicated by Gerben J. Westerhof and Ernst T. Bohlmeijer (2012), whose study suggests that the process of narrating surpasses the structure of a story in its impact on mental health. They identify the nexus between narration and mental health in the balance between proximity and distance towards personal experiences in identity construction. In maintaining identity, the degree of identification with positive and negative experiences is crucial and requires rich processes of narration (Westerhof & Bohlmeijer, 2012, pp. 109–111, 122–123).

For the purpose of this chapter, I will follow Westerhof and Bohlmeijer's practice of understanding mental health in relation to the balancing between closeness and proximity to personal experience in life narratives. Narration in this chapter denotes narrative means used to mediate experience and identity. Therefore, the features analyzed are discursive distance and evaluative distance between the narrating I and their former self as well as positioning at the levels of story, interaction, and identity. Discursive distance is linguistically discernible, whereas evaluative distance and positioning are interpretative categories based on linguistic cues. Together these features cover the semiotic, rhetorical, and cognitive aspects of the ways of narrating one's life.

In literary studies, analytical methods for the study of a first-person narrating I and their relationship to their former self have a long tradition. The narrator may approximate the former experiencing I as self-quotation or self-narration. The discursive movement between past and present can be linguistically identified in the narration, which makes evident the contribution literary studies can make to the study of the ways of narrating proximity and distance (Cohn, 1978, pp. 14, 17; cf. Palmer, 2004, pp. 9–13, 53–54). Also, the narrating self may express evaluative continuity and sameness with their former self or a psychological distance from that—that is, there can be a consonant or a dissonant narrator. While consonant narrators align themselves with the perspective of the self in the story events of the past, dissonant narrators assume intellectual or moral distance from their former selves (Cohn, 1978, pp. 145–158). The analytical model rests on the basic distinction in literary narratology drawn between story content and discursive expression, which posits that the story is the *what* in a narrative that is depicted, discourse the *how* (Chatman, 1978; see also Abbott, 2007, pp. 39–40, Björninen et al., 2020; Genette, 1980, p. 27). The *how*, the narrative modes of telling one's story, has gained much more attention in literary narratology than in the social sciences oriented towards narrative. Gerontologist Kate de Medeiros (2014, pp. 11–12) gives an impressive overview of different approaches to narrative in her book on narrative gerontology but does not concentrate on the story versus discourse distinction.

The theory and methodology of narrative discourse modes have been developed mostly for the analysis of literary texts, especially novels. In the move to introduce these methods to nonfictional interview materials, I am building on the theory of cross-fictionality that I have developed together with Jarmila Mildorf. Cross-fictionality denotes fictional modes of representing the mind characteristically used in a nonfictional narrative environment. Those modes range from direct thought presentation to mental verbs summarizing cognitive operations and to forms that discursively mix several subjects (Hatavara & Mildorf, 2017a, 2017b). Cross-fictionality as an approach is best suited to study instances of third-person narration, where questions of storytelling rights and epistemological privilege are highlighted. In a similar fashion, however, the many discursive modes of telling in a life interview can benefit from the model that enables one to draw distinctions between the narrator using discursive modes attached to their perspective or indicating another point of view, either another person or a former self. Here is where I believe the semiotic understanding of narrative with its emphasis on discursive modes of articulation can contribute to inter- and multidisciplinary narrative studies in the field of (mental) health: Literary studies provide concepts to more precisely analyze the "*how* we narrate" rather than the "*what* we narrate" that shapes our identities and affects our actions.

Narrative analysis of conversational narratives, interviews, and other nonfictional texts has concentrated mostly on storylines and story contents. One notable exception is positioning theory, where identities are studied in situated narrative interaction and in relation to both story content and narrative discourse (see Bamberg, 2004; Deppermann, 2013, p. 2). Positioning theory as developed by Michael Bamberg (1997, 2004) helps one to understand how the distinction between story and discourse levels can also be discerned in social interaction. Narrative positioning refers to (1) positions taken and given in the story—the content of what is discussed, (2) positioning in the situation—where people participate in social interaction, and (3) positioning related to identities and normative discourses (Bamberg, 1997, p. 337; 2004, pp. 136–137). Therefore, the model considers three aspects of narrative: *what* is told, *how* it is told, and *how* it relates to identity. More diverse models on how these levels interact have also been developed (cf. Deppermann, 2015, pp. 377–380 and *passim*). This chapter combines the literary model of representing the mind with positioning theory in order to be able to analyze *how* life stories are narrated in an interview and especially how experience is related to identity, which has been indicated as crucial to mental health.

Before introducing my material and starting the analysis, it is important to notice that this chapter does not aim at providing an overview of how life stories are narrated or claiming any one-to-one correspondence between story content and storytelling modes. From a literary–narratological point of view the ever-changing relation between some narrative features and interpretative outcomes is part of the research tradition. One of the clearest statements against one-to-one correspondence between any form and function in narratives comes from Meir Sternberg (1982), whose "Proteus principle" denies such easy "package deals" in the interpretation of narratives; any narrative form may gain several and changing functions. Nonetheless, since it does matter how one narrates, it is well worth to examine particular cases to better understand how the ways of narrating may affect mental well-being. After all, if *how* we narrate is what matters to our self-understanding and our actions, these ways require closer analysis than has been conducted this far. In the following, I will analyze the discursive and evaluative relations two interviewees have towards their past selves and their life as well as how the narrative modes used function between the three levels of positioning: story, interaction, and identity.

Life Narratives of the Oldest: Mental Health Discussed

The materials analyzed come from a research project called Vitality 90+ at Tampere University, Finland. The project has a large corpus of oral life stories and narrative interviews with a total of 245 persons aged 90+ in Tampere in

1995 and in 2012. The study investigates trends and predictors of health and functioning, quality of life, formal and informal care and services, very old age as a stage of life, subjective experiences of long life, as well as the biology of longevity. Besides life story interviews, the data include mailed surveys, register data, functional performance examinations, and blood tests. The interviews have a loose thematic structure that includes asking about the life events from childhood to the present and clusters of model questions surrounding the topics of important things in life, hobbies and everyday life, thoughts about old age, estimation of one's own health and mood, possible illnesses and ways of maintaining health, and thoughts about the present in relation to one's life experience. The interviews were conducted by several researchers and students, and they vary greatly in form and content even though all follow the pattern of first asking about life events and then addressing the themes.

For the purpose of this chapter, I have read and listened to the 45 interviews conducted in 2012. From the material, I have selected two cases to be analyzed more closely in respect to the ways in which the respondent's life is narrated. Both interviews were conducted by experienced health science researchers. Typically for the material, the two men interviewed do not talk much about mental well-being or problems thereof, even when directly asked. It is also worth noticing that the generation these interviewees belong to experienced World War II as it was fought between Finland and Russia. Both men served in active duty, but they do not talk about the war much; this is also typical of the whole material. I have chosen the two narratives to be analyzed because they offer two quite opposite views on how to tell someone about mental difficulties in the life span of more than 90 years. Based on an initial analysis, one can say the two interviewees exhibit different types of identification between distance and proximity with their past experiences, and this can shed light on the conclusions that Westerhof and Bohlmeijer (2012) draw on the basis of their narrative psychology approach.

The first interviewee, whom I call Simo, has an overall frame of reference in his life story in his Christian faith. From that perspective, he offers the events of his life as already thought through and interpreted as a clear life course. Strong hindsight determines how past events are related in the moment of telling, which hints towards what Westerhof and Bohlmeijer (2012, p. 111) see as overidentification: There is little room for alternative storylines, and the particular personal experience of finding faith functions as a nuclear script. By contrast, in the second interview, a person I call Oskari relates short episodes in his life, often without any clear indication of their significance for him or signs of strong agency in the happenings. He often proposes himself as a victim of circumstance, overwhelmed by events and other people's intentions, coming close to what Westerhof and Bohlmeijer (2012, p. 111) designate as underidentification. Oskari also discloses at the end of the interview that he has never before told the events of his life or his ideas on life to anyone. While Simo often repeats that he has led an ordinary life, a life that has been quiet, happy, and healthy, Oskari tells about the difficult and even violent relationship with his parents and his wife, often refers to his overall dark mood, and expresses surprise at his own longevity.

Both interviewees are male, and both have two children; Oskari is a widower and Simo is married for a second time. He has one child from each marriage. Simo's wife is also present in the interview, which of course might have many effects on the way Simo tells his life. She does not talk much, though, but at times provides pieces of information Simo forgets in the moment, fills in gaps in other ways, or affects the trajectory of how questions are asked.

When asked about his experience with old age, Simo says that he has been surprised that old age sometimes feels mentally hard, and continues: "It is like, I can't say negative, but at times depression enters this living" (01.04.42). Shortly afterwards he mentions that he was prescribed first some downers, then antidepressants when he had "a really bad this kind of depression." His wife changes the subject to Simo never before needing any medication, and mental health is not picked up again as a subject. Whereas Simo talks directly about depression, using the concept himself without being provided it first, Oskari tells about his mood only after being asked about permanent medication:

OSKARI: Well, no. I don't have any such medication I would necessarily need to take every day, that they would matter. But I have that coronary artery, have had one clog, medication for the coronary artery. And then the sleeping pills, and then there is the medicine for cholesterol, and then a peace of mind pill.
INTERVIEWER: Yes, you have that.
OSKARI: Right. But nothing much more then. So, I don't have, five pills I take in the morning, two in the afternoon. And then the sleeping pill, there's the mind in that. I mean the kind of medicine to stabilize sleep, it is not a mood medicine. It is in order to stabilize sleep. (1.25.10)

Here Oskari is searching for the right word to describe the medicine he is taking and first talks about peace of mind, then about mood and about stabilizing sleep. He denies explicitly that his medicine is for mood control but explains that it helps with his sleep.

Both interviewees refer to medication for mental health, but Simo openly and with clear vocabulary, Oskari more indirectly and hesitantly and seemingly in search for the right words. What is more, he repeatedly uses negatives in the example above. When asked about medication, he first says "no," followed by a "but" and several uses of an "and." The interviewer changes into "yes" of Oskari having medication, but he soon switches to "nothing much more" again. This happens both when he talks generally about his need for medication—which he first says he does not have and then lists eight daily pills—and when he speculates about the nature of his evening pill.

The same type of difference between the narratives of the two men continues throughout the interviews. While the interview of Simo presents a case where a life story is well verbalized and organized from the beginning until the present, told to inform the interviewer, the interview of Oskari is a process of making sense of the events in his life also for the narrator himself. He keeps searching for words and expressions to portray his life events. In the next two sections, I will analyze the interviews separately before moving to a comparison of the two.

Simo's Narrative: A Retrospective Life Story

Simo had been in the same job for a long time; he worked as an independent chimney sweeper in a small coastal city. At the beginning of the interview, he refers to the job as not being very prestigious but continues: "It was a well-paying job, when there was a sober, respectable man doing it." Here, Simo defines himself in positive terms. He does not use the first person to say *I was a sober, respectable man* but instead tells about a quality of the job as its good pay, and then explains that as a result of a personal character trait. Grammatically, Simo uses the third person when he talks about himself as having been "a sober, respectable man" doing his job. Therefore, it is only the context that indicates that Simo is classifying himself when talking about "a man." In this description of his former self, Simo uses third-level positioning—the script of a sober, respectable man as a good provider for the family—to position his past self in the story level (level one). His past experiences are summed up to reveal a permanent personality trait, self-positioning Simo as a "respectable man" in the past and still at the present (level two; cf. Deppermann, 2015, pp. 378–379). Besides this evaluative consonance with his former self, Simo discursively takes a distance from his former self as "a man," thus linguistically appearing as a dissonant narrator.

This combination of discursive distance and ideological consonance as well as direct references to third-level positioning of self into social roles and scripts is prevalent throughout the interview. Simo repeatedly summarizes his life: While talking about joining the church of Divine Service of the Advent he says "life has been very peaceful and healthy"; after talking about his children he outlines "this is about it, the kind of peaceful life." In this way he again very explicitly draws from third-level positioning to summarize a certain type of life he has always led, suggesting full consonance with his former self. At the same time, he refrains from narrating particular experiences he has had in the past. It is difficult to tell whether he would feel proximity or distance towards his experience in the past as the script of a peaceful life overcomes any singular experience, and stories that would portray past experience are mostly not articulated in the interview.

When the interviewer asks Simo about his future plans and wishes for life Simo turns the subject towards his wife, Kaija. Even though she is nine years younger than Simo she appears to have more problems with her physical health.

SIMO: I always think of ways how to help and take care of Kaija, since she has these difficulties. The kind of prosaic life in a way, but with a spiritual basis.

INTERVIEWER: So, supporting and helping each other, you have managed anyway.

SIMO: You, that is my . . . In our summer house, there is a photo of a husband and a wife, and we grow old supporting each other, it says under the card. (1.00.21)

Here, Simo describes his life with his wife by referring to a card with a photo of a married couple, prototypically only referred to as "a husband" and "a wife." His words do not reveal if the photo portrays himself with his wife or someone else, but at least the phrase he quotes clearly originates from something like a greeting card. With the reference to the photo and the phrase

Simo places his happy marriage in a larger cultural frame, representative of an ideal relationship. This brings to a head his most widely used narrative practice of resorting to widespread generalizations of his life as ordinary and peaceful. In terms of positioning, Simo jumps right into the third-level evaluation and resorts to an existing cultural item, a card, to summarize his relationship with his wife. Even when Simo talks about his present life at the beginning of the excerpt, he uses an iterative temporal adverbial "always." This again generalizes his life into a continuum with consonance governing the whole "peaceful life."

Two very short deviations from this overall happy and peaceful life can be found in the interview, and both are linked to the war Simo participated in. The first example, as seen below, is from quite the beginning of the interview when Simo gives a short overview of his life span, the second a little bit later when he explains that he had two children from two marriages:

Then I went to the war in 1941, and got out in December 1944. Then started that, it was a little problematic that period after coming back from the army, I had that kind of difficulty to settle. It went by as I worked at the railroad engineering, dad got me that. His cousin was the boss, but he had died in the Winter War in that bombing. And then I met Kaija, and we have been married, 60 years soon. (02.27)

One child, yes. I have [a child] from the first marriage after the war, I got married right after. It was a mistake, I wasn't able to stay put and then [she] wasn't suited for that and then she divorced me, and there is one girl from that marriage. She is 64 now, and she has been in contact, has visited here as well. (17.05)

In the first example Simo searches for words for a short while when talking about his return from the war—the events of the war itself are completely omitted, with only the start and end years given. The hesitation in the second sentence is preceded by and continued with facts that contain exact numbers in years. Even when hesitating, Simo is able in hindsight to label his past experience as "problematic" and "difficulty to settle." No details on his past experience are given, nor hints of the types of difficulties he had. The only details are the years given and the fact that Simo's father's cousin had been the boss at Simo's workplace before being killed in the war. In the end, Simo returns to his second marriage and the time span of almost 60 years offers a closure to the story of temporary difficulties.

The first marriage is discussed in the second example above. Simo evaluates the short marriage soon after the war as a mistake and gives a reason for the divorce. No internal states of mind or past thoughts are given, but a concise account of what happened and an explanation of it from the current perspective. Again, all is well as the first wife is in contact and visits Simo and Kaija. In these last two examples dissonance from the former self is evident both discursively and ideologically as Simo uses hindsight to reminisce about his difficulties and a mistaken marriage, carefully displaying change and continuity from his former self (cf. Deppermann, 2015, p. 379).

Later in the interview, the interviewer asks about the most important things in Simo's life. Simo talks about the big role religion has played in his life and concludes with a summarizing line, after which the interviewer tries to ask for more:

SIMO: Inner life in balance, and death doesn't feel scary.
INTERVIEWER: So, has it been this religion, when you've had hard times in your life, that has helped you to cope?
SIMO: Hard times, you mean?
INTERVIEWER: Yes, when you've had difficulties. Or obstacles in life, how have you coped?
SIMO: Well, I did have a little after returning from the war, I had a little drinking problem. And then this made it so that I started thinking a little and studying things. The kind of a pretty ordinary life, that nothing particular has happened to me. [laughter]
INTERVIEWER: What about the years in the war, what kind of an experience were they?
SIMO: Well, that then, not that delightful at all. I was at [a place] all the time, and especially the last surge. There I got wounded a little. That was an experience of its own, one that you wouldn't like to talk much about. (40.58)

Here again Simo jumps into the evaluative, generalizing statement about the status of his inner life without providing access to his intimate thoughts on the story level of past events. On the level of the interaction in the interview (level two), Simo is struggling to follow the interviewer's line of asking as difficulties in life are expected to have happened, and he asks for clarification on the suggested "hard times." His investment in the happy, peaceful life (level three) hinders his ability to even consider hardship in life. After the interviewer clarifies that she really means difficulties in life, Simo mentions the period after his return from the war. This time, he gives a more informative answer, and from the dissonant position of the narrating self positions his former self in the category of an alcoholic. Furthermore, he makes evident that he has changed since. In order to make that clear, he uses a familiar script of a former alcoholic recovered with the help of religion. Next, he returns to his claim of ordinary life with "nothing particular" having happened—the laughter perhaps indicating an uneasiness in the interview interaction at the time.

The interviewer is not fully content with the acclaimed ordinariness and tries to ask more about the war, which presumably had been a difficult experience. Simo resorts to a negative expression "not that delightful," which indicates his strong aim at giving a "delightful" portrayal of his life. He also resorts to a passive expression in the end, stating "you" as unwilling to talk about the war. In between those two expressions Simo tells a little about what had happened in the war, but again without any details of what it was like for him to live through the events. Besides strong hindsight prevailing over past experience, Simo refuses to discuss or describe difficult experiences.

Oskari's Narrative: Stories of a Life Unfolding

Oskari was a sheet-metal worker, first in the same place for about 20 years but then short periods in several places after getting on to early retirement. He had spent the first seven years of his childhood with his grandparents. He remembers his mother once visiting and having a discussion with his grandmother:

> I remember nothing else from the conversation, but this stuck to my mind. As mother then said to her own mother, that is my grandmother, that yes it really has to. Meaning me, well, with that. And I got a little upset, and I thought. I thought how have I really been that disobedient here now, that because of that it really has to now. It was said with emphasis, as well, but grandmother answered nothing. (9.15)

This little story is informative of a situation where a little boy was upset listening to a conversation where his mother forces his grandmother to take care of him, apparently against the grandmother's will. This interpretation, however, is left for the audience to make, since Oskari gives no more interpretation of the episode apart from his own emotions of being upset and puzzled. Oskari only tells about past positionings on the story level (level one), and any interpretative positioning on level three is left for the interpreter to make in regard to a parent's and a grandparent's obligations towards a child.

In the example above, Oskari discursively uses direct discourse of the people acting in the past events, quoting verbatim both his mother ("yes it really has to") and himself ("how have I really . . ."). Right at the beginning he refers to partial epistemological dissonance from his own past self as he claims to remember "nothing else," but then quotes his mother's words in the dialogue and his own former thoughts giving details of the past events. The temporal marker "now" is repeated twice in his thoughts in the fifth sentence, and the deictic marker "here" is also used to indicate location and discursive origin in the past world. In between these two quotations from two past actors, his mother and himself, he uses indirect discourse of the narrating I to reveal his emotion in the past. Discursively, this quotation moves between the narrating self and the narrated self in several ways. It also indicates a consonant self narrator feeling empathy towards himself as a child.

From the perspective of positioning theory, Oskari moves between positioning levels one and two. The very first sentence positions him in the interaction meta-narratively (level two; cf. Deppermann, 2015, pp. 379–380) as someone who tries to tell all he remembers but also makes evident the importance of what is to come as a permanent recollection for both his former and present self. Positioning towards the interviewer is also evident between the quoted sentences as Oskari explains that his mother's words were a reference to himself. In what follows, Oskari positions himself as a child on the story level (level one; cf. Deppermann, 2015, p. 377) wondering about his mother's and grandmother's evaluations of himself.

A little later, Oskari tells that living with his mother and father after he had turned seven years old was hard since they disliked him, and especially his father was ill-tempered and violent. When asked why he still had lived at home several years after coming of age, he explains:

Well, I stayed. I didn't leave, that's right. I started having this idea and this mentality, since I always often heard, it was father who started it. I mean when they had a fight, you could easily hear the word, that you are crazy. And so did I hear, as well. My mother said, as well, that are you a little crazy, Oskari, and so did father. And I started seriously to wonder at school age, and I thought to myself, am I really crazy? Is there something wrong with me, since they always say so? (24.45)

In this part of the interview, Oskari again assumes the past point of view of himself as a child and discursively repeats his thoughts at the time. The last sentence and part of the sentence preceding that are in the form of quoted inner monologue of Oskari's thoughts when he was at school. Before that, Oskari summarizes his thoughts and feelings that had grown over a period of time in the discourse of the narrating self but with the experiential perspective of the former self. He portrays his developing fear of being crazy from "started having" to the iterative "always often" and all the way to seriously giving thought to the issue. What is more, Oskari also quotes verbatim the words both his parents allegedly said, first as a collective, then each one individually, rephrasing parts of the past discussion (level one).

In this example, Oskari positions himself in between his parents as a witness to their fighting on the story level. On the level of the interview interaction (level two), he reflects ("I mean," "you could," "so did I") on his continuing effort to evaluate his state of mind. Right after the last quotation, he gives an even more direct explanation of his past thoughts: "It grew on me, that they said again and again the same, that I won't cope, that I don't understand things." Here, Oskari evaluates his former self in a way that creates a sympathetic yet emotionally dissonant relation: He now understands he was indoctrinated and emphasizes the nature of the indoctrination by repeating the words of his parents once again. The choice of the first-person pronoun in the parents' question that he reiterates ("am I really crazy?") emphasizes his submission at the story level (level one) to what his parents had said to him.

Often the moments of change in Oskari's life are narrated in a way that makes them seem vividly recalled but at the same time fully out of his control as a past agent. Events leading to his marriage start with a visit to a bar with an older male friend:

And we sat there the two of us, and I guess we had some drinks there. And then from next there a person came there in front of me. And I don't remember her words now, that she used. But what she meant was, don't go together with an old man like that, get yourself some woman. I didn't answer anything. I did understand the issue, but where would I at that moment get one, I mean it will necessarily take some time. (49.29)

Here, Oskari first tells about an instructive statement from a stranger. He says openly he does not remember the exact words but rather the meaning and significance of the words. Interestingly, the discursive form of what he relates after the introductory clause "what she meant was" is in the form of direct discourse and as such functions as a kind of hypothetical quotation of the exact words that the person could have used. Oskari then goes on to tell about his lack of action and his reasoning. Discursively, he both mixes the language of the narrating I with his former thoughts ("would" instead of *will* and "that" instead of *this*) and uses direct quoted monologue of his experiencing I at the end of the example. From the point of view of positioning, on the story level (level one) Oskari is a recipient of a seemingly good piece of advice he does not know how to follow. On the level of telling (level two), Oskari makes an effort to remember, "now" at the interview moment, what had happened, and he addresses the interviewer with an explanation ("I mean") relevant both in the past and at the present moment. It seems as if the script of a young man meeting a woman and getting married (level-three positioning) is so encompassing that there is no way of questioning the advice, neither in the past story nor in the interactive situation of the telling.

Close to the end of the interview, the interviewer asks about the highlights of Oskari's life, events with positive importance for Oskari, and he answers:

Well. I have had very little of them, one needs to really search for them. But in the end, after all, there is this apartment, and there are other things, as well. But this is a good example this apartment, we lived in [a neighborhood in Tampere], so did we. We had the same size as this is, but it was an apartment. And we had no trouble in there, it was a good place to be. A shop right next door and a bus stop, and a short way to the city. But it once happened so that, when I got back from work again in the evening. And the wife was at home, so we didn't talk much about something else. She said first that you go and sign your name there in the paper. She said the name of the agency, where she had already been to in the morning. She said she had already signed. Go and sign your name, that we are going to get a new place. And I got totally terrified, that we still have an old mortgage to pay. And now to take a new mortgage, that what's going to happen now. But I didn't yell anything, I went and signed my name. Since I thought and I knew, since I knew her. That if I say I won't go. That it'll turn into such a terrible fight, that she won't give up, I will have to go and do it. I thought I'd rather do it willingly than forced. And I went and signed and I haven't regretted. And now we have lived here for nearly 30 years. (1.48.41)

This story exemplifies the type of identification Westerhof and Bohlmeijer (2012) classify as a victim plot, where "protagonists are being overwhelmed by events and have lost power to effect change" (p. 111). Oskari tells about coming home to a situation where his wife has already decided on buying a new flat and only gives Oskari the directions on what he needs to do to finalize what she has decided to do and already done for her part. Despite his total lack of agency in the related story world (level-one positioning), Oskari offers this story in the interview interaction (level-two positioning) as a highlight in his life. When Oskari gives details on the niceness of the old flat and of his doubts, the reader expects something to go wrong with the new place or Oskari to make his wife change her opinion and convince her to stay in the nice apartment they have. Quite unexpectedly, Oskari tells that he was too frightened to do anything but what his wife had told him and to sign the papers to buy the new place. This, at least, leads the reader to expect a catastrophic ending. On the contrary, however, the resolution portrays Oskari as very happy with the outcome he has just told he was forced into. The reader is left to wonder why Oskari tells this story about being oppressed and forced to act against his reasoning and fear as a highlight in his life. It is almost as if he uses no hindsight at all to make this story a proper narrative but chronicles the phases of events as he experienced them in the past, unfolding one part at a time without a narrative design.

Discursively and in the light of positioning theory, this example resembles the previous ones from Oskari's interview. Again, Oskari gives both direct quotations from the past story world, this time his wife's. He also tells about his own emotions ("totally terrified") and gives direct quotations of his own past thoughts. Discursively, Oskari shifts between his former self experiencing the happenings and his narrating self making sense of the past. This time, his thoughts in the past also give information on his wife's mind as he says he knew her so well that he was able to come to a conclusion without a fight between them even though he felt tempted ("I didn't yell anything"). On the story-level positioning (level one), Oskari renders both what his wife said and what he did and did not do himself. On the level of the interview interaction (level two), Oskari self-positions his experiencing self either as just plain compliant with his wife or as a wise husband coping with a marital situation in the best possible way. Understood in the latter sense, the story may be interpreted as telling us about a highlight in Oskari's life. The fact that the new place was and is apparently comfortable as well, and that they did not get in trouble with the mortgage, is just a side effect in this story. In a sense, Oskari as a narrator exhibits both dissonance from his former self, since his fears were proved wrong, and consonance with his past self, since he can proudly say he did not participate in a fight.

Ways to Narrate a Life (Story)

In this final section of my chapter, I will examine the analytical findings concerning Simo's and Oskari's interviews and relate those to some of the assumptions previous studies on narratives and mental health have suggested. In this chapter, I set out to analyze how the narrators discursively and evaluatively relate their narrating self to their former self and what kind of positionings they used in the process of narrating their lives. As an analytical frame I have used the conclusions Westerhof and Bohlmeijer (2012, p. 123) have reached in their study on identification in life stories. They argue that flexible ways of having distance and proximity to one's past experience is the key to mental health. I also aimed at introducing a novel interdisciplinary methodology based on the cross-fictional approach to discourse narratology and on positioning theory to study the ways people narrate their lives.

The analyses of the two life interviews shows that the methodological combination of narrative discourse modes and positioning theory can be complementary in life story interviews. The former enables the linguistically based analysis of the ways of discursively and evaluatively mediating the present narrating self with the former experiencing self and the latter the study of how the three levels of positioning function in the telling of one's life. Together they help to analyze the ways the interviewees narratively mediate and organize their past experiences and their present identities. What is more, my analysis demonstrates that different ways of narrating may be connected with different levels of positioning: Oskari's narration, rich with several modes of representing past thoughts of himself and others, operates mostly on the first and second levels of positioning, whereas Simo, with his discursively monological narration, often refers directly to level-three positioning and is heavily influenced by hindsight.

Simo's narration indicates discursive distance from past experience, which is rarely addressed at all and never discursively made present. Evaluatively, he shifts between dissonance and consonance with his former self: He is a redeemed alcoholic traumatized by war and at the same time has led a completely ordinary, peaceful, and happy life throughout. The latter positioning is repeatedly emphasized by Simo. Oskari's narration shifts discursively between past and present in deictic markers, tenses, and quotations from past thoughts and talk; he both approximates past experience linguistically and evaluates and describes his past experience from the later point of view in, for example, the use of mental-state vocabulary like "terrified." He uses several discursive modes, also those mixing the points of view of past and present self. Oskari also moves between dissonance and consonance in his evaluation of his former self, mostly exhibiting a sympathetic relation to his past self. In Oskari's narration, the positioning levels one and two, the story and interaction with the interviewer, are prevalent as the effort to make sense of past experience at the time of telling becomes highlighted. Generally, Simo quite openly offers the interviewer third-level interpretations of his life, whereas Oskari leaves interpretations implicit.

One perspective on these results is provided by Gary Saul Morson in his model of narrative temporalities. Morson (1994, pp. 6–14) makes a distinction between narratives as causally organized sequences of past events or as a hypothesis of what might have happened. Foreshadowing and sideshadowing both present a sequence: In the first, all events are determined by the beginning, but in the second, it is the outcome, the present moment, that determines the narrative and organizes the sequence. The hypothetical mode is called "sideshadowing," which allows for speculating on possibilities, seeing several options in the past. From this point of view, sideshadowing might be seen to allow a rich possibility for narrating a story, foreshadowing would have closed the process of narrative sense making already, and backshadowing may be used to explain (away) past happenings in a way suitable to the moment of telling.

Simo tells a coherent story with an overall frame of a happy life. The one deviation in the cause of the life events, the period after the war with alcoholism and a failed marriage, has been fully merged into the frame as an impetus for finding religion and a sound way of living again. Yet, Simo's narrative resources are rather narrow and stable. Simo exhibits mostly distance from his former experience with a strong aim at maintaining an identity narrative of a happy life of a respectable, sober man. By contrast, Oskari does not provide a coherent life story with meaningful, causal sequences. His narrative is full of little stories vividly exposing his past experiences but not always with a clear connection to each other or to an evolving life narrative. Therefore, it seems the two interviewees demonstrate quite opposite ends on the continuum of exceptional and ordinary, individual and scripted (cf. Hyvärinen, 2016). Simo's narrative mode is mostly backshadowing, whereas Oskari's shifts between foreshadowing and sideshadowing.

This more open and incoherent narrative by Oskari may be linked to the fact that in the course of the interview, he twice mentions that the interview is the first time he has told about his life, exposing everything. Therefore, it is his first time of narratively organizing his life for articulation. Bruner (2004, p. 694) argues that life stories are dependent upon language use and cultural conventions that guide the telling of life narratives. For this reason, life narratives have the power to organize memory and to structure perceptual experience to the extent that "we *become* the autobiographical narratives by which we 'tell about' our lives" (Bruner, 2004, p. 695, emphasis original). Life stories become habitual and start to structure experience itself, which in the end means that life is not constituted of lived experiences but rather is formed by telling and interpreting one's life (Bruner, 2004, p. 708). In the light of Bruner's idea, it may be argued that Simo has integrated his life (story) as one of a "sober, respectable man" with a "peaceful life," whereas Oskari portrays more episodic, experiential happenings and events from the course of his life and has not (yet) formed a habitual narrative of his life.

Kuisma Korhonen (2013, p. 266) has emphasized the difference between narrative as a product or a form and narration as a process in his research on cultural trauma, also emphasizing the inevitable bond between the psychological and the cultural. He builds his argument on research that has shown the therapeutic effect of narrative to rely more on the process than on the product of narrative action. According to Korhonen (2013, pp. 278–281), the important narrative skill is to learn to become the narrator of one's own story, to accept the changing contents of a life narrative of one's own, and to find one's own words and expressions for one's memories and emotions. He argues that stories that offer ready-made solutions and plots that pretend to adhere to the world may be harmful in repressing some other stories and interpretative possibilities.

Judging by the results in this chapter, the *ways* of narrating do deserve more attention. An important distinction cutting across narrative discourse modes and narrative positioning is the question of coherence. As Matti Hyvärinen and his colleagues have argued, coherence should not automatically be considered a virtue and an indicator for a good and healthy life story (Hyvärinen et al., 2010, pp. 1, 6–7). This also has to do with the important distinction between story and discourse, the *how* and the *what* of narratives: The performative and evaluative functions of narrative may surpass the importance of the narrative account (Hyvärinen et al., 2010, p. 11). My two examples in this chapter showcase two very different ways of narrating. Most importantly, the analysis of the different ways of narrating their lives point towards very different conclusions on the mental well-being of the two interviewees than is evident from the content of the interviews. Based on content analysis, it might be easy to conclude Simo is very happy (as he keeps saying) and manages to narratively organize a complete life narrative. Oskari, on the other hand, keeps telling about his dark mood and difficult life experiences without producing a life narrative with a clear sense from beginning to end. However, if Westerhof and Bohlmeijer as well as Korhonen and Hyvärinen are correct in placing flexible ways of narrating ahead of the content of the narrated story in regard to positive effects on mental health, Oskari would seem to be someone with more resources for well-being than Simo. His proven ability to use many discourse modes, shifts between dissonance and consonance, and not only distance from but also approximations to his past experiences may suggest he is better equipped to cope with changing contents and contexts of his life narrative than is Simo, who discursively remains in the moment of narrating and strongly holds on to one overall interpretation of his identity. Empirical research on the possible relation between the ways of narrating and mental well-being lies mostly ahead.

References

Abbott, H. P. (2007). Story, plot, and narration. In D. Herman (Ed.), *The Cambridge companion to narrative* (pp. 39–51). Cambridge University Press.

Bamberg, M. (1997). Positioning between structure and performance. *Journal of Narrative and Life History*, 7(1–4), 335–342.

Bamberg, M. (2004). Positioning with Davie Hogan: Stories, tellings, and identities. In C. Daiuete & C. Lightfoot (Eds.), *Narrative analysis: Studying the development of individuals in society* (pp. 135–157). Sage.

Barthes, R. (1977). Introduction to the structural analysis of narratives. In *Image-music-text*, transl. S. Heath (pp. 79–124). Fontana.

Björninen, S., Hatavara, M., & Mäkelä, M. (2020). Narrative as social action: A narratological approach to story, discourse and positioning in political storytelling. *International Journal of Social Research Methodology*, 23(4), 437–449.

Blix, B. H. (2016). The importance of untold and unheard stories in narrative gerontology: Reflections on a field still in the making from a narrative gerontologist in the making. *Narrative Works*, 6(2). https://journals.lib.unb.ca/index.php/NW/article/view/25799

Bruner, J. (1987/2004). Life as narrative. *Social Research*, 71(3), 691–710.

Chatman, S. (1978). *Story and discourse*. Cornell University Press.

Cohn, D. (1978). *Transparent minds*. Princeton University Press.

de Medeiros, K. (2014). *Narrative gerontology in research and practice*. Springer.

Deppermann, A. (2013). Positioning in narrative interaction. *Narrative Inquiry*, 23(1), 1–15.

Deppermann, A. (2015). Positioning. In A. de Fina & A. Georgakopoulou (Eds.), *The handbook of narrative analyses* (pp. 369–387). Wiley Blackwell.

Genette, G. (1972/1980). *Narrative discourse*. Cornell University Press.

Hatavara, M., & Mildorf, J. (2017a). Hybrid fictionality and vicarious narrative experience. *Narrative*, 25(1), 65–82.

Hatavara, M., & Mildorf, J. (2017b). Fictionality, narrative modes, and vicarious storytelling. *Style*, 5(3), 391–408.

Hatavara, M., & Toikkanen, J. (2019). Sameness and difference in narrative modes and narrative sense making: The case of Ramsey Campbell's "The Scar." *Frontiers of Narrative Studies*, 5(1), 130–146.

Herman, D., Jahn, M., & Ryan, M. (2005). Introduction. In D. Herman, M. Jahn, & M. Ryan (Eds.), *Routledge encyclopedia of narrative theory* (pp. ix–xi). Routledge.

Hutto, D. D., Brancazio, N. M., & Aubourg, J. (2017). Narrative practices in medicine and therapy: Philosophical reflections. *Style*, 51(3), 300–317.

Hyvärinen, M. (2008). "Life as narrative" revisited. *Partial Answers*, 6(2), 261–277.

Hyvärinen, M. (2016). Expectations and experientiality: Jerome Bruner's "canonicity and breach." *Storyworlds*, 8(2), 1–25.

Hyvärinen, M., Hydén, L., Saarenheimo, M., & Tamboukou, M. (2010). Beyond narrative coherence: An introduction. In M. Hyvärinen, L. Hydén, M. Saarenheimo, & M. Tamboukou (Eds.), *Beyond narrative coherence* (pp. 1–15). John Benjamins.

Hyvärinen, M., & Watanabe, R. (2017). Dementia, positioning and the narrative self. *Style*, 51(3), 337–356.

Korhonen, K. (2013). Broken stories: Narrative vs. narration in travelling theories of cultural trauma. In M. Hyvärinen, M. Hatavara, & L. Hydén (Eds.), *The travelling concepts of narrative* (pp. 265–286). John Benjamins.

Morson, G. S. (1994). *Narrative and freedom: The shadows of time*. Yale University Press.

Palmer, A. (2004). *Fictional minds*. Nebraska University Press.

Sternberg, M. (1982). Proteus in quotation-land: Mimesis and the forms of reported discourse. *Poetics Today*, 3(2), 107–156.

Van Tassel, D. D. (Ed.). (1979). *Aging, death, and the completion of being*. University of Pennsylvania Press.

Westerhof, G. J., & Bohlmeijer, E. T. (2012). Life stories and mental health: The role of identification processes in theory and interventions. *Narrative Works*, 2(1). https://journals.lib.unb.ca/index.php/NW/article/view/19501

9

Narrative Ethics and Dementia

Critical Comments and Modifications

Daniela Ringkamp

Introduction

Contemporary approaches in personal identity theory and in medical ethics sometimes draw on narrative methods to establish the identity of persons suffering from dementia. Due to the symptoms of the disease,[1] which is accompanied by a severe loss of memory and language skills, narrative means are regarded as an adequate method to support the construction of personal identity, especially with the condition of Alzheimer's disease.[2] According to proponents of this perspective, for example Marya Schechtman, Elisabeth Boetzkes Gedge, and Jeffrey Blustein, the personal identity of dementia sufferers can be constructed through *external* narratives: Having the life story of a patient narrated by relatives or caretakers helps everyone involved to cope with changes in the patient's personality and is of importance in processes of decision-making, when the person concerned is no longer able to articulate stable preferences.[3] Narrative approaches are also essential in the everyday care of dementia patients and in biography work, as they address the implicit memory of the patients and help them to meet the challenges of the disease (Toffle & Quattropani, 2015).

Even though this individual approach should be appreciated and biography work with dementia patients should be enhanced, I would like to draw attention to some critical aspects of the concept of narrative identity as it is developed by its proponents. These critical aspects do not aim to undermine the concept of narrativity as such. Rather, this chapter challenges the implementation of narrative accounts in a certain version of personal identity theory and in medical ethics. There are—as shown in the second part of this chapter—several problems that go hand in hand with external narratives, and these problems make it difficult to regard them as a solid basis

Daniela Ringkamp, *Narrative Ethics and Dementia* In: *Narrative and Mental Health*. Edited by: Jarmila Mildorf, Elisabeth Punzi, and Christoph Singer, Oxford University Press. © Oxford University Press 2023.
DOI: 10.1093/oso/9780197620540.003.0010

for solving problems in medical ethics or for developing a stable identity of dementia sufferers. Nevertheless, in other contexts, for example in literature, linguistics, media studies, and the everyday care of dementia patients, narrative means can be a useful tool for analyzing strategies of speaking about dementia and interacting with persons suffering from dementia.

In the first part of the chapter, I will briefly point to the concept of personal identity as it is grounded in the tradition of John Locke and I will integrate narrative accounts within this field. In the second part, I will discuss advantages and disadvantages of modeling the identity of dementia patients through external narrative means. In this context, I will point to the relational structure of external narrative accounts, which makes it necessary to consider the first-person experiences of dementia patients and other features that complicate the application of narrative to dementia theory. These critical aspects will be reinforced with reference to the approaches of Galen Strawson and Peter Lamarque, who both discuss problems of conceiving personal identity through narrative concepts. I will conclude with some remarks concerning the substance and complexity of narrative accounts, which, however, should ultimately not be discarded as such. The extent to which a sensible use of narrative means in dealing with dementia can be achieved will be shown in a brief discussion of Jonathan Franzen's short story "My Father's Brain" at the end of the chapter.

The Concept of Identity: Narrative Approaches

The philosophical concept of diachronic identity concerns the relation of an entity (objects, living beings, and so on) to itself over the course of time. A fundamental distinction in this context is the distinction between what is called "numerical" identity and "qualitative" identity (de Grazia, 2005, p. 13, p. 89). If we consider the numerical identity of an entity, we refer to the "persistence of a single entity" (de Grazia, 2005, p. 13, p. 89)[4] as such, as an extended being. For example, the tree that is growing in front of my house goes through various changes: It is this specific tree, not the one growing next to it, that bears fruits in the process of its development and loses its leaves in the course of the year. A qualitative identity, in contrast, considers the qualitative properties and characteristics of an entity, for example the specific colors of the leaves or the composition of the bark. This distinction can be transferred to human beings. On the one hand, we can point to an individual as such, who can be identified in a numerical way by pointing to this person's day of birth, his or her biographical descent, and the day of death if the person is not alive anymore. On the other hand, we can point to the qualitative properties of an individual, to his or her preferences, character traits, emotional reactions, and all other aspects that constitute this person in his or her personality. This distinction between numerical and qualitative identity is also given in our ordinary language about dementia. When, for example, a wife says about her husband, who lives with dementia, that he is not the person she married a long time ago, she points to the deep changes in his character, which are a symptom of the illness and which concern the *qualitative* identity of the patient. At the same time, however, she may say that in spite of all this, he is still the person she married: In this case, she points to the *numerical* identity of her husband.

Narrative accounts of personal identity concern the qualitative notion of identity and pick up a specific problem, which was mentioned by John Locke in his famous definition of personal identity. Locke was confronted with the question of how far it is possible for a person to conceive of oneself as a continuing self in the course of time, by undergoing various changes in character traits, living conditions, and so on. In answering this question, Locke provides a definition of identity as well as a definition of the concept of a person, which is still relevant in the current philosophy of person and personhood:

> This being premised, to find wherein personal identity consists, we must consider what PERSON stands for; which, I think, is a thinking intelligent being, that has reason and reflection, and can consider itself as itself, the same thinking thing, in different times and places; which it does only by that consciousness which is inseparable from thinking, and, as it seems to me, essential to it; [. . .] and as far as this consciousness can be extended backwards to any past action or thought, so far reaches the identity of that person; it is the same self now it was then; and it is by the same self with this present one that now reflects on it. (Locke, 1690, XXVII, p. 9)[5]

The concept of a person, however, is not sufficient to define "the idea of a man in most people's sense" (Locke, 1690, XXVII, p. 8). To specify what is indicated by Locke as a "man in most people's sense," the idea of a person has to be complemented by "the same successive body not shifted all at once" (Locke, 1690, XXVII, p. 8). This is why, strictly speaking, Locke's idea of human beings not only refers to the concept of people as persons, but also considers bodily aspects in which "the same immaterial spirit" (Locke, 1690, XXVII, p. 8) is integrated. Nevertheless, the reference to the physical condition of mental elements is rather rare; instead, Locke emphasizes and appreciates the person who perceives and reflects on his or her own inner mental states. Therefore, it is psychological continuity and the capability of having first-person memories that enable a person to situate oneself in one's own life, in one's biographical past, present and future, and to do this, a person must have sufficient rational abilities and cognitive skills to identify oneself. This emphasis on cognitive skills and on the capability of judgment can also be seen in a further definition of personal identity, which is no less than "the sameness of a rational being" (Locke, 1690, XXVII, p. 9).

External narrative accounts of personal identity address the problem of qualitative identity and take up Locke's concept of personhood. In contrast to Locke, however, they do not emphasize the perspective of one's inner psychological continuity or rational capabilities. We do not identify ourselves as beings with certain mental states, but we are embedded in social contexts in which we interact, we shape our own lives, and it is this specific life story that constitutes our identity. Therefore, according to Marya Schechtman, personal identity can be conceived as a story:

> According to the narrative self-constitution view, the difference between persons and other individuals [. . .] lies in how they organize their experience, and hence their lives. [. . .] Some, but not all, individuals weave stories of their lives, and it is their doing so which makes them persons. On this view a person's *identity* [. . .] is constituted by the content of her self-narrative, and her traits, actions, and experiences included in it are, by virtue of that inclusion, hers. (Schechtman, 1996, p. 94)

Schechtman's reference to the story of a person's life serves as an argumentative framework for a holistic approach to an individual biography. As a continuum between past, present, and future, a life narrative enables one to conceive of the identity of a person as a unified whole. Whereas, according to Schechtman, identity in psychological continuity accounts is "a relation between independently definable time-slices, in a narrative the parts exist in the form they do only as abstractions from the whole, and so the whole is, in an important sense, prior to the parts" (Schechtman, 2014, p. 100). The life story of an individual as a whole ensures the continuity of personal identity and guarantees the unity of self in the course of time.

Proponents of narrative approaches also emphasize that developing a life story requires fewer cognitive abilities than psychological continuity accounts. Telling a life story depends not only on biographical memories of a single person, but also on others who interact with the person and contribute important parts to their life story. This is especially mentioned by Martina Schmidhuber, who is an advocate of narrative identity accounts: It is "difficult to fix personal identity merely on memories. Even in early childhood, one's identity is fundamentally influenced by others, even though one may not remember this as an adult. [. . .] Since others shape a person and influence her identity [. . .], it is evident that all persons are dependent on one another" (Schmidhuber, 2013, p. 307; my translation).[6] Narrative approaches are situated in a relational setting, in which the construction of a life story is an interactive project (Gedge, 2004, p. 446). The life story of an individual is always dependent on and influenced by the actions and opinions of others. And the importance of other persons also explains the extent to which narrative approaches can be transferred to dementia patients:

> Infants and the demented cannot self-narrate, but other people can and do form narrative conceptions of them. In keeping with present aims, the claim is not about the way in which others can form narrative conceptions of what infants and the demented are *like* [. . .], but rather about the way in which they can begin or continue an *individual* life narrative that anticipates or recalls the unfolding of that *individual* life. Bringing past and future into the present, as it were, on behalf of the person who cannot do it herself. (Schechtman, 2014, p. 104)

If a person is no longer able to tell his or her own story, it is the task of others to continue the life story of a person living with dementia, to report changes in preferences, character traits, and so on: "[P]roxy decision-makers should regard themselves as the *continuers* of the life stories of those who have lost narrative capacity" (Blustein, 1999, p. 21). It is important to note that in this context, it is a nonfiction narrative that is the central tool for figuring out the identity of a patient. There are of course other options to establish narrative access to the self of people living with dementia, for example experimental and fragmented passages in novels that aim to illustrate the inner experiences of such people for persons who do not share the same experience, but these are not at the center of those accounts favored by Schechtman, Blustein, and others. Instead, oral life stories, which may guarantee a high degree of authenticity, are the core element of external narratives.[7]

Neither Schechtman nor Blustein gives a concrete example of a narrative that illustrates the possibility of retelling the life story of a person living with dementia. However, the extent to which it is possible to continue the life story of such a person through others is demonstrated by Martina Schmidhuber, who refers to the biographical report of Gabriele Zander-Schneider, *Sind Sie meine Tochter? Leben mit meiner alzheimerkranken Mutter*.[8] Zander-Schneider cared for her mother, who experienced dementia, and explained the changes her mother went through, as well as her own way of dealing with this. A brief extract from Zander-Schneider's report, which is mentioned by Schmidhuber, narrates the following incident:

> A lilac is blooming at the edge of a property. Already, when approaching it, the aromatic smell is wafting towards me. "Isn't this great? Do you also smell this?" "Yes, yes," mother answers and looks in the other direction. I try it again when we are standing in front of the bush and pull down a branch slightly further, so that it is possible to press your nose into the splendid blossom. "Mother, come on, smell it once again." I know that she has always loved such odours, but I also know that the loss of the senses of smell and taste is typical for Alzheimer's disease. Mother is standing next to me and looks at me. I demonstratively press my nose into the blossom. "Come on, try it."—"Yes," she says, and laughs at me without understanding. It is pointless. As much as I would like to give her a pleasure, she doesn't understand me. "What a pity," I think with sadness, and release the branch.[9] (Zander-Schneider, 2006, p. 95; my translation)

It is especially the changes in her mother's character that are mentioned by the daughter; they not only describe the progress of the disease but also the problems and losses that dementia entails for the relatives and friends of the patient concerned. Therefore, Zander-Schneider's report can be seen as a typical example of the relational character of external narratives: They explain the loss of characteristics and the changed perceptions of the person living with dementia as well as the challenges these changes imply for one's social surroundings.

Narrative Identity, Ethics, and Dementia: Some Problems

Proponents of external narratives mention several advantages of retelling the life story of patients suffering from dementia, beginning with an appreciation of their personhood and individual value (Blustein, 1999, p. 28), and also referring to the importance of proxy decision-making (Blustein, 1999, p. 22) and of allowing for a good life for dementia patients in the later stages of the disease. In what follows, I would like to discuss some further aspects that are brought forward by advocates of external narratives and that have partly already been mentioned. These aspects concern the following points:

1. Narrative reconstructions of a life story that are performed by others and not by the dementia patient do not require advanced cognitive capabilities of a person suffering from dementia. Therefore, even in the later stages of dementia, when a person is no longer able to communicate verbally and there are no stable preferences, it is possible to continue his or her life story through the narrations of other people.

2. This leads to an appreciation of the present condition of dementia patients and allows one to overcome the criterion of first-person psychological continuity and of remembrance, as mentioned by Locke (Schechtman, 2014, pp. 105, 107). Not gradual change but rather the realization of a person's overall values and preferences helps one to evaluate the current condition of patients suffering from dementia or of persons in a persistent vegetative state.

3. The relational structure of narrative accounts reflects our dependence on social surroundings. Each of us is more or less dependent on other persons, and this dependence also shapes the structure and the content of our life story, which is the central feature for defining personal identity. We are all characterized by mutual dependence, and this dependence on others is reflected in a situation when other persons continue to tell the story of our life.

4. It is possible to adhere to identity as a diachronic, unified whole, while at the same time acknowledging the present condition of a patient. This leads to a more stable definition of identity than is developed by Locke—identity is conceived of as diachronic holism, as pointed out by Schechtman, and some problems of Locke's account can be overcome, for example the question of whether I am the same person in unconscious states, in deep sleep, in a persistent vegetative state, or

before birth. Generally speaking, other persons are in a position to begin or to continue my life story when I am unable to do so. Like a sonata or any other piece of music, which only gains perfection if we listen to it as a whole, the qualitative identity of a person is adequately considered if we respect its origin, formation, and development as a whole (Schechtman, 2014, p. 107).

5. Finally, as Elisabeth Boetzkes Gedge and Jeffrey Blustein point out, external narratives are a useful instrument for proxy decision-making, which is necessary to identify the interests of dementia patients, who are not able to articulate their preferences, in the final stage of the disease.

I would like to contrast these aspects with some general critical remarks that foreground a number of problems that also concern their implementation in medical ethics and personal identity theory. Based on this criticism, I will try to offer a new perspective on the supposed advantages of external narrative accounts at the end of the chapter.

First of all, external narratives do not overcome the criterion of psychological continuity and memory as such. Indeed, a person living with dementia does not have to remember former experiences and his or her life story. However, other persons must be in a position to recollect that person's life story and to remember the major events and experiences in his or her life. Therefore, the criterion of psychological continuity is only transferred from the person experiencing dementia to people in his or her family and wider social environment.

This also shows that even external narrative accounts presuppose advanced cognitive abilities, for example the capability to reflect on the person's past, to anticipate the person's preferences and wishes, and to show a certain amount of judgment. Again, it is not the person diagnosed with dementia who has to possess these abilities, but those who retell the life story can only do so in a condition of sufficient cognitive skills and soundness of mind.

Proponents of external narrations do not discuss the concept of narrativity as such. At first glance, this does not seem to be problematic: Studies about the concept of narrativity are normally relegated to linguistics or literary research, whereas advocates like Schechtman and Blustein are merely interested in philosophical identity theory and its relation to medical ethics. Nevertheless, a closer look at the concept of narrativity helps us to clarify some important aspects also for external narrations. Of course, I cannot discuss the literary concept of narrativity in detail here. However, there are, as Peter Lamarque points out, some minimal conditions a narration must fulfill to count as a narrative. First, a narration must be told by a narrator; second, it sets at least two events in a temporal sequence (Lamarque, 2004, p. 394). Besides these minimal features, there are no specific requirements concerning reference, truth, and subject matter. For Lamarque, this leads to the fact that "[v]ery little of substance can be inferred from the premise that a piece of discourse is a narrative" (Lamarque, 2004, p. 394).[10] Moreover, as there are no specific requirements concerning reference and truth, the fictional or nonfictional character of narrations gives rise to some questions. As Lamarque mentions, even fact-based narratives like biographies or historical narratives "involve both selection and ordering of fact" (Lamarque, 2004, p. 398); they include interpretation and evaluation and never represent an event "as such" or "as it really took place."

What do these considerations imply for external dementia narrations? Of course, we know many famous narrations from literature that not only fulfill the formal criteria of narrations, but also contain stylistic devices and rhetorical features and tell a compelling story that affects the reader and gives rise to political or social reflections. There are also experimental narrations that aim to break down the traditional concept of narrativity. The existence of these ambitious narrations should not mislead us into believing that everything that is told or written down might for the same reasons count as a narrative. Even though they might fulfill some formal criteria, there may be reasons for not designating everything that is told in external dementia narratives as a narrative per se. If we take up Blustein's "continuer" view, for example, we just learn that other persons should continue the life story of persons with dementia. There are no details or instructions about whether continuing the life story of those who are no longer able to do so should meet any criteria concerning content, concept, or style. Therefore, the continuer view is rather general and merely illustrative. It can be questioned if Blustein is really interested in *narrations* or if it is merely important for him to learn something about the values and preferences of the person living with dementia. If the latter is important, it is enough to tell something about a patient's character, ideals, and moral concept, but this telling need not necessarily count as a narrative.[11] A similar problem is also apparent in Schechtman's position, for example when she holds that the sentence "Father was always a natty dresser and would be mortified" instructs relatives and nursing staff to make sure he is dressed neatly (Schechtman, 2014, p. 105). It can be doubted whether this sentence really counts as a substantial narrative that meets more than the minimal conditions mentioned by Lamarque.

External narrations emphasize the relational character of personal identity and stress the importance of the social environment of a person with dementia. Of course, each of us is embedded in social contexts from our early life on; many of us retain multiple social contacts throughout our whole life, and these contacts also form our self-understanding and the way we perceive the world. Nevertheless, some problems may arise if the notion of relational integration is overemphasized or isolated from other circumstances. As other persons continue to tell the life story of a person with a dementia diagnosis, there is a risk of paternalistic influences by those who continue the narration. These influences can operate consciously or unconsciously, but in both cases, the values and preferences of a person with dementia are falsified. Perhaps the other persons believe that they know what is better for this person, they may not correctly reflect the person's present preferences (which is indeed difficult to do), or they may intentionally misunderstand the patient's first-person expressions. So, the imposition of external values cannot be ruled out, and, as Couser points out, external influences can even be so severe that they violate a person's privacy (Couser, 2018, p. 6). Moreover, as other persons continue to tell the life story of a person living with dementia, it is not clear at all if they really tell the story of another person or rather their own story. This has serious consequences for the question of personal identity: Is it really the identity of a dementia patient that is built up, or is it the identity of the storyteller, of the relatives, caretakers, or others, that is central? If, for example, Gabriele Zander-Schneider regrets that her mother is no longer able to smell the fragrance of lilac, it is not clear at all if this is important for her mother or for herself. So, in her biographical report, we learn much about the personal affection of the daughter, who observes the progress of the disease and her mother's character changes. However, biographies, as Lamarque holds, are based on value judgments, and this entails some problems (Lamarque, 2004, p. 400). Zander-Schneider's report merely appreciates the daughter's perspective, and it is debatable whether it really provides access to dementia "as such" and offers objective insight into the mother's identity.

Finally, if the importance of narrations by relatives and caretakers are strongly coming to the fore, there is a danger of disregarding the verbal or nonverbal expressions of people with dementia. However, these are important if we are to gain access to the current condition of a person suffering from dementia, and continuing the life story of a patient is impossible if the narrator only recognizes a person's past and not the present situation. Proponents of external narratives regard narrations as an adequate means to manage the loss of a patient's cognitive capacities. At the same time, they dissociate themselves from positions that strengthen the notion of inner psychological continuity and advanced cognitive skills as a condition for developing personal identity. This should consequently lead to an appreciation of those episodic first-person statements a dementia patient is still able to perform, for example the nonverbal articulation of preferences through gestures, facial expressions, movements, and bodily reactions. Many problems in medical ethics, for example decision-making in a state of progressive dementia, arise because the patients concerned seem to have different experiences in this state of dementia than they did before, when they were in a state of advanced cognitive competence. The question concerning the validity of these episodic experiences cannot be adequately answered if the first-person expressions in the current situation of dementia are disregarded.[12] Of course, the fragmented, verbal and nonverbal expressions of dementia patients can be picked up by other persons. However, first and foremost, it is the person living with dementia who expresses himself or herself.

The potential risk of disregarding the first-person expressions performed by the patients themselves in a state of dementia illustrates another problem. According to Schechtman, diachronic holism is a central feature of external narratives. It is, however, not clear at all what "diachronic holism" implies and the extent to which holistic access to a person's identity allows for considering episodic and fragmented expressions. It seems as if, for Schechtman and others, that there is a fixed concept of a person's identity, which can also be told by others, and this concept is still valid in the person's state of dementia. In this context, it is not only unclear if Schechtman confuses cause and effect: Schechtman assumes that personal identity can be established by narrations in general. This, however, is not very convincing, since narratives do not produce a unity of the self, but rather presuppose it (Lamarque, 2004, p. 406). Moreover, as I already mentioned, external narrations run the danger of disregarding the first-person expressions and the current state of a dementia patient. This criticism can be continued: The adherence to a concept of identity as a whole not only disregards the first-person expressions of persons suffering from dementia but also ignores the complex, diverse, and inconsistent ways in which a person builds up his or her identity. In light of this, Lamarque emphasizes that

[t]he impression given by the term "narrative" is of a complete, rounded story with a beginning, middle and end that helps make sense of complex events. The model is historical narrative or the complex narratives of fiction. But personal narratives virtually never attain completeness, closure, or unity. [. . .] The whole idea of a "life-narrative" is far too literary and grandiose. (Lamarque, 2004, p. 405)

So, is there really a kind of diachronic holism that constitutes our identity, or are we ultimately episodic individuals who change our opinions and value judgments in the course of time? Galen Strawson strongly argues for what he calls episodic individuals, who do not consider themselves as "something that was there in the (further) past and will be there in the (further) future" (Strawson, 2004, p. 430). Even though some of the criticism Strawson raises against the concept of diachronic unity in personal identity is merely provocative, there are still some important points to consider, especially with regard to the personal identity of dementia patients. Dementia is characterized by the loss of long-term memory, by an increasing loss of self-perception and biographical knowledge. Still, dementia patients experience emotional excitement, they interact with their social environment, and they also express, even though in a discontinuous way, value judgments and preferences. Due to the circumstances of the disease, the question arises as to whether a greater emphasis on episodic experiences is more adequate than a strong adherence to identity as a diachronic and unified whole. Although Strawson does not discuss dementia or other mental illnesses in the context of his approach, it may be fruitful to refer to his position.

Narrative Identity: Modifications

Nevertheless, despite all these critical aspects, external narratives should not be abandoned wholesale. However, to obtain access to the inner perspective of dementia patients, external narrative accounts must be revised in fundamental aspects. First of all—and this is essential not only for narrative accounts but also for every theory of identity that aims to represent the present situation of persons suffering from dementia—the perspective of diachronic unity must be diminished. Of course, in care settings, it is important to know about a person's previous interests, values, and character traits. But this should not prevent us from recognizing changes in thinking and behavior and to appreciate the episodic nature of perceiving, which is characteristic for dementia. These episodic elements have to be placed at the center of those approaches that aim to investigate the identity of dementia patients. Moreover, episodic experiences are articulated not only verbally but also through a variety of expressions like movements, reactions, facial expressions, and so on, and these forms of articulation must be integrated into an account of narrative identity. According to Katja Crone, even nonnarrative, implicit and qualitative characteristics of mental life must be considered (Crone, 2017, p. 14), and authors like Thomas Fuchs and Michela Summa, who emphasize the importance of body memory for personal identity, also discuss gestures and nonreflected movements as a way of bodily expression (Summa & Fuchs, 2015). It is also essential that—in the case of an external narration of the life of a dementia patient—the narrator reflects on his or her position as the person who tells the life story of a patient. He or she must be aware that narrative access to another person's life story is never objective but is influenced by the narrator's own perspectives and interpretations.

The extent to which such a revised concept can be applied is exemplified by Jonathan Franzen in his short story "My Father's Brain" (2002). In the story, Franzen tells about his father's Alzheimer's disease and presents his confrontation with the father's character, the course of the disease, and how he himself dealt with the symptoms. At the end of the story, Franzen writes:

> Hour after hour, my father lay unmoving and worked his way toward death; but when he yawned, the yawn was *his*. And his body, wasted though it was, was likewise still radiantly *his*. Even as the surviving parts of his self grew ever smaller and more fragmented, I persisted in seeing a whole. I still loved, specifically and individually, the man who was yawning in that bed. And how could I not fashion stories out of that love—stories of a man whose will remained intact enough to avert his face when I tried to clear his mouth out with a moist foam swab? I'll go to my own grave insisting that my father was determined to die and to die, as best he could, on his own terms. (Franzen, 2002, p. 36)

What is interesting here is that Franzen reflects on his role as narrator: It is he himself who insists that his father wants to die his own way. And even though Franzen takes a holistic perspective toward his father's life, he expressly mentions that it is he, the son, who does so. The numerical identity of the father's body remains untouched, and the construction of the qualitative identity is situated in a social setting in which Franzen is the narrator of his father's story. But even though Franzen may be of importance, he could not write the story without the first-person expressions of the father. This is why proponents of phenomenological approaches of identity like Fuchs and Summa remark that external narrative accounts presuppose the first-person actions and articulations of a person with dementia himself or herself. If the identity of a dementia patient should be illustrated by external narrations, as is claimed by Schechtman, Schmidhuber orBlustein it is essential not only to reflect on the role of the narrator, but also to take full account of the expressions and reactions of a patient, especially when they are not verbal. This can be a first step toward solving the difficulties that external narrative accounts entail.

Notes

1. I use the term "disease" to describe the medical aspects and implications of dementia and the term "illness" to refer to the personal feelings and emotions patients have in dealing with the symptoms of dementia.
2. Along with frontotemporal dementia, vascular dementia, and dementia with Lewy bodies, Alzheimer's disease is one of the four main types of dementia. Alzheimer's disease progresses slowly in three stages—mild, moderate, and severe. The symptoms range from slight forgetfulness and disorientation at the beginning to severe deficits in memory skills, loss of speech, inability to carry out everyday activities, loss of awareness of recent experiences, and a complete nursing care dependency in the last stage. More than 60% of the dementia patients suffer from Alzheimer's disease (Alzheimer's Association, n.d.). In 2015, 46.8 million people worldwide were affected by dementia, and it is anticipated that the rate will increase up to 74.7 million patients in 2030 (Prince et al., 2015).
3. As the narratives are mainly told by other persons and not by the patient himself or herself, I will refer to them as *external* narratives.
4. DeGrazia explicates the difference between numerical and qualitative identity with reference to identical twins: "[E]ven if two twins were qualitatively identical, they would be numerically distinct" (De Grazia, 2005, p. 13).
5. This definition of the concept of the person has raised many questions, some of which were already discussed by Locke himself—for example, whether the interruption of someone's stream of consciousness leads to the emergence of a new person or not. However, I will not discuss these problems in this chapter.
6. The original quote is: "*Es ist „problematisch, personale Identität lediglich an Erinnerung festzumachen. Denn bereits in der frühen Kindheit wird die eigene personale Identität*

grundlegend von anderen geprägt, meist ohne dass sich die Person im Erwachsenenalter daran noch erinnern kann. [. . .] Dadurch, dass andere die Person immer mitprägen und ihre Identität beeinflussen, wird [. . .] deutlich, wie abhängig alle Personen [. . .] von anderen sind."

7. Gedge endorses imaginative dialogues between a proxy decision-maker and the demented patient as a kind of biographical speaking. These imaginative dialogues must fulfill norms of adequacy: Proxy judgments have to tell coherent stories of the life of a patient (Gedge, 2004, p. 442).

8. This is the original German title; the English translation would be "Are You My Daughter? Living with My Mother, Who Suffers from Alzheimer's Disease" (my translation).

9. The original quote is: *"Am Rand eines Grundstücks steht ein Fliederbusch in voller Blüte. Schon einige Meter davor weht mir der intensive Geruch entgegen. 'Ist das nicht herrlich? Riechst du das auch?' 'Ja, ja', antwortet Mutter und schaut in eine völlig andere Richtung. Ich versuche es noch einmal, als wir direkt vor dem Strauch stehen, und ziehe einen herabhängenden Zweig noch etwas weiter herunter, sodass man die Nase direkt in eine der prächtigen Blüten drücken kann. 'Mutter, komm, riech doch auch mal.' Ich weiß, dass sie solche Gerüche immer sehr gemocht hat, weiß aber auch, dass der Verlust des Geschmacks- und Geruchssinns zu Alzheimer dazugehören kann. Mutter steht neben mir und schaut mir zu. So stecke ich selbst demonstrativ die Nase noch einmal tief in den Flieder hinein. 'Komm, probier es mal.'—'Ja', sagt sie, und lacht mich verständnislos an. Es hat keinen Zweck. Sosehr ich ihr auch eine Freude machen will, sie versteht nicht, was ich meine. 'Schade', denke ich traurig und lasse den Zweig wieder los."*

10. Galen Strawson strengthens this perspective and takes it further: If the only clear criterion for a narrative is a temporal sequence between two events, then ordinary actions like taking a cup from the cupboard and making coffee can count as a narrative. For Strawson, this is trivial, as our daily life entails many of these ordinary activities (Strawson, 2004, p. 439).

11. A further objection Lamarque raises against narrative accounts of personal identity is a confusion between life and narrative: The "merging of life and narrative is a mistake. A narrative, being a story, must be narrated, but a life need not be narrated" (Lamarque, 2004, p. 402). This confusion between life and narrative as two completely different subjects can also be opposed to Blustein's position.

12. This is also mentioned by Maartje Schermer, who points out that "there remains a problematic tension between continuing a person's life story and attending to a person's actual preferences or needs" (Schermer, 2003, p. 40).

References

Alzheimer's Association. (n.d.). *Stages of Alzheimer's*. https://www.alz.org/alzheimers-dementia/stages

Blustein, J. (1999). Choosing for others as continuing a life story: The problem of personal identity revisited. *Journal of Law, Medicine & Ethics, 27*, 20–31.

Couser, G. (2018). Illness, disability, and ethical life writing. *CLCWeb: Comparative Literature and Culture, 20*(5). https://doi.org/10.7771/1481-4374.3482

Crone, K. (2017). Strukturen der Identität und des Selbstverständnisses von Personen. *Deutsche Zeitschrift für Philosophie, 65*(1), 1–15.

De Grazia, D. (2005). *Human identity and bioethics*. Cambridge University Press.

Franzen, J. (2002). My father's brain. In *How to be alone: Essays* (pp. 7–38). Picador.

Gedge, E. B. (2004). Collective moral imagination: Making decisions for persons with dementia. *Journal of Medicine and Philosophy, 29*(4), 435–450.

Lamarque, P. (2004). On not expecting too much from narrative. *Mind & Language, 19*(4), 393–408.

Locke, J. (1690). *An essay concerning human understanding*. Alex Catalogue.

Prince, M., Wimo, A., Guerchet, M., Ali, G., Wu, Y., & Prina, M. (2015.) *World Alzheimer report: The global impact of dementia: An analysis of prevalence, incidence, cost, and trends*. Alzheimer's Disease International. https://www.alz.co.uk/research/WorldAlzh eimerReport2015.pdf

Schechtman, M. (1996). *The constitution of selves*. Cornell University Press.

Schechtman, M. (2014). *Staying alive: Personal identity, practical concerns, and the unity of a life*. Oxford University Press.

Scheermer, M. (2003). In search of the "good life" for the demented elderly. *Medicine, Health Care and Philosophie, 6*(1), 35–44.

Schmidhuber, M. (2013). Verlieren Demenzbetroffene ihre personale Identität? In G. Gasser & M. Schmidhuber (Eds.), *Personale Identität, Narrativität und praktische Rationalität: Die Einheit der Person aus metaphysischer und praktischer Perspektive* (pp. 295–311). Mentis.

Strawson, G. (2004). Against narrativity. *Ratio, 17*(4), 428–452.

Summa, M., & Fuchs, T. (2015). Self-experience in dementia. *Rivista Internazionale di Filosofia a Psicologia, 6*(2), 387–405.

Toffle, M. E., & Quattropani, M. C. (2015). The self in the Alzheimer's patient as revealed through psycholinguistic-story based analysis. *Procedia—Social and Behavioral Sciences, 205*, 361–372.

Zander-Schneider, G. (2006). *Sind Sie meine Tochter? Leben mit meiner alzheimerkranken Mutter*. Rowohlt.

10

Narrative Experiments with Medical Categorization and Normalization in B. S. Johnson's *House Mother Normal*

Sara Strauss

Introduction

Despite increasing knowledge about age-related syndromes such as Alzheimer's disease and other types of dementia, they still often result in the social exclusion, stigmatization, and isolation of the persons affected. Although specialist literature and numerous campaigns by governmental and nongovernmental organizations, like the Alzheimer's Society and the Mental Health Foundation, inform people about the symptoms of these diseases and offer their support to patients and relatives, in a sense the patients are silenced within society (Alzheimer's Society, n.d. a; American Psychiatric Association [APA], 2013; Ames et al., 2017; Mental Health Foundation, n.d.). What contributes to their isolation and silencing is the difficulty to express what it means to live with dementia. Dementia causes a severe loss of patients' cognitive and linguistic faculties; people at an advanced stage are unable to give a voice to their inner sentiments, nor to their most urgent needs and demands. Along with the gradual progression of the disease, memory impairments and aphasia sooner or later lead to a complete loss of language in the person affected (Alzheimer's Society, n.d. b, p. 7; APA, 2013, p. 613). This loss of speech and the inexpressibility of the patient's thought processes constitute key problems for conveying an inside perspective of a person with dementia. Despite all their achievements in spreading knowledge about dementia, this is where specialist literature and media campaigns that inform about medical conditions reach their limits. These works usually center on the methods of diagnosis, the typical symptoms, and especially the economic issues of care.[1] What these informative texts and campaigns

Sara Strauss, *Narrative Experiments with Medical Categorization and Normalization in B. S. Johnson's* House Mother Normal In: *Narrative and Mental Health.* Edited by: Jarmila Mildorf, Elisabeth Punzi, and Christoph Singer, Oxford University Press. © Oxford University Press 2023. DOI: 10.1093/oso/9780197620540.003.0011 cannot convey is an inside perspective into living with dementia. Yet, it is precisely this first-person perspective that typically inspires people to identify with another person. By imagining the point of view of a fictional character with dementia, narratives can elicit such processes of identification in the reader and thereby arouse empathy with a dementia patient (Nussbaum, 1995, pp. 5–7). By these means, literature can help to transcend boundaries of social isolation and stigmatization.

Recent studies in the fields of philosophy, sociology, and narrative psychology have examined autobiographical narratives by patients with neurodegenerative diseases with regard to their meaning-making processes, their sense of self, and the limits of language and narrative coherence (Hydén & Brockmeier, 2008). It is, however, not only autobiography but also narrative fiction that can contribute to a better understanding of dementia. As a mode of discourse, narratives play a crucial role in the disciplines of literary and cultural studies. These disciplines analyze both fictional and factual narratives as representations that reflect cultural and social contexts in the real world. Against this background, this chapter refers to narrative as the telling of a story as well as to the narrative text as the product of this process of telling, for example a novel, short story, or further literature in prose writing. It examines B. S. Johnson's novel *House Mother Normal* (first published in 1971) as a fictional dementia narrative that enables processes of make-believe. By assuming the first-person perspective of several characters with age-related neurocognitive impairment, *House Mother Normal* hypothetically tells the experience of dementia from within. From a narrative studies point of view, this chapter is interested in the way in which this mode of storytelling makes it possible for readers to identify with the characters portrayed. As James Phelan states, "[N]ovels explore the concrete particularity of ethical dilemmas faced by fully realized characters, and those explorations harness the cognitive power of the emotions" (Phelan, 2014, p. 541). By stimulating readers' powers of imagination and their emotions, fiction can enable outsiders to get a sense of what it means to live with a neurocognitive disease.

At the same time, the inexpressibility of the experience of dementia through language poses fundamental challenges to literary representation. Authors of narrative fiction meet the difficulty of representing the situation of mentally confused, disoriented, or aphasic characters with the help of experimental techniques. Therefore, a strong focus of this chapter is also on Johnson's experiments with formal elements and narrative techniques, such as interior monologue, fragmentation, disruptions, and silences, to convey an inside perspective of the reality of dementia patients. Thus, the chapter also explores the extent to which fictional narratives can offer a change of perspective, for example to mental health practitioners, and raise awareness of the limited medical and economically driven discourse about dementia.

Categorization and Normalization of Mental Health and Pathology

As regards definitions of mental health, within the context of this chapter mental health is understood as a culturally constructed concept whose classification varies depending on the values of different cultures and social groups. In its most general sense, it refers to a person's cognitive and emotional state of well-being that enables the person to act autonomously in everyday life. Alzheimer's and other forms of dementia, by contrast, impair the person's capacity to lead an autonomous life. What can be and often has been criticized about discourses on mental health and ill health is their focus on categorization and diagnostic scales and their normative tendencies. Especially in the case of neurodegenerative syndromes like dementia and Alzheimer's disease, scales are used to predict the prevalence and likely progression of the mental decline. Patients' cognitive abilities are measured in contrast to "normal" aging. The APA emphasizes the challenge this implies: "The differential diagnosis between normal cognition and mild NCD [neurocognitive disorder], as between mild and major NCD, is challenging because the boundaries are inherently arbitrary. Careful history taking and objective assessment are critical to these distinctions" (2013, p. 610). In comparison to the performance of persons without dementia and depending on the degree to which each patient's autonomy is impaired, the individuals are then grouped into the three phases of mild, moderate, and severe dementia (Kurz et al., 2016, p. 19). Of course, an early diagnosis is vital for a treatment of the disease and maintaining the patient's autonomy as long as possible: "[N]ot only does diagnosis lead to access to treatments and services, but also it encourages individuals to make important decisions and plans at a stage in the disease process at which this is still feasible" (Kane & Thomas, 2017, p. 39). Yet, the prevalence and the temporal development of the symptoms differ from patient to patient since they depend on further factors specific to each individual, for example their education, intellectual involvement, or physical health and exercise (Gatz, et al., 2001; Stern, 2012, p. 1007). What is more, the normative categorization of patients often confuses the patients and their relatives alike:

> [P]atients and their families often struggle to translate abstract neuro-psychological concepts about past, present, and future loss . . . into their everyday lives. . . . Diagnoses are of course associated with distinct normative story lines about what people might reasonably expect over the time continuum. But . . . affected individuals and their families find the meaning of cognitive scores to be confusing. . . . Nevertheless, medical professionals, and researchers in particular, treat people as straightforwardly categorizable on the basis of their neurological and neuropsychological profiles. (Medved, 2014, p. 91)

In a similar vein, the Alzheimer's Society warns against a disregard of individuals and their experience for the sake of categorization:

> While it can be helpful . . . to have some awareness of the likely progression of a person's dementia, it is important to realise that everyone's experience will be different. It is much more important to focus on trying to live well with dementia, meeting the needs of the person at that time, than to focus only on which stage they are in. (n.d. b, p. 1)

Thus, a standardized assessment of the patient's condition and their categorization into normative scales might result in a disregard for individual deviation from set criteria. Of course, this normative classification within "boundaries [that] are inherently arbitrary" (APA, 2013, p. 610) fulfills an economic function in the medical industry: It is used as a quantitative measure to gauge how much care is necessary at certain stages of dementia and the costs associated with it.

Individual Experience and Normative Categorizations of Mental Health and Pathology in *House Mother Normal*

In his novel *House Mother Normal*, Johnson contrasts normative classifications of mental health with inside perspectives into living with neurodegenerative disease. Johnson's experimental work portrays eight care home residents at different stages of dementia. In metatextual elements that "function . . . as an ironic introduction to each new character" (Bernaerts, 2014, p. 299), the narrator provides pathological categorizations of the elderly people's conditions. These are followed by first-person renditions of the characters' individual experiences of life in the care facility. Through unmediated interior monologues, Johnson attempts to give an inside perspective into the consciousness of people with cognitive impairments. In the following analysis, this chapter will examine Johnson's use of narrative fragmentation, disruptions, and silences as a way to convey the situation of a fictional elderly woman at the onset of neurocognitive disorder and of three other characters with mild to severe dementia. Contrasting these perspectives with the meta-narrative introduction and epilogue of the head nurse raises questions as regards the normalizing function of categorizations of mental health and pathology.

In Johnson's novel, Sarah Lamson, aged 74, is a nursing home resident with dementia at such an early stage that it cannot yet be detected through the typical tests at the care facility. It is only by means of the setting and the fragmentation of Sarah's interior monologue that the reader can conclude that she has mild cognitive impairment. In order to diagnose neurodegenerative disorders, patients usually undergo a cognitive assessment of their memory, their mental abilities, and their spatial and temporal orientation. At the fictional care home in *House Mother Normal*, residents are asked to respond to 10 questions for the diagnosis of dementia—for example, "Where are you now? What is this place? What day is this?" (Johnson, 1986, p. 6). The person's mental ability is then measured by the number of correct answers to these questions. Before giving voice to the fictional characters' interior monologues, a meta-textual frame narrative introduces each patient with a chart informing the reader about their social, physical, and mental condition (Johnson, 1986, pp. 7, 29, 51, 73, 95, 117, 139, 161, 183). These charts state the person's age, marital status, and the number of correctly answered questions during the cognitive test. This assessment is complemented by a quantitative evaluation of the elderly person's physical abilities—for example, "sight 60%[,] hearing 75% . . . [,] smell 50% [and] movement 85%" (Johnson, 1986, p. 7). Johnson here points to the excessive reliance on statistical data and quantitative measurements in the medical sector and health care industry. By leading the detailed quantification of impairments to absurdity, he cautions against a normative comparison of patients, just as the Alzheimer's Society warns:

Health professionals often use scales to measure the . . . changes [of a person's behavior and mood]. . . . Some of these scales were developed specifically for Alzheimer's disease and work better for that than for other types of dementia. Assessment of the extent of someone's dementia should take account of these scales but should also take a broader view of the person, including their capabilities and needs. (n.d. b, p. 2)

The fact that some scales are more suitable for assessing Alzheimer's disease than other forms of dementia becomes apparent when one considers the differences in symptoms and progression of impairments caused, for example, by Lewy body dementia or vascular dementia. In the case of Lewy body dementia, physical changes, such as "[s]lowness, gait imbalance and other parkinsonian movement features," are very prominent and "are more likely to be an important cause of disability early in Lewy body dementia than in Alzheimer's" (Alzheimer's Society, n.d. c). By contrast, as vascular dementia is caused by several minor or major strokes that obstruct the cerebral blood flow, its effects vary depending on the regions of the brain affected:

Memory loss may or may not be a significant symptom depending on the specific brain areas where blood flow is reduced. Vascular damage that starts in the brain areas that play a key role in storing and retrieving information may cause memory loss that is very similar to Alzheimer's disease. (Alzheimer's Society, n.d. d)

Johnson's representation of dementia features people with diverse symptoms and at various stages of cognitive impairment that may hint at different types of dementia. These, however, remain undiagnosed by the usual routine in the fictional nursing home and receive no medical treatment. Here, numerical data and pathological listings of disorders supersede considerations of the residents' individual experience of illness and their quality of life.

What is more, the bureaucratic system of the medical facility even denies elderly people the status as individual persons when identifying all of them by means of an abbreviation. In her meta-narrative introduction, the head nurse, the so-called House Mother (Johnson, 1986, p. 5), explains: "We no longer refer to them as inmates, cases, patients, or even as clients. These particular friends are also known as NERs, since they have no effective relatives, are orphans in reverse" (Johnson, 1986, p. 5). This remark subverts the historical evolution in clinical medicine and psychology to classify persons with mental health issues: from their early criminalization and internment as "inmates, cases" to the latter more sympathetic attitude towards "patients, or even as clients" (Johnson, 1986, p. 5). Johnson creates an ironic effect when the head nurse prides herself and the institution on transcending this advancement and now referring to patients by the assumedly neutral acronym "NERs" (Johnson, 1986, p. 5). The cold, distancing categorization as "NERs" points to the fact that the residents are not valued as individuals with unique identities but are only recognized with regard to their social relations or the lack thereof. The loss of these familial relations coincides with a presumable loss of identity and worth within society.

The characters' interior monologues, by contrast, disclose that their feelings of identity persist despite experiences of illness. Sarah Lamson, for example, strongly identifies as a mother and widow of a traumatized war veteran and as an emancipated woman running her own pub (Johnson, 1986, pp. 8–21). The absence of "effective relatives" (Johnson, 1986, p. 5), however, makes these elderly people particularly vulnerable and leaves them dependent on the health care system, the care facility, and the medical professionals and managing staff in authority. As will be seen towards the end of the analysis, the fictional characters can no longer protect themselves from violations of their human rights, which makes them vulnerable to neglect, exploitation, and abuse.

In contrast to this first impersonal, quantifying, and normative introduction to each care home resident that "serve[s] as alienation effect" (Havemann, 2011, p. 168), the narrative that follows foregrounds each patient's individuality. As is typical of interior monologue, the narrative mimics the characters' random, illogical, and chaotic thought processes (Palmer, 2005, pp. 570–571). It is, among others, through fragmentation, incomplete sentence structure, confusing adverbial references, and unexplained allusions that literary devices like interior monologue and stream of consciousness try to imitate the associative structure of human consciousness (Strauss, 2013, pp. 44–51). These narrative techniques, then, illustrate how mental processes are shaped not only by each person's cognitive faculties but also by their individual experience, memories, and spontaneous associations. The unexplained elements and blank spaces left to the reader point to the fact that a person's mental life is only partly accessible to the outsider. Thus, these narratives subvert normative ideas about human cognition.

In *House Mother Normal*, Johnson employs interior monologue to represent the fictional characters' consciousness at different stages of dementia. Although the assessment chart that precedes Sarah Lamson's interior monologue lists a number of "patholog[ies]" (Johnson, 1986, p. 7), her mental and physical condition is difficult to differentiate from "normal" aging because most of the elderly woman's impairments can be considered rather common at her age. The chart states a movement rate of 85%, "incipient hallux valgus[,] osteo-arthritis[,] suspected paraphrenia" and a perfect score in the cognitive test (Johnson, 1986, p. 7). Sarah's interior monologue confirms her good condition, but it also shows that she preferably immerses herself into her memories instead of living in the present and that these reminiscences are occasionally disrupted. Apart from the daily routine at the care home, her mind is constantly preoccupied with recollections of her distant past during World War I and II. Sarah's identity is strongly shaped by her roles as a widow of three husbands and as a single mother working hard to make a living for herself and her son. In her interior monologue, she recalls different unconnected experiences that made her a self-reliant woman and are therefore crucial for her formation of self. Overall, the elderly woman's interior monologue conveys a preoccupation with the past. Her identity and life course have strongly been influenced by the experience of the two world wars. Formally, her stream of consciousness is still characterized by coherent thought processes, but the typesetting of the novel suggests that she occasionally struggles to remember the incident correctly or to find the right word to express her experience. Sarah's interior monologue is then interrupted by pauses and longer silences. These silences and disruptions indicate her incipient loss of language as well as her efforts at retrieving her memory. While the representation of Sarah's thoughts exposes the fluent transitions between forgetfulness caused by "normal" aging and mild cognitive impairment, it is the format of her interior monologue, the blank spaces and disruptions, that reveal her memory slips and thereby the onset of pathological mental decline.

As in Sarah Lamson's personal history, the wars and their aftermaths also play a vital role in the memories of the other elderly people in the residential facility. As a former soldier in World War I, Charlie Edwards, for example, still has to come to terms with the fact that "[he]'d got used to the noises people made" (Johnson, 1986, p. 44) when he killed them to defend his own life. Having been disabled in the First World War and unserviceable in World War II, his retrospectives are characterized by the guilt he feels when he asks himself, "Why wasn't I killed like most of my mates?" (Johnson, 1986, p. 44).

The experience of the two world wars thus marks an essential phase in the lives of the Lost Generation and reveals much about their identities and the issues that unremittingly preoccupy them during their later life. In this way, *House Mother Normal* emphasizes how crucial it is for society to retain the memory of the experience of the elderly in order to understand them and their motives, but it also accentuates the importance of cultural memory for society as a whole. As such, it calls out for more respect for the elderly and a more considerate attitude that takes into account individual person's identities and protects them from discrimination and abuse.

It is through the format of the characters' interior monologues that *House Mother Normal* conveys the harm dementia causes to the memory of the individual. Thus, Johnson employs fragmentation, jumps in time, unexplained causalities, ruptures, and silences to represent the erosion of the characters' cognitive abilities and the disorientation caused by dementia. He presents Sarah's and the other patients' reminiscences in a nonlinear narrative, which mimics the spontaneity and impulsiveness of their flashbacks. The individual fragments that constitute Sarah's interior monologue are stripped of any chronological order. The elderly woman's recollections move abruptly between scenes from her life as a young woman during World War I, to her time as a governess in France between the wars, and to later adult life as a self-employed pub owner during World War II (Johnson, 1986, pp. 16–19, 21, 22). For the reader, the context of the scene can merely be reconstructed when he or she considers the fragment in comparison to other incidents recalled by the character. For instance, although Sarah Lamson is able to completely recall certain events from her adult life, the memories of her infancy are abruptly disrupted: "We kids used to run about in felt slippers then, they were the cheapest, a cut above the barefoot kids. It was our way of [*sic*]" (Johnson, 1986, p. 22). Sarah's line of thought remains unfinished. Instead, after a silence, which Johnson represents through blank lines, her consciousness turns to her current activity of pushing another care home resident in his wheelchair: "Tired of pushing. But still carry on. Slog, slog." (Johnson, 1986, p. 22). Dementia patients usually remember best what was stored early in their memory because "older memories are consolidated more firmly than newer ones" (Milwain, 2011, p. 188), so that recollections of childhood and the distant past disintegrate later than the most recent ones. Nonetheless, the disruption of Sarah's childhood reminiscences exemplifies that the cognitive loss does not follow a chronological order and differs from person to person. Due to a failure in her powers of concentration, the flashback to Sarah's infancy is interrupted and remains incomplete. Instead, her consciousness moves to her present situation in the care home.

Both psychology and narratology have described such fragmented narratives caused by neurocognitive degeneration or trauma as "broken narratives": "'[B]roken narratives' not only revolve around a crucial event which typically defies direct representation or straight-forward narration, their brokenness is also often reflected in the texture and on the level of narrative discourse" (Nünning & Nünning, 2016, p. 59; see also Hydén & Brockmeier, 2008). While Sarah Lamson's experience of incipient dementia and her recollection of two world wars and life with a traumatized husband defy straightforward narration, the author reflects this brokenness in the nonlinear structure of the interior monologue and in the typesetting of his novel. The "broken narrative" thereby challenges the reader to reconstruct the story of Sarah's life, just as dementia challenges the patient to remember her life correctly. Due to the high degree of fragmentation, the changing focalizers (i.e., characters whose perspective is alternately adopted), and the narrative's many blank spaces and open ends, the novel does not allow for one truthful interpretation but offers different versions of the care home residents' experiences.

By portraying Sarah Lamson's consciousness, Johnson not only presents a character in an early phase of dementia but also exposes the difficulty of diagnosing the onset of a progressive disease like dementia and differentiating it from "normal" aging. He thus alerts readers to the challenge that normative mechanisms of medical classification pose to the practitioner. Joseph Kane and Alan Thomas sum up this challenge and stress the importance of combining clinical proficiency with expertise in recognizing individual deviation from classificatory norms:

> If the ongoing evolution of the dementia concept has taught us anything, it is that exceptions to criteria exist, and that the application of core concepts to individual patients is a nuanced clinical skill best conducted by an experienced practitioner, rather than a series of items on a checklist or administration of diagnostic criteria. (2017, p. 39)

While the fragmentation, disruptions, and silences indicate Sarah's struggle for words and the dissolution of her memory and therefore suggest her mild cognitive impairment, other fictional characters in *House Mother Normal* experience the effects of advanced dementia. George Hedbury and

Rosetta Stanton, for example, are fully affected by loss of memory and language. The neurodegenerative disease has progressed to such a degree that they show cognitive as well as physical symptoms. Due to severe impairments in the ability to control their muscles, patients in an advanced state of neurodegenerative diseases are often unable to walk, are bedridden, or can no longer swallow food (Alzheimer's Society, n.d. b, pp. 6–7). What is more, Alzheimer's and other types of dementia coincide with a gradual loss of linguistic faculties, ultimately resulting in aphasia (APA, 2013, p. 613).

Johnson's novel attempts to evoke the steady progression of the disease and its corrosive effects on communication through its experiments with linguistic representation, narrative form, and fragmentation. The characters' "broken narratives" thereby expose "[t]he problem [. . .] of the limitation of verbal patterns as conveyors of thought" (Scholes & Kellogg, 1966, p. 199). While the means of linguistic expression for representing the illogical chaotic nature of human consciousness as such are already limited, it is even more difficult to give voice to the inner life of people affected by (mental) disease. In her study of illness memoirs, Kathlyn Conway problematizes patients' "confrontation with the limits of language and literary form for representing pain, suffering, and awareness of mortality" (2007, p. 3). Beyond its insufficiency for a literary expression of suffering, in *On Being Ill* Virginia Woolf highlights the practical shortcomings of language for an effectual communication between patient and medical staff:

> Finally, to hinder the description of illness in language, there is the poverty of the language. English, which can express the thoughts of Hamlet and the tragedy of Lear, has no words for the shiver and the headache [. . .] but let a sufferer try to describe a pain in his head to a doctor and language at once runs dry. (2008, p. 102)

These limits of expression are even more nuanced in the case of neurodegenerative diseases. Here, aphasia renders it impossible for the patients themselves to express what it means to live with dementia.

In *House Mother Normal*, George Hedbury, for instance, experiences symptoms of severe dementia and aphasia. Johnson represents his mental decline through a disintegration of language. George's interior monologue mainly consists of monosyllabic or disyllabic words that are separated from each other by blank spaces and that, at first sight, seem to be unrelated. Although the patient's consciousness is still symbolized by grammatically correct words, sometimes even short phrases, the reader can only guess at their logical coherence. Nonetheless, Johnson once again shows that the elderly man's mental activity not only entails random, illogical thoughts but that the separate words convey meaning in consideration of the character's personal identity. In consequence of his cognitive degeneration, George experiences physical impairments and is dependent on a wheelchair. Despite the disintegration of his thoughts, his interior monologue reveals that he is well aware of his present condition. His physical disability concerns him so much that the first word of his interior monologue is "Lame" (Johnson, p. 140). He is also conscious of all the daily activities in the care home, in which he must participate passively, for example the physical exercise during which Sarah Lamson pushes him around in his wheelchair. George's interior monologue reveals that he is wheeled around much faster than is pleasant for the old, disabled man: "moving moving! / everything's moving! /? / moving / stopped good" (Johnson, 1986, pp. 153–155). The quotation in the original actually extends over two pages, with blank spaces and blank lines in between. Long silences between George's thoughts show that he is incapable of concentrating on anything else while being moved around. Instead, he is entirely absorbed in the unsolicited impressions that penetrate him. The question mark conveys the confusion this fast movement causes in the elderly man, until he is finally relieved when the movement stops.

While Johnson already shows how the faculty of linguistic expression gradually disintegrates in George Hedbury's consciousness, he experiments further with the limits of language and its signifying processes in the interior monologue of 94-year-old Rosetta Stanton. Most of Rosetta's stream of consciousness is not represented by meaningful words but by sound combinations, for example: "Galluog . . . lwcus . . . ynad" (Johnson, 1986, p. 163). Johnson thus not only mimics the fragmentation of the human mind in the course of dementia but also demonstrates that aphasia poses another challenge for a reliable categorization of patients into the classificatory system prevalent in the health care sector. In addition to the idea that an assessment of patients by quantitative measures proves problematic, the limitations to communication between client and medical professionals and the lack of time needed to engage with each patient individually render the traditional mechanisms of categorization unreliable and at times arbitrary.

While Johnson's work contrasts normative approaches to psychiatric disorders with first-person insights into the experience of neurocognitive disease throughout, it further problematizes normalizing conceptualizations of mental health in the house mother's epilogue. Although the meta-textual introduction by the head nurse establishes her as the narrator of the frame narrative and the person in authority in the care home (Johnson, 1986, pp. 5–6), the epilogue digresses from this order of diegetic levels. Here, intradiegetic and extradiegetic levels of the text merge: The head nurse is at once a fictional character within the story world and a narrator who steps out of the conventions of storytelling through meta-textual commentary. Just like those of the elderly residents, the house mother's interior monologue is preceded by a chart informing readers about her personal, social, and medical condition. In contrast to most patients in the institution, the head nurse is comparatively young and achieved a perfect score in the cognitive test (Johnson, 1986, p. 183). However, her assessment chart and the following interior monologue disclose that it is she who is in severe need of psychiatric and medical treatment. While the fragmented narratives of the residents hint at bewildering events throughout the daily routine, the house mother's epilogue finally reveals that this confusion is not attributable to the elderly people's mental decline but to her inconceivable, malevolent actions. Her stream of consciousness proves that the head nurse exploits the aged for their remaining workforce, exerts physical violence to discipline them, and sexually abuses them. Thus, the carer forces the elderly to regularly witness her exhibitionist performances and erotic zoophilism. Whereas the house mother's diagnostic chart provides the medical explanation that her reasoning might be affected by a "[dormant] malignant cerebral carcinoma" (Johnson, 1986, p. 183), the ensuing narrative discloses that it is a misapprehension of power that motivates her evil, criminal acts against those that are dependent upon her. In sole charge of the management of the care facility, the head nurse indulges in the control she has over the aged, socially isolated, and defenseless residents: "My children. From this dais / I am monarch of all I survey. This is my Empire. / I do not exaggerate, friend. They are dependent / ... Nothing is more sure than that I am / in control of them. And they know it." (Johnson, 1986, p. 190). Through its unconventional line breaks, the head nurse's epilogue receives a poetic form that creates rhythm and emphasizes crucial words like "dais," "monarch," "Empire," or "dependent." It is through this experimental combination of narrative and lyrical modes that Johnson exposes the house mother's megalomaniac personality traits.

By demonstrating an extreme case of abuse of authority, Johnson draws attention to the importance of employing skilled and reliable medical professionals and carers. Especially with regard to the growing demands and scarce resources in the health care sector, heightened attention should be paid to staff's adequate training and to a continuous and rigorous monitoring of care institutions. The fictional insights into the consciousness of characters with dementia reveal that what is required of the medical and caregiving staff is, first and foremost, empathy. This ability to empathize can only unfold its potential if the bureaucratic system of health care politics allocates enough time for carers to engage with their patients. A close interaction with patients and their life stories is necessary in order to comprehend that their individual conditions might deviate from classificatory norms.

Finally, it is especially in the para-text of the novel's title that Johnson contests cultural conceptualizations of "normality." By naming the fictional character in authority and narrator of the frame narrative "House Mother Normal" (Johnson, 1986, title page), the author points to the relation between normalization and power. Though the cognitive assessment of the house mother categorizes her as "normal" in contrast to the residents with age-related mental impairments, her actions are not only marked by non-conformity but also constitute criminal acts in which she abuses those dependent on her. The implied readers here feel compelled to clearly distance themselves from these actions and consequently question the notion of "normality" and its medical and cultural conceptualization.

Conclusion

B. S. Johnson's *House Mother Normal* contrasts different views on mental health and classifications of illness. It juxtaposes and connects a meta-textual frame narrative replete with medical categorizations and quantitative clinical criteria with interior monologues that represent the patients' inside perspectives. With the help of the interior monologues, the author draws readers' attention to the personal identity of each character and to their individual experience of dementia. By facilitating processes of identification with the fictional characters, the novel thus counters mechanisms of stigmatization and social exclusion of people with dementia. It is through fragmentation, silences, and disruptions that Johnson represents the elderly people's "broken narratives." Along with the progression of the disease, these "broken narratives" demonstrate the patients' growing aphasia. In verbalizing these narratives in experimental fashion, Johnson points to the inability of language to adequately represent the experience of dementia. And by opposing the age-related mental impairment with the evil, abusive behavior of the so-called House Mother Normal, the author also ironically questions established mechanisms of medical categorization and their normalizing functions as regards health and pathology. In a similar vein, Gay Becker concludes about such "broken narratives," which she terms "narratives of disruption" (1997, p. 10), that they disclose "that cultural notions of normalcy can be contested" (1997, p. 46).

By conveying a first-person perspective on life with dementia, fiction thus offers another view on neurocognitive disorders than specialist literature directed at professionals and media campaigns that focus on spreading knowledge and information among the general public. As such, fictional narratives can provide mental health practitioners with the possibility to change perspectives and imagine the experience of cognitive impairment from within. At the same time, literature has an affective dimension usually absent in expository texts. It enables the reader to identify with the characters and thereby arouses feelings of empathy. These feelings and processes of identification elicited in the story world can effect positive changes in mental health practitioners' actions in the real world.

It is through foregrounding the difficulties arising from the health care sector's reliance on normative categorization that Johnson's novel exposes the challenges this implies for medical professionals, psychologists, carers, politics, and society as a whole. Since the health care industry is oriented towards an economic and bureaucratic management of scarce resources, it requires practitioners to resort to categorizations, quantitative assessments, and statistical data. Limited financial resources, a shortage of skilled nursing staff, and perceived lack of time when it comes to treating an increasing number of elderly patients impede an engagement with the person as an individual. In this regard, in addition to medical and psychiatric expertise, Johnson's novel foregrounds empathy as an indispensable skill for respectful treatment of people living with psychiatric disorders. The combination of medical knowledge and psychiatric and social skills, however, can only realize its full potential when the political and social circumstances allow health care providers the time needed to focus on the requirements of the individual patient.

Note

1. Although the Mental Health Foundation focuses its projects in an exemplary way on individual life stories and on improving the situation of people who experience mental

health problems, the foundation resorts to economic issues in order to raise awareness about age-related mental impairments. The subtitle to the section on "Mental health in later life" on the foundation's website reads: "The total cost of dementia to the UK is £26.3 billion." Placing this information in the most prominent position as a subtitle indicates that it is primarily the economic impact that is necessary to attract attention to the importance of mental health in old age (Mental Health Foundation, n.d.).

References

Alzheimer's Society. (n.d. a). *Alzheimer's Society: United against dementia*. https://www.alzheimers.org.uk/

Alzheimer's Society. (n.d. b). *The progression of Alzheimer's disease and other dementias: Factsheet 458LP*. https://www.alzheimers.org.uk/sites/default/files/migrate/downloads/factsheet_the_progression_of_alzheimers_disease_and_other_dementias.pdf

Alzheimer's Society. (n.d. c). *Lewy body dementia*. https://www.alz.org/alzheimers-dementia/what-is-dementia/types-of-dementia/lewy-body-dementia

Alzheimer's Society. (n.d. d). *Vascular dementia*. https://www.alz.org/alzheimers-dementia/what-is-dementia/types-of-dementia/vascular-dementia

American Psychiatric Association. (2013). *Diagnostic and statistical manual of mental disorders* (5th ed.). American Psychiatric Publishing.

Ames, D., O'Brien, J. T., & Burns, A. (Eds.). (2017). *Dementia* (5th ed.). CRC Press.

Becker, G. (1997). *Disrupted lives: How people create meaning in a chaotic world*. University of California Press.

Bernaerts, L. (2014). Minds at play: Narrative games and fictional minds in B. S. Johnson's "House Mother Normal." *Style, 48*(3), 294–312.

Conway, K. (2007). *Illness and the limits of expression*. University of Michigan Press.

Gatz, M., Svedberg, P., Pedersen, N. L., Mortimer, J. A., Berg, S., & Johansson, B. (2001). Education and the risk of Alzheimer's disease: Findings from the study of dementia in Swedish twins. *Journals of Gerontology: Series B, 56*(5), 292–300. https://doi.org/10.1093/geronb/56.5.P292

Havemann, M. (2011). *The subject rising against its author: A poetics of rebellion in Bryan Stanley Johnson's oeuvre*. Georg Olms.

Hydén, L.-C., & Brockmeier, J. (Eds.). (2008). *Health, illness and culture: Broken narratives*. Routledge.

Johnson, B. S. (1986). *House mother normal*. New Directions.

Kane, J. P. M., & Thomas, A. (2017). What is dementia, and how do you assess it? Definitions, diagnostic criteria and assessment. In D. Ames, J. T. O'Brien, & A. Burns (Eds.), *Dementia* (5th ed., pp. 33–43). CRC Press.

Kurz, A., Freter, H. J., Saxl, S., & Nickel, E. (2016). *Demenz: Das Wichtigste: Ein kompakter Ratgeber*. Deutsche Alzheimer Gesellschaft.

Medved, M. I. (2014). Everyday dramas: Comparing life with dementia and acquired brain injury. In L. Hydén, H. Lindemann, & J. Brockmeier (Eds.), *Beyond loss: Dementia, identity, personhood* (pp. 91–106). Oxford University Press.

Mental Health Foundation. (n.d.). *Our work: Mental health foundation*. https://www.mentalhealth.org.uk/our-work

Milwain, E. (2011). Understanding behavioural change in dementia. In S. Curran & J. Wattis (Eds.), *Practical management of dementia: A multi-professional approach* (2nd ed., pp. 185–196). CRC Press.

Nünning, A., & Nünning, V. (2016). Conceptualizing "broken narratives" from a narratological perspective. In A. Babka, M. Bidwell-Steiner, & W. Müller-Funk (Eds.), *Narrative im Bruch: Theoretische Positionen und Anwendungen* (pp. 37–86). V & R Unipress.

Nussbaum, M. C. (1995). *Poetic justice: The literary imagination and public life.* Beacon Press.

Palmer, A. (2005). Stream of consciousness and interior monologue. In D. Herman, M. Jahn, & M.-L. Ryan (Eds.), *Routledge encyclopedia of narrative theory* (pp. 570–571). Routledge.

Phelan, J. (2014). Narrative ethics. In P. Hühn, J. Pier, W. Schmid, & J. Schönert (Eds.), *Handbook of narratology* (Vol. 2, pp. 531–546). De Gruyter.

Scholes, R., & Kellogg, R. (1966). *The nature of narrative.* Oxford University Press.

Stern, Y. (2012). Cognitive reserve in ageing and Alzheimer's disease. *Lancet Neurology, 11,* 1006–1012. https://doi.org/10.1016/S1474-4422(12)70191-6

Strauss, S. (2013). *"This bright inward cinema of thought": Stream of consciousness in contemporary English fiction.* WVT.

Woolf, V. (2008). On being ill. In *Selected essays* (ed. D. Bradshaw) (pp. 101–110). Oxford University Press.

11

Mental Illness Representations in the German Mass Media

The Case of Depression

Marina Iakushevich

The World Health Organization (WHO) considers depression to be one of the most widespread mental illnesses worldwide:

> Depression is a common illness worldwide, with more than 264 million people affected. Depression is different from usual mood fluctuations and short-lived emotional responses to challenges in everyday life. Especially when long-lasting and with moderate or severe intensity, depression may become a serious health condition. It can cause the affected person to suffer greatly and function poorly at work, at school and in the family. At its worst, depression can lead to suicide. Close to 800,000 people die due to suicide every year. Suicide is the second leading cause of death in 15-29-year-olds. (WHO, 2020)

For this reason, it is comprehensible that this mental health problem is present in the media discourse. In the German mass media, including print and online newspapers, TV, and radio, depression has been a topic discussed intensively from the 1970s until now. Since the 1980s, medical experts in Germany have spoken of global epidemics of depression; depression is called a *Volkskrankheit* (folk disease).

In this chapter, I want to discuss the role of narrative in the media discourse on depression in Germany. To begin with, I introduce some general concepts used in linguistic discourse analysis and especially the concept of narrative as I will use it in the following analysis. My textual analysis focuses on metaphor because of its essential role in this discourse.

Marina Iakushevich, *Mental Illness Representations in the German Mass Media* In: *Narrative and Mental Health*. Edited by: Jarmila Mildorf, Elisabeth Punzi, and Christoph Singer, Oxford University Press. © Oxford University Press 2023. DOI: 10.1093/oso/9780197620540.003.0012

Discourse and Narrative: Linguistic Discourse Analysis

The term *discourse* has been used in different scientific disciplines such as history, sociology, anthropology, philosophy, political science, or linguistics (Gee & Handford, 2012, p. 5; Niehr, 2014, pp. 16–26). *Discourse* is also used in a common sense in everyday language, where it refers to a form of language use or ways of speaking (Niehr, 2014, p. 7; Spitzmüller & Warnke, 2011, p. 5; van Dijk, 1998, p. 1). Each of the disciplines focuses on one specific aspect of discourse, according to its theories and methodology. Some aspects are always present, such as language use, communication, and interaction (van Dijk, 1998, pp. 1–2). So, discourse analysis can be generally defined as "the study of language in use" (Gee & Handford, 2012, p. 1; Niehr, 2014, pp. 27–32; van Dijk, 1998, p. 2)—that is, the language use in one specific context, the context of society, culture, history, institutions, identity formation, politics, power, and all the ways in which language helps us to accomplish certain communicative purposes (Gee & Handford, 2012, p. 5; Spitzmüller & Warnke, 2011, pp. 13–17; van Dijk, 1998, pp. 13–16). The description of discourse as language use means that discourse is studied as a form of social interaction, as a way communication is related to its social context (van Dijk, 1998, p. 5). According to Felder, there is a systematic interconnection between language use and thoughts: Particular language phenomena can indicate social beliefs, social norms, and power (Felder, 2010, p. 13). For example, different grammatical constructions indicate different contexts of use; they are context-sensitive (Felder, 2012, pp. 117–118; Gee & Handford, 2012, p. 5; Harvey & Adolphs, 2012, p. 470; Semino, 2008, pp. 20–22; Spitzmüller & Warnke, 2011, pp. 123–124).

Discourse, as it is seen in German linguistics, is a net of texts or talk that are thematically, temporally, and semantically interconnected (Busse & Teubert, 1994, p. 14; Niehr, 2014, pp. 32–44; van Dijk, 1998, pp. 2–3). Texts and talk are manifestations of discourse and a point of departure in linguistic discourse analysis (Felder, 2012, p. 117; Foucault, 1990, p. 115; Gee & Handford, 2012, p. 5). The intertextual relations between texts and talk are the basis of discourse. Therefore, the analysis of these intertextual relations can shed light upon the structure of discourse: its topic, its actors and their opinions, their arguments and struggles over definitions. Felder (2010, p. 25) calls this *semantische Kämpfe* (semantic struggles) in order to stress contradictions that take place in mass media discourses. Discourse has to be analyzed on all linguistic levels: phonetics, lexis, syntax, semantics, pragmatics, text (Busse & Teubert, 1994; Felder, 2012; Spieß, 2011; Spitzmüller & Warnke, 2011).

In the analysis of mass media discourses, the specific context has to be considered:

Media discourse refers to interactions that take place through a broadcast platform, whether spoken or written, in which the discourse is oriented to a non-present reader, listener or viewer. [. . .] [M]edia discourse is a public, manufactured, on-record, form of interaction. (O'Keefe, 2012, p. 441)

The production of media discourse is driven, among other things, by the economic interests of the publishers (Burger & Luginbühl, 2014; Weischenberg et al., 2006, pp. 127–128). As a consequence, journalists have to take into consideration the tastes, interests, and common concerns of a mass media audience, in order to reach as many as readers as possible and to make profits for their employers (Cross et al., 2017, pp. 83–84). Given this context, it is understandable that themes and topics negotiated in newspapers, in TV shows, and on the internet are very close to the everyday life experiences and problems people have.

In Germany, media discourse increasingly draws on medical discourse. Some researchers even talk of a "medicalization" of the media discourse (Busch, 2015, p. 369). Even health professionals refer to the medicalization of social processes (Schneider, 2013). Although themes from medicine, medical research, and treatments have been present on the journalistic agenda in Germany since the 1950s, especially in the last two to three decades there has been an enormous increase in publications on health and illness (Cross et al., 2017, pp. 93–98 for social media; Kohring, 2005, pp. 27–28). Topics around health and illness, well-being, fitness, and therapies are very popular and abound in the media. One can find popular science articles, interviews with experts, and personal life stories of people experiencing health issues.

Media discourse is a place of knowledge transfer and knowledge making, where knowledge is expressed and regulated (van Dijk, 2012); it is also a place to create and negotiate social norms and values. Media discourses discuss the social and moral impact of illness and diseases in societies, and in doing so also reveal the complexity of prevalent concepts of health and illness. Media discourses do not try to communicate scientific facts and scientifically accepted truths in the way scientific communities do, but they negotiate medical content in an individualized and "attractive" fashion, drawing on personal interest stories (Busch, 2015, p. 370; Busch & Spranz-Fogasy, 2015, pp. 351–353; Fleck, 1980, p. 149 for popular science). Expert knowledge and expert authority are used by journalists in order to legitimize their reporting and to bolster their own authority.

Narrative in Mass Media Discourse

Another point that characterizes the mass media discourse on depression in Germany is the increasing number of narrative elements in those journalistic texts. In this section, I therefore want to discuss some relevant features of narrative first. "Narrative is a fundamental human way of giving meaning to experience," as Garro and Mattingly argue (2000, p. 1), and "narrative mediates between an inner world of thought-feeling and outer world of observable actions and states of affairs" (p. 1). It is understandable that narratives are present in everyday conversations and are very important for social interactions in many different contexts of everyday life (Ochs & Capps, 2001, pp. 7–8). Researchers in conversational narrative analysis stress the importance of the collaborative work of interlocuters in the process of storytelling (Norrick, 2000, p. 12; Ochs & Capps, 2001, p. 3). Moreover, life events can still be coherently ordered, explained, and brought into a logical order only through narrative, through telling and retelling stories of personal experience to other people (Ochs & Capps, 2001, p. 2). As regards written language, Mikhail Bakhtin, for example, considered readers to be also authors and the act of reading to be a dialogue between the reader and the text (Ochs & Capps, 2001, p. 3).

The vital role of narrative as a sociocultural practice and verbal technique for recapitulating experiences was already emphasized by Labov and Waletzky in 1967. In their pioneering work, Labov and Waletzky described the structure of oral narratives. It prototypically entails an orientation, a complication, an evaluation, a resolution, and a coda, with emphasis on a linear order of events (Labov, 1997, pp. 399–403; Labov & Waletzky, 1967, pp. 32–41). Norrick criticizes Labov and Waletzky's narrative theory because of the decontextualized interview style of the stories (Norrick, 2000, pp. 1–2). He pointed out that in conversational storytelling the entire context is important for recapitulating, constructing, reconstructing, and verbalizing experiences (Norrick, 2000, pp. 2–3). Thus, Norrick and some other researchers (Middleton & Edwards, 1990) postulate that local context can influence how events and characters are remembered and arranged in narratives. Although

Norrick makes these points for oral conversational contexts, his argument is also valid for the texts that are under study in this chapter: We have to consider the mass media context with its specific communicative purposes such as knowledge transfer, information, and entertainment, to name only some of them. These specific circumstances can explain why the stories told in the mass media texts are told in a particular way. Moreover, as I pointed out above, linguistic discourse analysis is the analysis of language in use (i.e., in concrete communicative situations); thus, narratives also need to be considered in their discursive contexts.

Labov and Waletzky's structure of narratives is represented in specific textual patterns, for example the thematic text structure (Brinker, 2010, pp. 60–65). Further, the textual manifestation of narratives can be found in specific language phenomena, such as temporal and personal markers that are observable at all linguistic levels: words and word combinations, grammatical structures like tense and aspect, grammatical constructions, text layout, and other semiotic resources like pictures, graphics, and so forth. Temporality is, in my opinion, one of the most important structural aspects in narrative texts. It is by definition crucial for narratives. Narrative can be seen as the situatedness of events in time and space: "*Grundlegende Dimension der Erzählung ist die Zeit als Abfolge von Ereignissen*" (Vogt, 2014, p. 96; for the relevance of the chronological order of acts in narrative structures see also Heinemann & Viehweger, 1991, p. 238).

So, the basis for this study will be newspaper texts that contain narrative elements. Mass media texts on depression often show one specific pattern: The text begins with a narrative part in which a personal story of depression is told. These narrative parts of the texts are always followed by expository passages, explanations about this mental illness, its symptoms, causes, therapies, and consequences—that is, the narratives are used for illustration. I analyze narrative passages from texts about depression in which persons with depression talk about their symptoms or others report those symptoms. For now, however, I will turn to metaphors as one important feature of those narratives.

Metaphor and Discourse

The importance of metaphor for linguistic discourse analysis has been stressed by many researchers (Böke, 1996; Kirmayer, 1992, 2000; Nerlich, 2005; Niehr, 2014; Semino, 2008; Spieß, 2011, 2014; Spitzmüller & Warnke,

2011; Wengeler, 2003). For instance, Brigitte Nerlich shows that one singular metaphor can structure the whole discourse (Nerlich, 2005). Elena Semino also stresses the central role of metaphors in the construction of meaning in literature, politics, science, and medicine, and she uses the term *discourse metaphor* for such instances (Semino, 2008). Metaphor is considered as "a pervasive linguistic phenomenon" and "central to many different types of communication" (Semino, 2008, p. 1). One important point identified in current metaphor research is the significance of the entire context in which a metaphor is used. In the dynamic multidimensional socio-cognitive model of metaphor (Hampe, 2017, pp. 3–23), metaphor is not seen as a static concept as it is traditionally described in conceptual metaphor theory (CMT) (Lakoff & Johnson, 1980) but as a dynamic concept, related to "socially emergent cognition" (Gibbs, 2014, p. 38). CMT had a huge impact on linguistics. Lakoff and Johnson (1980) showed the pervasiveness of metaphors in our everyday life and formulated basic conceptual metaphors that are conventional in thought and language. For example, the conceptual metaphor ARGUMENT IS WAR is linguistically realized by the expression *He attacked every weak point in my argument*. Through conceptual metaphors we can express abstract, complex, and unfamiliar areas of experience in terms of concrete, simple, and familiar concepts. In the example mentioned above, the complex concept ARGUMENT is experienced and expressed as a physical struggle between two subjects with different goals (Semino, 2008, p. 7).

Conceptual metaphors represent abstract concepts in terms of concrete, tangible, sensorimotor human experiences. Johnson (1987) argues that conceptual metaphors are based on bodily experience. Moreover, they allow for the communication of otherwise senseless and unspeakable suffering (Kirmayer, 1992; Low, 2005). On the other hand, our metaphors are also culturally produced. Our bodily sensations and movements are affected by culture; thus, metaphors can communicate bodily sensations as well as social, cultural, and political meaning (Turner, 1984).

CMT has been further developed by other scholars with respect to the context of language use. A number of studies show that metaphor use can vary according to context, register, or genre (Semino et al., 2013, p. 41). Linell (2009) speaks of "recontextualization"—in other words, the meaning of metaphors can be used very flexibly by different speakers or writers in different communicative contexts. For instance, Semino and colleagues (2013) discuss how the *gate* metaphor for pain is used in scientific papers and self-help books in order to explain scientific facts to laypersons and to experts and to show how different aspects of metaphorical meaning are actualized for different communicative purposes. Jensen (2017) shows with the expression *to sit down* how metaphoricity emerges in talk when many persons interact in a specific social situation. He argues that metaphors can emerge from the dynamics of human dialogue and their meaning can be interactively negotiated between persons within the constraints and affordances of their sociocultural environment. Deignan (2017) postulates that metaphors can be realized in text as well as in images. This aspect is highly relevant for mass media discourses, in printed or digital form, which entail all sorts of semiotic codes: texts, images (static and animated), graphics, music, tones, and so forth (Bateman, 2016; Hess-Lüttich et al., 2017).

According to the theoretical premises introduced in the sections above, I discuss some examples from my corpus in order to show the interplay of metaphor and narrative in the mass media discourse. For this purpose, I will draw on the view on narrative discussed above as well as Labov and Waletzky's theory of narrative. In my analysis, I will show what structures the stories about depression have and what influence they have on the mass media discourse in Germany. Because of the limited space in this chapter, the analysis will concentrate on one aspect of the textual structure: temporality. For this purpose, I analyze single words and word combinations typically used for depression and its symptoms.

Discourse Analysis of Selected Examples

In the following, I analyze a corpus of about 1,000 texts on depression in the period from 1951 to 2015 from the archives of the German newspapers *Die Zeit, Der Spiegel,* and *Frankfurter Allgemeine Zeitung* (*FAZ*) (printed and online versions), the so-called quality media. These three newspapers also call themselves "quality media" in order to emphasize the high quality of their journalistic work, their thorough investigations, and their sophisticated writing techniques.[1] The aim of the analysis is to show some features of the media discourse on depression in Germany: (1) the crucial role of metaphors and their verbal and visual representations in the constitution of the specific portrayal of depression in the German mass media and (2) the interplay of the surface language phenomena and narrative structures. As I pointed out above, the main assumption is that the context is important: The specific mass media context triggers specific metaphors that are traceable in certain language phenomena such as single words and grammatical constructions. More specifically, I discuss conceptual metaphors that are typically used for the portrayal of depression, as well as their discourse functions.

To begin with, I discuss the term *depression*. The German medical term *Depression* was introduced by Emil Kraepelin at the end of the nineteenth century. *Depression* comes from the Latin *deprimere*, which means to press or pull down (Duden, 2014, p. 474).[2] So, the German word *Depression* is a metaphor on a single-word level. The metaphor exemplifies very well the fundamental metaphorical process of thinking and speaking of one thing in terms of another. We think and speak about depression as if it were a physical body sensation, a feeling of something big and heavy that is pressing down upon us. Depression as a mental illness is a very individual, subjective experience that can be, especially for others, very abstract and hardly comprehensible. The metaphor helps people with depression to express their feelings and their inner condition in order to make them understandable for others. Moreover, the metaphor makes it possible to communicate about depression: In psychiatry, doctors often do not have any other access to a patient's feelings than the subjective descriptions of the patient himself or herself. Moreover, the current psychiatric diagnostic system (like DSM[1]-5) is symptom-based. Thus, it is not surprising that even medical terms are metaphorical.

The metaphorical nature of terms for mental illnesses was already pointed out in the 1980s. Feer (1987, p. 23) goes so far as to say that there is no other way to express the suffering of mentally ill people than by using metaphorical expressions. The complex inner psychic experiences of mentally ill people cannot be described and named with ordinary, literal language. As studies on metaphor have already shown, there are metaphors that are frequently and typically used by persons with depression, as well as highly individual metaphors (Semino, 2008, pp. 187–188). In the mass media texts I analyzed, I found first and foremost the conventional metaphors that go back to some basic metaphorical concepts as they are formulated by Lakoff and Johnson (1980) in CMT. These conventional metaphors seem to be more appropriate for mass media communication because they can easily be recognized and deciphered. Individual, creative metaphors can be suitable to describe a personal, unique experience; at the same time, however, they cannot always be easily understood and traced back by many people. Moreover, conventional metaphors, since they are culturally determined, implicitly also convey

---

[1] DSM-5 stands for Diagnostic and Statistical Manual of Mental Disorders, Fifth Edition.

cultural norms and goals (Low, 2005). In the following examples, I discuss several metaphors that correspond to the concept of pressing or pulling down as expressed in the term *depression*.

Depression Is a Heavy Burden

The media texts very often contain descriptions of the symptoms of depression. These descriptions are made from the perspective of people suffering from depression; they are subjective and individual. Nonetheless, we find the same conceptual metaphors that are consistent with the underlying cognitive concept of a heavy weight pressing down upon the person. These subjective experiences are verbalized in German as *gedrückte Stimmung* (depressed mood),[3] *niedergeschlagene Stimmung* (downcast, downhearted mood), and *bleierne Müdigkeit* (leaden tiredness). The person who suffers from depression feels as if a heavy burden, a heavy weight, were pressing upon him or her from above. Lead is a heavy metal, so the potential component of heaviness is also present in the expression *bleierne Müdigkeit* (leaden tiredness). In the expression *niedergeschlagene Stimmung* (downcast mood) it is obvious that the pressure, the burden, comes from above, such as in the following examples:[4]

1. [V]ersuchte Elizabeth, ihre **gedrückte Stimmung,** ihre Ängste und krankhafte Unruhe unter Kontrolle zu halten (*FAZ,* August 8, 1999, p. 13) (Elizabeth tried to get her **depressed mood,** her anxiety, and her pathological agitation under control.)
2. Die Trauerfeier für Robert Enke hat sie aufgewühlt, noch immer ist sie frisch, die Erinnerung an dieses schwarze Loch, in dem sie über Jahre saß. Wo zunächst nur ein dumpfes Gefühl der Trauer war. Und **bleierne Müdigkeit** (*Zeit Online,* January 19, 2009) (The funeral service for Robert Enke has stirred her up, it was still very fresh, this memory of the black hole in which she has been sitting for years. Where at first there was only a dull feeling of grief. And a **leaden tiredness.**)

In these examples, the very complex, subjective, and individual mental dispositions of people with depression are verbalized through more concrete bodily sensations of carrying a heavy burden. As examples four through eight will show, these text passages are written from the perspective of the persons who suffer from depression. On the one hand, they are expressions of the subjective feelings and sensations that are linguistically realized in conventional metaphors. At the same time, the metaphorical expressions *gedrückte Stimmung* (depressed mood), *niedergeschlagene Stimmung* (downcast, downhearted mood), and *bleierne Müdigkeit* (leaden tiredness) are also medical terms. They are used by psychiatrists in their medical professional discourse to describe and to evaluate the symptoms of depression. The metaphors make it possible for sufferers to externalize individual experiences, to communicate their feelings and make themselves understood, especially because, as I mentioned above, there is often no other way for ill people to communicate their very subjective and abstract inner psychic processes than through metaphors (Feer, 1987; Semino, 2008, pp. 175–176).[5] There are no literal equivalents for the metaphors mentioned above; the symptoms of depression are always expressed in metaphorical language. Some studies show that these metaphors are also used by patients in psychotherapy. For instance, McMullen and Conway (2008) analyzed audiotaped psychotherapy sessions in the United States and found that sufferers of depression overwhelmingly use the metaphor DEPRESSION IS WEIGHT to describe their experience to their therapists. Used in the newspapers, these conventional metaphors generalize individual experience by presenting it in an easily accessible way. So, in the mass media context journalists use these metaphors to focus on the personal experiences of the ill persons they write about and at the same time to inform their readers about typical symptoms of depression. For newspaper audiences, metaphor is an appropriate way to approach this subjectivity and to learn about depression.

In the context of mass media, the verbal means are often supported by other semiotic codes, such as images, pictures, graphics, and so forth. In the analyzed newspapers, in their printed or online versions, photographs and pictures are used to concretize the subjective feelings described in the texts. The pictures can be seen as material representations of abstract feelings and emotions of people with depression. In *Spiegel Wissen* (January 2011, p. 14), we have a photograph[6] that shows a young man kneeling on his right knee. He tries to hold with his hands a board above his head on which five persons are standing; only their legs can be seen. This picture shows iconically[7] what a heavy burden can look like: A person tries to hold the burden that presses upon him from above. So, the photographer tried to find a concrete visual image for an abstract subjective feeling of the ill person. In this way, the picture helps to objectivize the subjective feeling and to make it understandable and accessible for the readers of the newspaper article.[8]

This picture and the verbal expressions discussed above are both consistent with the conceptual metaphor DEPRESSION IS A HEAVY BURDEN. They are also consistent with other basic metaphorical concepts such as SICKNESS AND DEATH ARE DOWN (Lakoff & Johnson, 1980, p. 24) and EMOTIONAL EXPERIENCE IS A PHYSICAL OBJECT (Lakoff & Johnson, 1980, p. 15; Semino, 2008, pp. 181–182). The sick person is pressed down by the depression and is lying down. The burden is so heavy that the person cannot stand upright and is surely not able to move. In this picture we can see what the embodiment of metaphors really means. The physical experience of carrying such a burden is compared to having a depression. On the other hand, the picture can be seen as a realization of the literal meaning of *gedrückt* (depressed) and *niedergeschlagen* (downcast, downhearted). This interplay of verbal text and image is very popular in mass media contexts (in newspapers as well as in advertising). It makes texts attractive for readers: The texts are aesthetically more appealing, and the pictures make the text more comprehensible (Burger & Luginbühl, 2014, pp. 441–442).

Above, I discussed metaphor as a cultural phenomenon. In the metaphors on depression used in the mass media discourse in Germany, we can observe the depiction of depression in some culturally typical ways. One important part of the media discourse on depression is a search for its causes. Some scientific studies introduced and discussed in the mass media found that the job conditions in modern Western societies seem to weigh upon many people's minds and bodies. Temporary job contracts, heavy workload and stress, the expectation of permanent availability thanks to computer and smartphones, and social pressure on the job and in one's private life can lead people into depression. For example:

3. *80 Prozent der Deutschen empfinden ihr Leben als stressig, jeder Dritte klagt über* **Dauerstress in Job, Haushalt, Schule oder Studium.** *Leistungsdruck* (*Spiegel Wissen*, Number 1, 2011, p. 13). (80% of Germans find their life very stressful; every third person complains of **permanent stress at work, at home, at school or university. Pressure to work harder.**)

It is very interesting to see in the picture discussed above that the burden of the depression comes from people standing on the shoulders of the young man and pressing him down. Obviously, in Western societies, the causes of depression are seen in the social environment the person lives in—one's job, school, university, or home and the people one must deal with.[9] At the same time, the picture shows that the sufferer is alone and excluded from the others, from the rest of society. This emphasizes once again the singularity of the experience of this mental illness. And it depicts depression as an individual problem of the person, at least from the person's own perspective.[10]

Depression Is a Fall

The next five examples represent another crucial metaphor in the mass media discourse on depression.

4. *Schon viermal **fiel** der stämmige Zweiundsechzigjährige **in schwere Depressionen**, die zwischen drei Monaten und fast einem Jahr dauerten. [. . .] „Man **fällt** langsam **hinein** und wacht auch langsam wieder auf ", erinnert er sich (FAZ, April 15, 2002, p. 49).* (Four times already the sturdy 62-year-old man **fell into heavy depressions** that lasted between three months and almost one year. "You **fall slowly into the depression** and you also slowly wake up," he remembers.)

5. *Sebastian Deisler, der Bayern-Profi und Nationalspieler, hat in dieser vermeintlich paradiesischen Welt mit psychischen Problemen zu kämpfen. Die Frage, ob er auch außerhalb des Profifußballs **in Depressionen verfallen wäre**, läßt sich nicht beantworten* (FAZ, December 24, 2003, p. 30). (Sebastian Deisler, the professional soccer player from Bavaria and member of the German national soccer team, had to cope with problems in this supposedly paradisiacal world. The question whether he would have **sunk into depressions** outside professional soccer playing cannot be answered.)

6. *Dann begann ein langer Weg. Gespräche, Selbsthilfegruppen, Mutter-Kind-Kur—es dauerte mehrere Monate, bis es ihr besser ging, und ein Jahr, bis die Krankheit geheilt war. „Es muss nicht sein, dass so viele Frauen **in diese Depression rutschen**—und so lange damit kämpfen", sagt Werner* (FAZ, July 18, 2007, p. 40). (Then began a long journey. Talks, self-help groups, mother–child health retreat. It lasted many months until she felt better and a year until the illness was cured. "It

is unnecessary that so many women **slide into this depression** and struggle with it for so long," Werner says.)

7. *Während manche Patienten rasche, unvorhersagbare Umschwünge ihrer Stimmung erfahren, erleben andere vornehmlich die Höhenflüge der Manie oder stürzen regelmäßig in Depressionen* (FAZ, February 21, 2007, p. N2). (While some patients experience rapid, unpredictable mood changes, others primarily experience manic flights to extreme altitudes or regularly **plunge into depressions.**)

8. *Die größte Anzahl Patienten in der Tannenwaldklinik beispielsweise seien Angehörige von Suchtkranken gewesen, die, von der familiären Situation chronisch überfordert, oft sukzessive in eine Depression gerieten* (FAZ, February 21, 2002, p. 64). (The majority of the patients at the Tannenwald clinic, for example, have been relatives of addicts who, chronically overstrained by their family situation, often **successively got into a depression.**)

The German verbs *fallen* (to fall), *verfallen* (to sink), *stürzen* (to plunge), *rutschen* (to slide), and *geraten* (to get into) have one common semantic feature: The movement happens suddenly, as in fall, plunge, and get into. This is not the case with slide and sink. But all the verbs have the same semantic feature of "losing control." If you fall, slide, sink, or plunge, you cannot do anything; you are will-less, powerless, and weak; you totally lose control of your whole body. The experience of getting depressed is often described as a total loss of control of one's entire life, the loss of one's sense of self. These expressions are consistent with the metaphor DEPRESSION IS LOSS OF CONTROL. Loss of control in a depression has a downward orientation, just like in the metaphor DEPRESSION IS A HEAVY BURDEN.

In text passages that depict the subjective experiences of depressed persons as weak, helpless, and passive, depression becomes an agent and is personified; it is always depicted as an active part, an aggressive attacker, an enemy that has to be fought. This is why the person suffering from depression has to fight against the illness:

9. *[M]achten Depressionen das Leben unerträglich* (FAZ, November 4, 1968). ([D]epressions **made life** unbearable.)

10. *Die Seelenfinsternis sucht Arme und Reiche heim, [. . .] wie viel gesunde, produktive Lebenszeit eine Krankheit ihren Opfern raubt* (Der Spiegel, Number 31, 1999, p. 181). (The darkness of the soul

afflicts the poor as well as the rich, [. . .] how much of a healthy, productive lifetime **the illness robs of her victims.**)

Metaphors that conceptualize depression as a heavy burden or as a fall implicitly convey the norms that are valid in a society. To be depressed implies
that the person fails to achieve the goals that were expected of him or her by
others. Thus, the ill person does not meet societal standards and imperatives
such as success, hard work, and private happiness. Some writers (e.g., Lutz,
1986) have observed that in Western and European-American societies,
being happy is considered the normal state and lacking power and control is seen as a negative. Persons with depression cannot cope with these
norms and are consequently evaluated negatively and stigmatized by others
(McMullen & Conway, 2008, pp. 176–177).

Depression Is Darkness

Being depressed, being in a state of depression, is depicted as getting into and
staying for an indefinite time in a dark room, a dark container, or a dark hole:

11. *Seelische Finsternis bleibt oft lange verborgen* (*Spiegel Wissen*, January
    2011, p. 7). (**The darkness of the soul** often remains undiscovered for
    a long time.)
12. *Aus dem Fernseher brabbelten Stimmen, sie lag einfach nur da,
    gefangen in einem großen, schwarzen Nichts* (*Spiegel Wissen*, January
    2011, p. 36). (Voices babbled from the TV, she simply lay there, **caught
    in the big, black nothingness.**)

Depictions of depression as darkness or as a dark hole the person fell into
are consistent with the conceptual metaphor that is usually used for many
mental illnesses, by sufferers as well as in medical terminology (Schuster,
2010, p. 211). Light and darkness metaphors are consistent with the conceptual metaphors (MENTAL) ILLNESS IS DARKNESS, (MENTAL) HEALTH
IS LIGHT. These metaphors overlap with the conventional metaphors
HEALTH IS UP, SICKNESS IS DOWN; GOOD IS UP, BAD IS DOWN
(Lakoff & Johnson, 1980, p. 15). Falling or sliding into a depression is also
coherent with these concepts. Each of these metaphors focuses on a different aspect of the subjective experience of getting depressed. Thus, there

is a cross-metaphorical correspondence between these metaphors (Lakoff & Johnson, 1980, pp. 7–9).

As I already discussed at the beginning of this chapter, the use of metaphors depends on the context. In order to give the personal, subjective perspective of people with depression, particular aspects of the metaphors are highlighted, verbally or visually. By choosing expressions like *to fall into depression, to slide into depression,* or *to plunge into depression,* people with depression are present in the mass media discourse; they become discourse actors (Spitzmüller & Warnke, 2011, pp. 172–187). The stories of depression are told from the perspective of the sufferers. The metaphors used in the discourse, as well as, for example, direct citations and narratives with a first-person narrator, are used in accordance with the needs of mass media discourse. With such stories, journalists can personalize abstract and complex medical topics and create human-interest content that can attract readers' attention. Personal stories about depression are to some extent informative because they demonstrate vividly the symptoms of this illness. Thus, it can be useful for people to the extent that they may recognize the symptoms and get help. On the other hand, these personal stories can satisfy a desire for sensation in journalists as well as in readers, especially if, for example, a well-known person tells the story of his or her depression (Dulinski, 2003).

Metaphor and Narrative in the Examples

The metaphors discussed in the section above play an important role in the narrative structures. The metaphor DEPRESSION IS A FALL is a subsequent metaphor to a more general conceptual metaphor DEPRESSION IS A JOURNEY. This metaphor is realized not only in single words or word combinations, but mostly on the textual level, as in the following example:

13. *Ohne ein Blatt vor den Mund zu nehmen, schildert die Autorin—mit vollem Bekenntnis zur mitunter resignativen Ausgangslage—ihr eigenes Erlebnis auf dem Leidensweg einer Depression. Auf ihm begegnete sie mehreren Ärzten (Zeit Online,* October 11, 1985). (Not to mince matters, the author depicts, with full commitment to her resigned starting point, her own experience **on the path of suffering from depression. On this path, she encountered many doctors.**)

The path of suffering is a metaphor that represents a mental illness like a process. This metaphor emphasizes the temporal aspect of the depression. It is an illness that does not disappear overnight; rather, it has a certain duration and takes a lot of time. In the next sentence, the metaphor is picked up again, but it can also be read literally: The illness is experienced as a path that has to be walked along and, at the same time, it can be a real path to a doctor. The expression *on the path of suffering* shows the internal, subjective perspective of the woman suffering from depression. The next sentence gives an external description of the events: *On this path, she encountered many doctors.* This creates a specific narrative texture that is also realized in the change of the verbal form (*depicts* is in the simple present, *encountered* is in the preterite). Thus, we see how metaphor and narrative are connected together: The aspects highlighted by the metaphor are also those that are crucial for narratives, and they are set into a temporal and experiential framework.

The aspect of temporality is also present in the conceptual metaphor DEPRESSION IS A FALL. The concrete realizations of the metaphor, like *to fall into a depression* or *to slide into depression* in the analyzed texts, mark the critical center of a story, the turning point, the moment that breaks and interrupts the previous course of the person's life. In Labov and Waletzky's theory (1967), this change of state constitutes a complication (Brinker, 2010, p. 61). The aspect of suddenness or abruptness is substantial in the subjective experience of depression, and at the same time it is substantial for the narrative structure of the story: "[A]ll narratives *depict a temporal transition from one state of affairs to another*" (Ochs, 1998, p. 189, italics in the original).

Another example illustrates the metaphor DEPRESSION IS A JOURNEY and at the same time the temporal aspect that is so crucial for people suffering from depression:

14. *Schätzungsweise drei Millionen Menschen in Deutschland leiden an einer Depression. Und die Tendenz ist steigend. Jede fünfte Frau und jeder zehnte Mann müssen im Lauf des Lebens mindestens **eine depressive Episode durchschreiten*** (FAS, August 8, 1999, p. 13). (Approximately 3 million people in Germany suffer from depression. And there is a tendency for these figures to rise. Every fifth woman and every tenth man have to **go through a depressive episode** at least once in their lives.)

To go through a depressive episode implies that the person with depression has to go by foot, and *to go through* implies that the person has to go through every part of the way and must not skip any part of it. Going by foot means going slowly; regarding depression, it might refer to the long duration of the illness. Thus, in this metaphorical expression we also find the aspect of temporality that is important for the experience of depression as well as for the narrative structure of the text. *Depressive episode* is also a medical term that emphasizes that depression is not always present; rather, it comes and goes.

Considering these examples, we can say that metaphors and metaphorical structures predetermine narrative textual structures, at least in the analyzed mass media discourse. Metaphors are helpful for mentally ill persons to communicate their individual experiences, and this makes metaphors attractive in narrative texts in mass media. This corresponds with the premises on the context sensitivity of metaphors postulated above. The mass media context triggers primarily conventional metaphors that are accessible for the mass audience.

In view of these results, we can see that narratives are an essential part of the German mass media discourse on depression. The stories about depression are told by sufferers to the journalists, who then use them in their popular scientific texts in order to inform the audience about this mental illness. As discourse actors, the journalists try to transfer the medical knowledge to their lay readers (Spitzmüller & Warnke, 2011, pp. 172–183). They use personal stories of depression to show that concrete cases can be useful for informing readers about symptoms and therapies of depression, a strategy very typical for newspapers (van Dijk, 1998, pp. 9–10). Personal stories are individual and emotional, and they are situated in the everyday life of the audience (Busch, 2015; Sandig, 2006). This personalization strategy is generally very popular in many areas of mass communication (Bentele et al., 2013, pp. 214–215).

Conclusion

In my examples, I tried to depict some important features of the German mass media discourse on depression. In particular, metaphors for symptoms of depression used by sufferers seem to play an important role in the newspaper texts. Metaphors of depression show on the one hand the pervasiveness of metaphorical concepts for some specific domains, like subjective experiences during an episode of mental illness. On the other hand, the examples analyzed also show that metaphorical concepts can be triggered by the context; different language speakers use different metaphors in different contexts. The metaphors used in the German mass media serve to create a specific media portrayal of depression from the perspective of the sufferers. Depression is experienced as a heavy burden that a person has to carry and that presses the person down. Furthermore, the moment of becoming ill is described as a fall, a sliding downward. Some people experience depression like a toilsome journey. Further metaphors are those of darkness and blackness, where depression is experienced like being in a black or dark room.

The analysis has also shown that metaphors of depression appear mostly in narrative texts. Different aspects of a metaphor seem to reinforce narrative structures; at the same time, metaphor can be constituted not only by a single word or a word combination, but on a more global textual level. And this text then has a narrative structure. So, metaphors are constitutive of narrative since they are manifestations of embodied experience. Concerning this point, we can agree with Labov and Waletzky (1967), who defined narratives as (oral) versions of personal experience.

Metaphors used in narrative texts seem to be very useful in the health communication of mass media. They make texts attractive for readers by visualizing experiences and concepts for them (if only in their mind's eye) and thus help in the process of transferring knowledge to a mass audience. For this purpose, conventional metaphors are more suitable. Some authors maintained that metaphors not only reflect the past but also define how we see our present and how we expect the future to be. This aspect may give new inspiration for further research.

Notes

1. It is also very interesting to see how these media present themselves for their audience on the internet. *FAZ* emphasizes the fact that it primarily explains things for the audience (see also the image film at http://verlag.faz.net/unternehmen/ueber-uns/f-a-z-unternehmensfilm-die-seiten-einer-zeitung-der-film-14302161.html).
2. For the history of the medical term *Depression*, see Schuster (2010).
3. For better understanding, I give a word-for-word translation of the expressions.
4. In all the following examples the relevant expressions are printed in bold letters; the respective English translation is placed in parentheses after the German citation.

5. One important point in this connection is also the social stigma that persons with mental illnesses are confronted with (Semino, 2008, p. 179), especially because mentally ill persons do not necessarily look ill.
6. For reasons of copyright, it is not possible to print this picture in this book.
7. Strictly speaking, this picture is not iconic in the sense that emojis are, for example. It has some iconic elements that are based on some similarity between the concept of the burden pressing on the person from above and the depicted young man who tries to stem a burden coming from above. For problems of iconicity, see Stöckl (2004, p. 50, pp. 65–66).
8. For perspectivity of images, see Kress (2012); for perspectivity of language, see Köller (2004).
9. It has been noted in some studies that depression sufferers tend to explain the disease as a consequence of circumstances beyond their control (Kangas, 2001; Semino, 2008, p. 184).
10. Semino (2008, pp. 178–190) found out that non-sufferers show a different perspective on the disease and use other metaphors.

References

Bateman, J. A. (2016). Methodological and theoretical issues in multimodality. In N.-M. Klug & H. Stöckl (Eds.), *Sprache im multimodalen Kontext* (pp. 36–74). De Gruyter.

Bentele, G., Brosius, H.-B., & Jarren, O. (Eds.). (2013). *Lexikon Kommunikations- und Medienwissenschaft*. Springer.

Böke, K. (1996). Überlegungen zu einer Metapherntheorie im Dienste einer „parzellierten" Sprachgeschichtsschreibung. In K. Böke, M. Jung, & M. Wengeler (Eds.), *Öffentlicher Sprachgebrauch: Praktische, theoretische und historische Perspektiven* (pp. 431–452). Westdeutscher Verlag.

Brinker, K. (2010). *Linguistische Textanalyse: Eine Einführung in Grundbegriffe und Methoden* (7th ed.). Erich Schmidt.

Burger, H., & Luginbühl, M. (2014). *Mediensprache: Eine Einführung in Sprache und Kommunikationsformen der Massenmedien*. De Gruyter.

Busch, A. (2015). Medizindiskurse: Mediale Räume der Experten-Laien-Kommunikation. In A. Busch & T. Spranz-Fogasy (Eds.), *Handbuch Sprache in der Medizin* (pp. 369–386). De Gruyter.

Busch, A., & Spranz-Fogasy, T. (2015). Sprache in der Medizin. In E. Felder & A. Gardt (Eds.), *Handbuch Sprache und Wissen* (pp. 335–357). De Gruyter.

Busse, D., & Teubert, W. (1994). Ist Diskurs ein sprachwissenschaftliches Objekt? In D. Busse, F. Hermanns, & W. Teuber (Eds.), *Begriffsgeschichte und Diskursgeschichte: Methodenfragen und Forschungsergebnisse der historischen Semantik* (pp. 10–28). Westdeutscher Verlag.

Cross, R., Davis, S., & O'Neil, I. (2017). *Health communication: Theoretical and critical perspectives*. Polity.

Deignan, A. (2017). Mapping and narrative in figurative communication. In B. Hampe (Ed.), *Metaphor: Embodied cognition and discourse* (pp. 200–219). Cambridge University Press.

Duden. (2014). *Die deutsche Sprache: Wörterbuch in drei Bänden*. Dudenverlag.

Dulinski, U. (2003). *Sensationsjournalismus in Deutschland*. Universitätsverlag Konstanz.

Feer, H. (1987). *Die Sprache der Psychiatrie: Eine linguistische Untersuchung*. Springer.

Felder, E. (2010). Semantische Kämpfe: Die Macht des Deklarativen in Fachdiskursen. In T. Fuchs & G. Schwarzkopf (Eds.), *Verantwortlichkeit—nur eine Illusion?* (pp. 13–59). Winter.

Felder, E. (2012). Pragma-semiotische Textarbeit und der hermeneutische Nutzen von Korpusanalysen für die linguistische Mediendiskursanalyse. In E. Felder, M. Müller, & F. Vogel (Eds.), *Korpuspragmatik: Thematische Korpora als Basis diskurslinguistischer Analysen* (pp. 115–174). De Gruyter.

Fleck, L. (1980). *Entstehung und Entwicklung einer wissenschaftlichen Tatsache: Einführung in die Lehre vom Denkstil und Denkkollektiv*. Suhrkamp.

Foucault, M. (1990). *Die Ordnung der Dinge: Eine Archäologie der Humanwissenschaften*. Suhrkamp.

Garro, L. C., & Mattingly, C. (2000). Narrative as construct and construction. In C. Mattingly & L. C. Garro (Eds.), *Narrative and the cultural construction of illness and healing* (pp. 1–49). University of California Press.

Gee, J. P., & Handford, M. (Eds.). (2012). *Routledge handbook of discourse analysis*. Routledge.

Gibbs, R. (2014). Conceptual metaphor in thought and social action. In M. Landau, M. Robinson, & B. Meier (Eds.), *The power of metaphor: Examining its influence on social life* (pp. 17–40). American Psychological Association.

Hampe, B. (2017). Embodiment and discourse: Dimensions and dynamics of contemporary metaphor theory. In B. Hampe (Ed.), *Metaphor: Embodied cognition and discourse* (pp. 3–23). Cambridge University Press.

Harvey, K., & Adolph, S. (2012). Discourse and healthcare. In J. P. Gee & M. Handford (Eds.), *Routledge handbook of discourse analysis* (pp. 470–481). Routledge.

Heinemann, W., & Viehweger, D. (1991). *Textlinguistik: Eine Einführung*. Niemeyer.

Hess-Lüttich, E. W. B., Kämper, H., Reisigl, M., & Warnke, I. (Eds.). (2017), *Diskurs—semiotisch: Aspekte multiformaler Diskurskodierung*. De Gruyter.

Jensen, T. W. (2017). Doing metaphor: An ecological perspective on metaphoricity in discourse. In B. Hampe (Ed.), *Metaphor: Embodied cognition and discourse* (pp. 257–276). Cambridge University Press.

Johnson, M. (1987). *The body in the mind*. University of Chicago Press.

Kangas, I. (2001). Making sense of depression: Perceptions of melancholia in lay narratives. *Health*, 5(1), 76–92.

Kirmayer, L. J. (1992). The body's insistence on meaning: Metaphor as presentation and representation in illness experience. *Medical Anthropological Quarterly*, 6, 323–346.

Kirmayer, L. J. (2000). Broken narratives: Clinical encounters and the poetics of illness experience. In C. Mattingly & L. C. Garro (Eds.), *Narrative and the cultural construction of illness and healing* (pp. 153–180). University of California Press.

Kohring, M. (2005). *Wissenschaftsjournalismus: Forschungsüberblick und Theorieentwurf*. Universitätsverlag Konstanz.

Köller, W. (2004). *Perspektivität und Sprache: Zur Struktur von Objektivierungsformen in Bildern, im Denken und in der Sprache*. De Gruyter.

Kress, G. (2012). Multimodal discourse analysis. In J. P. Gee & M. Handford (Eds.), *Routledge handbook of discourse analysis* (pp. 35–50). Routledge.

Labov, W. (1997). Some further steps in narrative analysis. *Journal of Narrative and Life History, 7*(1–4), 395–415.

Labov, W., & Waletzky, J. (1967). Narrative analysis: Oral versions of personal experience. In J. Helm (Ed.), *Essays on the verbal and visual arts* (pp. 12–44). American Ethnological Society.

Lakoff, G., & Johnson, M. (1980). *Metaphors we live by.* University of Chicago Press.

Linell, P. (2009). *Rethinking language, mind, and world dialogically: Interactional and contextual theories of human sense-making.* Information Age Publishing.

Low, S. M. (2005). Embodied metaphors: Nerves as lived experience. In T. J. Csordas (Ed.), *Embodiment and experience: The existential ground of culture and self* (pp. 139–162). Cambridge University Press.

Lutz, C. (1986). Depression and the translation of the emotional worlds. In R. Harré (Ed.), *The social construction of emotions* (pp. 63–100). Blackwell.

McMullen, L. M., & Conway, J. B. (2008). Conventional metaphors for depression. In S. R. Fussel (Ed.), *The verbal communication of emotions: Interdisciplinary perspectives* (pp. 167–181). Psychology Press.

Middleton, D., & Edwards, D. (1990). Introduction. In D. Middleton & D. Edwards (Eds.), *Collective remembering* (pp. 1–22). Sage.

Nerlich, B. (2005). A river runs through it: How the discourse metaphor CROSSING THE RUBICON structured the debate about human embryonic stem cells in Germany and (not) the UK. *Metaphorik.de, 8,* 71–104.

Niehr, T. (2014). *Einführung in die linguistische Diskursanalyse.* Wissenschaftliche Buchgesellschaft.

Norrick, N. R. (2000). *Conversational narrative: Storytelling in everyday talk.* John Benjamins.

Ochs, E. (1998). Narrative. In T. van Dijk (Ed.), *Discourse studies: A multidisciplinary introduction. Volume 1: Discourse as structure and process* (pp. 185–207). Sage.

Ochs, E. & Capps, L. (2001). *Living narrative: Creating lives in everyday storytelling.* Harvard University Press.

O'Keefe, A. (2012). Media and discourse analysis. In J. P. Gee & M. Handford (Eds.), *Routledge handbook of discourse analysis* (pp. 441–454). Routledge.

Sandig, B. (2006). *Textstilistik des Deutschen.* De Gruyter.

Schneider, W. (2013). Medikalisierung sozialer Prozesse. *Psychotherapeut, 58,* 219–236.

Schuster, B.-M. (2010). *Auf dem Weg zur Fachsprache: Sprachliche Professionalisierung in der psychiatrischen Schreibpraxis (1800–1939).* De Gruyter.

Semino, E. (2008). *Metaphor in discourse.* Cambridge University Press.

Semino, E., Deignan, A., & Littlemore, J. (2013). Metaphor, genre, and recontextualization. *Metaphor and Symbol, 28*(1), 41–59.

Spieß, C. (2011). *Diskurshandlungen: Theorie und Methode linguistischer Diskursanalyse am Beispiel der Bioethikdebatte.* De Gruyter.

Spieß, C. (2014). Diskurslinguistische Metaphernanalyse. In M. Jung (Ed.), *Methoden der Metaphernforschung und -analyse* (pp. 31–58). Springer.

Spitzmüller, J., & Warnke, J. (2011). *Diskurslinguistik: Eine Einführung in die Theorien und Methoden der transtextuellen Sprachanalyse.* De Gruyter.

Stöckl, H. (2004). *Die Sprache im Bild, das Bild in der Sprache: Zur Verknüpfung von Sprache und Bild im massenmedialen Text.* De Gruyter.

Turner, B. (1984). *The body and society.* Blackwell.

van Dijk, T. (1998). The study of discourse. In T. van Dijk (Ed.). *Discourse studies: A multidisciplinary introduction. Volume 1: Discourse as structure and process* (pp. 1–34). Sage.

van Dijk, T. (2012). Discourse and knowledge. In J. P. Gee & M. Handford (Eds.), *Handbook of discourse analysis* (pp. 587–603). Routledge.

Vogt, J. (2014). *Aspekte erzählender Prosa: Eine Einführung in Erzähltechnik und Romantheorie* (11th ed.). Fink.

Weischenberg, S., Malik, M., & Scholl, A. (2006). *Die Souffleure der Mediengesellschaft: Report über die Journalisten in Deutschland.* Universitätsverlag Konstanz.

Wengeler, M. (2003). *Topos und Diskurs: Begründung einer argumentationsanalytischen Methode und ihre Anwendung auf den Migrationsdiskurs (1960–1985).* Niemeyer.

World Health Organization. (2020). Depression. http://www.who.int/en/news-room/fact-sheets/detail/depression

PART IV

MENTAL HEALTH, LIFE STORYING, TRAUMA, AND ARTISTIC EXPRESSION

12

Narrating Shame in Contemporary Mental Distress Memoirs by Female British Authors

Katrin Röder

Introduction

At the beginning of her 2010 autobiography on obsessive-compulsive disorder (OCD) entitled *The Woman Who Thought Too Much*, British-Jewish poet and novelist Joanne Limburg (born in 1970) draws attention to the ubiquity of shame as a bodily, emotional, and social phenomenon across cultures: "Shame," she argues, "is an inescapable part of being human: without it, there would be little to stop us assaulting attractive strangers and defecating on tube trains" (Limburg, 2011, p. 1). Shame "acts as an internal social regulator, and most of the time, for most people, it does an unobtrusively good job. But shame can also be a bully" (Limburg, 2011, p. 1). In line with Helen B. Lewis (1971, pp. 426–429, 435), Limburg argues that in contrast to guilt, the feeling that "one has *done something* wrong," shame is

> the feeling that one is *being someone* wrong. [. . .] When we feel guilty, we want to right the wrong action; when we feel ashamed, we want to hide the wrong self away—or obliterate it. There are quite a few of my own selves I would obliterate, if I could: the unsuccessful, soiled selves that could never quite act or speak or look as they should; that drag shaming memories around with them. The youngest of these is myself in middle school. She is being told off in front of everybody, and her peers are enjoying it. (Limburg, 2011, p. 1)

Limburg describes the painful self-consciousness and the feeling of isolation that are created by shame:

Katrin Röder, *Narrating Shame in Contemporary Mental Distress Memoirs by Female British Authors* In: *Narrative and Mental Health.* Edited by: Jarmila Mildorf, Elisabeth Punzi, and Christoph Singer, Oxford University Press.

I had already spent several years as one of the class weirdos, [. . .] with my precociously serious manner, my penchant for long words, and my awkwardness at games. [. . .] often I was turned away. I can remember spending countless break-times walking round and round the perimeter of the playground all alone, head down, doing my best to look self-contained. I didn't feel the way I was trying to look: I felt lonely, and vulnerable with it. [. . .] My efforts to hide my soiled self had ended up with it being waved around in front of everybody [. . .] However I played it, I was different and that difference was felt as a stigma. (Limburg, 2011, pp. 1–4)

This chapter explores the connection between representations of scenes of shame (see also Hotz-Davies, 2007) and different forms of narrative fragmentations and silences in two contemporary British mental distress autobiographies, Limburg's *The Woman Who Thought Too Much* (2011) and Amanda Green's *My Alien Self: My Journey Back to Me* (2013). My approach to the concept of the "narrative" is drawn from literary narratology. In accordance with Gérard Genette, I use "narrative" to refer to "oral or written discourse that undertakes to tell of an event or a series of events" as well as to "the succession of events, real or fictitious, that are the subjects of this discourse, and [. . .] their several relations of linking, opposition, repetition, etc." (Genette, 1983, p. 25).

In my use of the term "scene", I follow Lauren Berlant, who states that

the scene is a suspension bridge, defined not by events but by wobbly atmospheres in proximity to a disturbance. [. . .] In the psychoanalytic sense, as in 'primal scene,' subjects become conscious of their nonsovereignty in an encounter with a threatening situation and get stuck in the affective atmosphere. That is what then constitutes the context for the becoming-event, the perturbing data that never quite makes it to knowledge. (Berlant, 2015, n. p.)

Apart from my application of the term "mental health" in contexts in which I refer to health care practitioners or social and human service providers, my use of the notion "mental health" follows the World Health Organization (2019) definition:

Mental health is defined as a state of well-being in which every individual realizes his or her own potential, can cope with the normal stresses of life, can work productively and fruitfully, and is able to make a contribution to her or his community. [. . .] Health is a state of complete physical, mental and social well-being and not merely the absence of disease or infirmity.

The chapter investigates shame as a form of communication and pursues the following questions:

1. Can the practice of addressing the shame and stigma surrounding mental distress air the difficulty of speaking or writing about this distress?
2. Does the practice of narrating scenes of shame related to aspects of mental distress imply a triumph over shame?

Theoretical and Narratological Approaches to Shame

Shame is defined as a negative affect (Tomkins, 1995a, p. 74) or social emotion (Brown, 2012, pp. 58–111; Damásio, 1999, p. 291; Tangney & Dearing, 2002, pp. 3, 5, 9, 13, 18) that both forms and disrupts identity through the performative stigmatizing interpellation "Shame on you!" (Mitchell, 2013, p. 312; Sedgwick, 2003, p. 36; Sedgwick, 1993, pp. 4, 13). As a highly self-conscious affect (Tomkins, 1995b, pp. 136–137) or emotion (Lewis, 2011, p. 2), it gives rise to a strongly relational concept of identity: The self in shame has internalized others' responses of derision and becomes aware of itself in relation to other people's responses of contempt (Tomkins, 1995b, pp. 138–139). Shame is both "peculiarly contagious and peculiarly individuating" (Sedgwick, 1993, p. 5); it can easily spread from individual to individual, and among stigmatized social groups,[1] it is a profoundly isolating affect that can lead to ostracization. For those who do not fit easily into heteronormative, predominantly White, ableist, and mentalist[2] societies (because they are, for example, queer, non-White, disabled, or in mental distress), shame "is simply the first, and remains a permanent, structuring fact of identity" (Sedgwick, 2003, p. 64). As shame is related to one's (imagined or real) visibility to others and to their (imagined or real) judgments and responses (Vanderheiden & Mayer, 2017, p. 8), it can lead to self-absorption and withdrawal. However, shame is irrevocably performative at the same time. It mantles "the threshold between introversion and extroversion, between absorption and theatricality, between performativity and—performativity," subverting expectations towards an autonomous, essentialist, unmediated, spontaneous, and "authentic" self-expression (Sedgwick, 1993, pp. 38, 64). Eve Kosofsky Sedgwick's performative concept of shame is based on Silvan Tomkins's affect theory, which is opposed to the notion of the core self (Sedgwick & Frank, 1995, p. 6) and which emphasizes the inseparable connection between shame and positive affects ("Interest-Excitement"; "Enjoyment-Joy"). Tomkins argues that shame only sets in after positive affect was activated (Sedgwick & Frank, 1995, pp. 22–23, 74). The shame response, Tomkins states, is "an act of facial communication reduction" (1995b, p. 137). "By dropping his eyes, his eyelid, his head, and sometimes the whole upper part of his body, the individual calls a halt to looking at another person [. . .] and to the other person's looking at him, particularly at his face" (Tomkins, 1995b, p. 134). Shame is a deeply ambivalent and affectively rich form of communication in which

> excitement or enjoyment is only incompletely reduced. [. . .] Because the self is not altogether willing to renounce the object, excitement may break through and displace shame at any moment [. . .] [T]he residual positive wish is not only to look at the other rather than look down, but to have the other look with interest or enjoyment rather than with derision. (Tomkins, 1995b, pp. 137–138)

Shame points to one's desires, ideals, ambitions, and hopes; it "alerts us to things, people, and ideas that we didn't even know we wanted" (Probyn, 2005, pp. ix, 14). It speaks through silences and disruptions of verbal communication that are characterized by the desire for (verbal) communication. The desire to raise the interest of the other is an important motivation for the writing of mental distress memoirs, which make readers dwell on the scenes of shame and which enable them to fill the silences and gaps by using their empathy and imagination. Limburg writes about her life with OCD and its relationship to readers' interest: "It's not an interesting life, but it is quite an interesting predicament" (2011, p. 10). Many passages in Limburg's and Green's texts support Tomkins's "optimistic" description of shame as a communicative strategy, but in some cases, their silences and fragmentations harbor the full, irreducible ambivalence of the desire for (verbal) communication and of ineffability. They illustrate that verbal communication breaks off because something is too painful, too shameful, too anxiety-provoking, and too dangerous to access and express in words.

The dominant part of critical literature describes shame as a negative emotion that must be overcome or removed because of its harmful impact on the individual's self-perception and development (Bouson, 2009, p. 183; Bouson, 2016, pp. 143–192; Lelwica, 2017, pp. 15–16, 47, 93). Furthermore, shame is defined as a social emotion that can be divided into a "healthy" form, which must be valued and promoted (because it supports social co-herence, a "sense of belonging," an "acceptable social value system and norm base" as well as individual autonomy, "a stable and positive identity," integrity, "self-actualisation," authenticity, self-improvement, social adap-tation, resilience, and efficiency [Vanderheiden & Mayer, 2017, pp. 16–18, 20–22, 26, 31, 33]) and a "pathological" (and purportedly "female") form (characterized by passivity, withdrawal, silence, and depression) that must be externalized, confronted, and reduced (e.g., in shame-based psychotherapy) (Vanderheiden & Mayer, 2017, pp. 18, 31).[3] Although such approaches draw attention to (in the former case) the damaging consequences of social op-pression and (in the latter case) to the harmful and dangerous aspects of withdrawal (especially to its connection to depression and suicidality), they run the risk of positing standards of individual autonomy, resilience, adapt-ivity, or efficiency that may be new sources of shame for those who are unable to achieve them. Because of the long history of the oppression and silencing of disabled people, activist Eli Clare states that he continues to "feel slivers of shame, silence, and isolation still imbedded deep in my body," arguing that for him and other disabled persons it may be impossible to reduce, let alone overcome, many "negative" aspects of shame, not least because the shame-inducing ableist and mentalist social structures are very much in place (Clare, 2015, p. 110). Ableist and mentalist shame-inducing structures are those that introduce and uphold the stigma of nonnormative, purportedly "abnormal" forms of embodiment and neurodiversity. As Bradley Lewis has shown, referencing Judith Chamberlain's *On Our Own: Patient-Controlled Alternatives to the Mental Health System* and Michael L. Perlin's *The Hidden Prejudice: Mental Disability on Trial*, mentalism is "the social stigma and oppression against mental difference" that prevails in the "biopsychiatric medical model [. . .] which dominates mental health treatment in the West" (Lewis, 2010, p. 160). Furthermore, as Lewis convincingly argues, the "binary between normal and abnormal" introduced and upheld by the biopsychiatric medical model of mental illness "shores up this psychiatrization [of neurodiversity, K. R.] by providing tremendous social and psychological pressure to stay on the side of normality, or sanity" (Lewis, 2010, p. 162).

Withdrawal is a response to the stigma and shame surrounding mental distress that may indeed lead to severe depression and suicidality (Sinha, 2017, pp. 252, 257–258), as Green's and Limburg's autobiographies show (Green, 2013, pp. 225–227, 243, 317, 353, 369, 416, 419, 431, 450; Limburg, 2011, pp. 111, 114, 215, 319, 321;). Limburg writes:

> The Mental Health Foundation addressed this dilemma in 2000, in a report it called 'Pull Yourself Together! A Survey of the stigma and discrimination faced by people who experience mental distress'. One respondent wrote: 'when I tried to kill myself 2 years ago I walked out of A&E on Saturday morning and went to work on Monday as if nothing had happened because I was scared to let anyone know'. The report goes on to say: 'There were many more reasons why people could not tell work colleagues than why they could [. . .] the most frequently reported reason for not telling work colleagues was fear of discrimination, stigma and prejudice'. They have good reason for their fear: there are psychiatrists who advise their patients against disclosing their histories on application forms. (Limburg, 2011, p. 5)

Similarly, Amanda Green draws attention to the problem of hiding when in severe mental distress:

> When I sought help professionally, the obstacle became the way I looked—because I "look alright" I can't be too bad. Yes, I do look alright—my skin does not portray the years of angst, turmoil, drugs and alcohol abuse—but if I was not alright I would stay indoors, as I often did, unable to get out for days. No-one would ever see me when I was not alright. But this is no reason to ignore someone's pleas for help. (Green, 2013, p. 353)

However, far from being always "pathological," withdrawal in shame (the face[s] turned away, the loss of representability) might be a response that allows for an unpredictable transformation of the subject (Munt, 2008, p. 103), an aspect of shame that is also shown in Limburg's and Green's texts.

Many theoretical approaches regard shame as a social problem that must be solved on an individual or interpersonal level only (Sinha, 2017, pp. 253, 262, 269). According to Silvan Tomkins, however, shame can be processed (but not fully overcome) in ways that question its sociopolitical and cultural sources (oppression, alienation) and that motivate individuals to sympathize with and help others.[4] Feminist and queer scholars discuss shame as a socio-political resource that may point to the necessity of social change:[5] Marcianna Nosek, Holly Powell Kennedy, and Maria Gudmundsdottir (2010) point out that shame is a seismograph of socio-political inequality, showing that women who experience mental distress during their menopause feel shame, become silent, and withdraw because of the prevailing social discourses on menopause and aging and because they are neither offered enough social support nor enough life choices. In accordance with Sedgwick, Kaye Mitchell shows that shame has a strong socio-political, embodied (and often erotic or sexual) dimension: When represented in literature, auto/biography, and the media, scenes of shame are captivating and mesmerizing; they exert a power that makes narrators, characters, and readers return to them continually. Shame can become "a near-inexhaustible source of transformational energy" that gives rise to unexpected and non-essentialist forms of subjectivity and identity (Sedgwick, 1993, p. 4). Narrative representations of scenes of shame can comprize becoming-events, e.g. unexpected transformations of narrating and narrated "I"s, and can facilitate surprising narrative connections.

As a reduced, disrupted form of verbal or nonverbal communication, shame is defined as "an interruption of and impediment to communication that is itself communicated" (Tomkins, 1995b, pp. 134–138). It creates a fragmented, at times opaque, oral or written narrative that comprises temporal segments in which "subjects become conscious of their nonsovereignty in an encounter with a threatening situation and get stuck in the affective atmosphere" and that withholds information about the most painful, dark, humiliating experiences (Berlant, 2015, n. p.). In autobiographical narratives like Limburg's and Green's, such information is alluded to through textual gaps that can be graphically conspicuous (as in the case of Green's *My Alien Self*) and through implicit as well as explicit ellipses—that is, temporal elisions, chronological lacunae, or lateral omissions in the narrative continuity that either indicate the lapse of narrated time (explicit ellipses) or not (implicit ellipses, Genette, 1983, pp. 106–108). In addition to temporal ellipses, the texts by Green and Limburg contain "paralipses," omissions of "some important action or thought of the focal hero, which neither the hero or the narrator can be ignorant of but which the narrator chooses to conceal from the reader" (Genette, 1983, p. 196)[6] or allusions to pieces of information that the narrator (and even the author) may lack altogether. As my analysis investigates literary autobiographies, it draws on concepts from literary narratology ("ellipsis" and "paralipsis"). However, I will not use the notions "narrator" and "protagonist" but employ the terms "narrating 'I' " to refer to "the narrator [...] who tells the autobiographical narrative" and "narrated 'I' " to signify "the subject of history," "the object 'I' " or "the protagonist of the narrative" (Smith & Watson, 2010, pp. 72–73). I use "narrative" in a broadly narratological sense as outlined above. Autobiographical narratives that are strongly infused with shame do not give full insight into a person's interior state. For this reason, it is imperative for readers as well as for professional listeners in clinical contexts (i.e., psychologists, psychiatrists, and general practitioners (GPs)) to pay attention to narrative lacunae because they often point to deep-lying, painful forms of distress that authors and clients find too shameful to share directly or uninhibitedly.

Shame, Mental Illness, and Gender

Bradley Lewis's problematization of the stigmatization of neurodiversity through the biopsychiatric medical model of mental illness as well as Limburg's discussion of the report of the Mental Health Foundation (MHF) have shown that in mentalist societies, mental distress is a shame-inducing condition that stigmatizes the persons affected (Lewis, 2010, pp. 160–162; Limburg, 2011, p. 5). In *The Woman Who Thought Too Much*, Limburg elaborates on how in the history of psychology and psychiatry, persons with obsessions and compulsions were pathologized and stigmatized—that is, how they were regarded as suffering from " 'psychaesthenia', a deficiency in psychic (that is, mental), energy," from "degeneracy" or from "a more-than-averagely frenzied id, a weak, frightened ego, and a rather over-zealous, or 'sadistic' superego, which draws its violent power directly from the id," in short, from a "crazy illness [Freud, ibid.]" (Limburg, 2011, pp. 92–96). However, the pathologizing and stigmatization of persons with obsessions and compulsions is not a thing of the past. Biopsychiatry and neuroscience have insisted that obsessions and compulsions are caused by an "abnormal brain," a "dysfunctional basal ganglia," an "abnormal serotonin system" that must be medicalized or is in need of a behavioral " 'manual gearshift' " (to use Jeffrey Schwartz's term) in order to function "normally" (Limburg, 2011, pp. 288, 295–296).

Limburg's and Green's autobiographies show that in addition to its general medicalization of mental distress, medical discourse pathologizes behaviors that are linked with femininity. As feminist critics have argued, the female body has been medicalized for a long time in Western societies (e.g., through the "diagnosis" of "hysteria") in ways in which the male body has not—that is, femininity (in contrast to masculinity) was regarded as "pathological" in itself (Ussher, 2013, p. 63). Reading Limburg's and Green's books, one cannot but note that this medicalization of the female body is still not overcome in psychiatric practice today, a fact that is emphasized by Jane M. Ussher in her discussion of the gender bias in psychiatric nosology (Ussher, 2013, p. 64). As Hilary Mantel has fittingly observed in her review of Limburg's memoir that discusses Limburg's depiction of how mental distress in women is pathologized, "perhaps the trouble was womanhood? [. . .] Is Limburg's malady social, then? One GP tells her 'It comes from thinking too much'" (Mantel, 2010).[7] Green's and Limburg's autobiographies are texts that relate to the long history of this stigmatization and shaming of the female body through its medicalization. However, precisely because of this long history, both authors challenge this stigma by writing about it, by airing the problems related to this medicalization of the female body. Today, the majority of persons diagnosed with borderline personality disorder (BPD) like Sandra M. Dean (alias Amanda Green) are women (Ussher, 2013, p. 64; Wirth-Cauchon, 2001, pp. 5, 56, 66, 78, 87). There is a more equal distribution among genders when it comes to the diagnosis of OCD (Limburg's diagnosis as well as Green's) (Lochner et al., 2004). According to the 2016 MHF report, however, British women are almost twice as likely as men to be diagnosed with anxiety disorders and are more likely to be diagnosed with OCD than men (MHF, 2016, pp. 15, 18).[8] Suicidality among women with mental illnesses is lower than among men (among men it is increasing) (MHF, 2016, p. 22).

Writing about shame has a strong impact on concepts of gender identity. In women, it is regarded as having a "defeminizing effect" that can free a transformational energy that disrupts normative concepts of femininity (Mitchell, 2013, pp. 309, 312, 325). Limburg's and Green's texts on shame are characterized by such transformational energy—that is, by the impulse to externalize (to write about) the shame connected to the psychiatric medicalization of neurodiversity, to make it a part of discourse. In this way, their memoirs do not triumph over shame but instead transform their audience's assumptions about mental distress and challenge shame-inducing social norms. They disrupt mentalist, severely gendered concepts of mental illness as well as the highly damaging stereotypes that endorse the pathology of the "shameless," "mad" writer who disregards or is ignorant of moral norms.

Although Limburg and Green both accept their diagnoses (Green, 2013, p. 289; Limburg, 2011, pp. 8 17–18, 29, 140),[9] they show the arbitrariness and fluidity of such classifications, question the binarism of "mental health" versus "mental illness" (Green, 2013, pp. 295, 434; Limburg, 2011, pp. 72–73, 315–316), and focus on the social causes of mental distress: in Limburg's case bullying, oppression of mental difference, rigid gender norms, oppression of women, antisemitism, and the pressure to perform her identity in accordance with gendered, mentalist social expectations (Limburg, 2011, pp. 1–4, 33–35, 61–67, 72–73) and in Green's case a rape, the stigma of growing up with a mother diagnosed with schizophrenia, bullying, lack of social support, and an invalidating social environment (Green, 2013, pp. 13, 30, 71–77, 351, 427–428).

Shame in Female Authors' Mental Distress Autobiographies

Mental distress autobiographies are not spontaneous disclosures of their authors' states of mind. Rather, they are carefully constructed responses to a long history of oppression, humiliation, silencing, invalidation, and objectification—that is, to experiences of being written about and of being categorized, diagnosed, and medicalized by psychiatrists and other health care professionals as well as by laypersons. According to Katie Rose Guest Pryal,

> [t]he psychiatrically disabled have long suffered exclusion from public life. Historically, doctors have isolated the psychiatrically disabled in asylums [. . .]. Today, the psychiatrically disabled continue to be denied civic participation: they are dismissed as criminals, committed patients, or simply unreliable observers of their world. [. . .] Psychiatric disabilities, even mild ones, or ones that respond well to treatment—mark a person as unreasonable [. . .], producing an unreliable ethos for the mentally ill. (Guest Pryal, 2010, pp. 479–480)

Authors of mental illness autobiographies challenge this rhetorical exclusion; they seek to break or at least lift the silence, to share their stories, and to fight stigma (Green, 2013, pp. 10, 27, 392; Green, 2014, pp. 56–57; Limburg, 2011, p. 11). The act of breaking public silence is very challenging for authors, not only because writing about mental distress can be retraumatizing and can trigger distress in the authors themselves as well as in their readers (Green, 2013, pp. 7, 14), but also because the authors put themselves (and their families and friends) at risk by acknowledging their personal history of mental illness, a fact that might lead not only to a questioning of the "reliability" and "truth" of their narratives but also to ostracization, discrimination, assaults, loss of career options, and other social disadvantages. "Amanda Green" is a pseudonym adopted by Sandra M. Dean (as she announced in a post on her website on November 3, 2014 that is no longer accessible, because she wanted to avoid stigmatization; Green,2014, p. 46). Limburg states that outing oneself by writing an autobiography on mental distress is a risk ("you'll think hard beforehand about how much you have to lose"), but she also argues (not without irony) that as the mentioning of her profession (poet) "is usually quite enough by itself to interrupt the flow of easy social intercourse," the risk may not be so great after all (Limburg, 2011, pp. 5, 10–11). In addition to the stigma of writing about mental illness in general, Limburg states that especially among literary authors, writing autobiography is considered a shameful occupation. Autobiography is regarded as a second-rate choice, something you do if you cannot produce a "proper" novel: "Novels were what proper writers wrote, and to write a memoir instead seemed, by contrast, like a failure of imagination, of creativity. It was a lesser form [. . .] and a narcissistic form at that; it was an act of unadulterated exhibitionism" (Limburg, 2011, p. 320). Limburg's friend, a novelist and "life-writing sceptic," encourages her to write a memoir that does not follow the conventional plot line with a redemptive ending. Not least in response to this suggestion, Limburg embraces the shamed genre, infusing it with creativity, imaginativeness, poetry, novelty, sensitivity, humor, and daringness.

Joanne Limburg's *The Woman Who Thought Too Much* (2010)

Limburg studied sociology, political science, and creative writing. She is a successful poet, novelist, and autobiographer. *The Woman Who Thought Too Much* was shortlisted for Mind Book of the Year Award in 2011. It is written in an essayistic style and is marked by a tentative approach to mental distress. Limburg uses thematic chapter headings ("Shame," "Nightmares," "Avoidance," "Losses") that are arranged in a largely (but not strictly) chronological order. The text includes different narrative voices (voices of persons describing their compulsions and obsessions quoted from the Padua Inventory, a self-report measure of obsessive and compulsive behaviors, voices of GPs, psychiatrists, therapists, teachers, classmates, parents, friends, etc.) expressing different viewpoints on OCD and other mental illnesses. Limburg uses quotations from the Padua Inventory at the beginning of every chapter and excerpts from diagnoses and medical reports on herself as well as from psychiatric literature (e.g., by Sigmund Freud, Melanie Klein, Marion Milner, and Judith L. Rapoport). She quotes passages from feminist literature (especially from Simone de Beauvoir's *The Second Sex*), pop and rock songs (e.g., by Morrissey, Eels, and Dan Hicks), nursery rhymes, novels (e.g., from Virginia Woolf's *Jacob's Room*), and from Samuel Johnson's *Prayers and Meditations*. In addition, Limburg references Dante's *Divina Commedia*, Sylvia Plath's poetry, the odes on melancholy by Coleridge and Keats, movies and plays (e.g., *The Aviator*, *As Good As it Gets*, *Dirty Filthy Love*), and Camus's writings on suicide.

In the first chapter (entitled "Shame"), the narrating "I" describes her early experiences at school as a silent, introverted, serious child with a stammer who pronounced that she had "a broken heart" after her grandmother's death. As a consequence of this admission of difference she was bullied and called "mad" by one of her playmates (Limburg, 2011, pp. 2, 18, 22). Although Limburg gives no final explanation of the cause of her distress, her memoir points to its social origins, describing it as a response to rigid gender and beauty norms: The narrating "I" relates how she thought of herself as "a boy deep down," experiencing the pressure to wear female underwear as a "punishment." She expresses resistance against being a "nice Jewish girl" and against becoming a traditional, "good Jewish woman" who is content with being a housewife (Limburg, 2011, pp. 34–35, see also pp. 26–37). Furthermore, Limburg's narrating "I" internalizes the negative social images of women as deficient, considering her female body not only as "humiliation enough in itself" but also as failing the requirements of female beauty norms (Limburg, 2011, p. 42). She depicts her compulsive self-harming (skin-picking) as a sign of her empathetic identification with the victims of patriarchal oppression, the victims of violence against women as well as with the victims of antisemitism (Limburg, 2011, p. 57). The narrating "I" gives very detailed descriptions of her episodes of skin-picking and her feelings of shame. Hilary Mantel praised Limburg's memoir for its honesty but felt the need to protect its author: "Can a writer be too honest? At times you want to close this book to protect its subject from your scrutiny" (Mantel, 2010). However, the scenes about skin-picking are not spontaneous disclosures of the "truth" about the author that was hidden in shame, although many readers may be voyeuristically attracted by the text precisely because they expect to find this "truth" in it. The scenes are carefully constructed and convey their transformational energy by giving rise to unexpected narrative connections as well as unusual representations of mental distress in women: Initially, the narrating "I" refers to the self-description of OCD sufferers as "conscientious," shy, rule- and "law-abiding," introverted, acceptance-seeking, "'reward-dependent'" persons (Limburg, 2011, p. 8). However, by verbalizing and dwelling on the narrated "I"'s scenes of skin-picking that happened in the year before her long-planned jaw operation, which she expected with "horror" (Limburg, 2011, p. 55), the narrating "I" creates a depiction of herself as a person with OCD who is not exclusively shy or introverted. Although (or precisely because) she does not simply overcome or master her shame, she surprises her readers with stirring, daring, and unsettling reflections and narrative connections that invite a plenitude of affective responses, ranging from empathy, interest, excitement, vicarious shame, anger, and fear to disgust:[10]

> At any time [. . .] my hand might absently push my sleeve up; then I will rub up and down my upper arm, scanning for any rough bits, any bumps, any scabs or bits of dry skin. [. . .] sometimes I would make a bigger cut, one which somehow I could not allow to heal. There is a crater-shaped scar above my left eyebrow, which I made the summer I was seventeen; that was the summer my great-aunt Ann told me that I was a pretty girl, that I had classic features, but I insisted that I could not possibly be described that way—not when I was Marked [. . .]. That was also the summer when I had a volunteer job in the office of an organization which campaigned for the rights of Soviet Jews. (Limburg, 2011, pp. 55–57)

In the following passage, the narrating "I" dwells on the shame and heightened self-consciousness that the narrated "I" experienced:

> From the start, I was disgusted with my skin habit—"You were *picking*, weren't you!"—and ashamed in general of the way that I seemed to be wasting my life, [. . .] picking and ruminating. [. . .] I was aware that the picking gratified me in some way and this seemed worse than just

little-girl disgusting; it had to be sexually perverse. It didn't hurt while I was doing it, and often I seemed to be in a kind of trance [. . .]. While I did so I would sometimes be distantly aware of a desire to get rid of irritating abnormalities, to get what the cosmetic adverts call the "impurities" out of my skin . . . (Limburg, 2011, p. 58)

Limburg's courses of studies in psychology encouraged her to read her habit as a sign with a deeper interpersonal, cultural, and political meaning (resistance against female beauty norms and against unbearable social and cultural conditions, identification with the victims of antisemitism), as something "terrible and exciting," something "dark and interesting," that she could intimately share (or not share) with her friends, as the narrating "I" describes retrospectively with a considerable amount of self-irony:

There was my disfigured soul mirrored in my skin, and if anyone could see it and accept it, then they would accept and understand me totally and utterly [. . .]. Now and then I would tell another girl about the picking, for attention, and for sympathy, and to be told that I shouldn't do it. I also hoped, I think, that perhaps they would say that nobody as beautiful as I should despoil herself in this way—which of course they never did. [. . .] I took great pride in my deep, dark and interesting sufferings and was appalled by the thought of someone ripping them away from me. I believed my fears and my depression: they were there to tell me that I was living in unacceptable social and cultural conditions and only when these were lifted could I experience any real happiness. (Limburg, 2011, pp. 60–62)

By quoting from Simone de Beauvoir's passages on a girl's self-harming behavior, Limburg establishes a semantic frame that generates a high degree of ambivalence. According to de Beauvoir, the girl's

sado-masochistic aberrations involve a basic insincerity; if the girl lets herself practice them, it means she accepts, through her repudiation, the womanly future in store for her; she would not mutilate her flesh with hatred if she had not first recognized herself as flesh. (Limburg, 2011, pp. 62–63)

Limburg's narrative sequence on the shame of self-harming, a shame probably felt the more intensely because of the very fact that it is a habit so severely censured by her role model de Beauvoir, unleashes unexpected transformational energy and shows that the body marked by compulsory skin-picking is a multivalent, often contradictory form of (self-)contact and communication as well as of a failed or disrupted communication. Limburg does not argue that self-harm is a precondition for or a necessary side effect of political activism. Instead, she shows that she understood self-harm as a highly ambiguous sign of (internalized) oppression and resistance a sign of sexual desire and of its absence (a sign of the desire for purity), a sign of vulnerability and of (the desire for) invulnerability, a sign of the desire for contact and of a desire for demarcation, a sign of fear, disgust, shame, pride, interest, excitement, and release. I would like to suggest that Limburg challenges de Beauvoir's reading of women's self-harming behavior as evidence of their insincere feminist position, of their inability to live up to feminist conviction, and of their inability to see themselves as anything other than "flesh" (Limburg, 2011, pp. 62–63). Limburg releases the transformational energy of her scene of shame by externalizing her shame—that is, by writing about it, by bringing it into discourse: She dwells on the embodied details of her compulsions ("the shame of not being able to control yourself like a normal, sensible person would"; Limburg, 2011, p.10), highlights her own shameful self-awareness as well as her own political consciousness (about oppressive gender and beauty norms, antisemitism), and thereby challenges de Beauvoir's shame-inducing representation of self-harm in women. Limburg's autobiography creates an image of a woman who, according to de Beauvoir's description, could not exist—that is, a portrait of a feminist (or, as Limburg herself emphasizes with self-irony, of a "teenage fundamentalist") who cannot stop herself from engaging in self-harming behavior (Limburg, 2011, p. 65).

Limburg describes many instances in which she experienced severely gendered forms of humiliations. Her GP simply stated that her depression was caused by "thinking too much" and could be overcome if Limburg found a boyfriend (Limburg, 2011, p. 99). She retorts years later, using this label ironically in the title of her book. A similar strategy of resistance can be found in the scene in which the narrating "I" describes the narrated "I" 's difficulties of establishing trust and a real communication with her psychoanalyst. When she told her analyst about her self-hatred, she was put down. This subversion of trust resulted in an act of withdrawal on the narrated "I" 's side that is turned into a verbal act of resistance by the narrating "I":

I said at one point that I was not only cruel to my own body, but that I had hypercritical thoughts about other women's although I never voiced them, in compensation for my supposed super-unkindness. "So *I* can breathe a sigh of relief, then!" she said. From that moment on I never entirely trusted her. But I couldn't quite admit this to myself, let alone to her. I just kept turning up and saying only what I thought would be safe for her to hear. One day, I spent at least a minute watching in fascinated horror as a huge, hairy spider crept across the floor, between her legs and then under the chair. She didn't ask why I was staring at her feet like that and I didn't tell her. (Limburg, 2011, pp. 106–107)

Limburg gives many examples of scenes in which she and other people in mental distress hide in shame: At the beginning of her chapter entitled "Avoidance," she quotes American psychiatrist Judith L. Rapoport's statement "When it gets bad, the patients hide" and adds her own reflections. Although she subscribes to Rapoport's observation, Limburg emphasizes that her silences in such situations are not related to the intention to willfully deceive or to withhold information but to a deep insecurity about her condition: "When people ask me how I am, I usually do the correct thing and say, 'Fine, thanks.' I'm never sure if I mean it though" (Limburg, 2011, p. 176).

In the final chapter, entitled "Losses," readers are confronted with a form of silence that strains the communication between narrator and reader. Here, shame (defined as the disrupted communication by Silvan Tomkins, see above) becomes a radical silence between brother and sister that severs the conversation as he was not able to express his problems towards her. The memoir ends not only with a paralipsis—that is, with Limburg's brother's omission of the reasons for his suicide in the imagined phone call between him and the narrated "I"—but with a silence that resonates with readers as they come to share the author's lack of knowledge about these reasons:

A couple of weeks after my brother died, I had a dream about him. I was at one of the innumerable dream versions of my mother's house, when the phone rang. She picked it up, listened, and turned white. "It's your brother," she said. I told her to give the phone to me, took it into the downstairs toilet, and locked the door. Then we had one of our normal, bantering conversations, and laughed together, entirely as if nothing had happened. We kept this up for five minutes or so, and then there was a pause. I felt something change, in the dream atmosphere, and in me, and then I asked him, "So why did you do it?" There was a silence. "Do *what*?" he asked, as if he really didn't know. "*You* know," I said. There was another silence and when he spoke again, he sounded as he had done in our last waking conversation: guarded, offhand, evasive. "I got distracted," he gabbled. "Things were distracting me. Look—I have to go now—bye!" Then he hung up, and I think that's as much of an answer as I'm ever going to get. (Limburg, 2011, pp. 320–321)

Limburg's text provides readers with some pieces of information about her brother's life in the United States that allow them to speculate about the reasons of this suicide (e.g., about the impact of his adult attention-deficit/hyperactivity disorder diagnosis, his medication with amphetamines and his symptoms of withdrawal, pressure to perform at work, the fear that he will not get tenure due to his diagnosis, his debts, and his depression), but it gives no final answer to the question why he committed suicide (Limburg, 2011, pp. 317–318). The ending of the memoir suggests that there was no way to bridge certain shame-related distances that existed between Limburg and her brother. These distances and gaps in communication manifest themselves strongly at the end of the memoir, but they can be felt throughout. Limburg's brother has a shadowy form of existence in the book; it is not fully silenced, but readers learn very little about him: "My brother haunts the book, but mostly by his absence," she writes in her recent memoir *Small Pieces: A Book of Lamentations* (2017, p. 115).

Limburg's autobiography shows that neither her mental distress nor her shame is overcome at the end. Commenting on her relationship with her husband, she admits that her anxieties are still intense ("Love makes us so vulnerable") and that they became worse during pregnancy and led to a miscarriage because of the enormous stress they caused her (Limburg, 2011, pp. 205, 227, 235.) After she gave birth, her husband had to do most of the work at home and earn the money, whereas she regarded herself a failure because she did not dare to take care of her son because she feared that she could harm him (Limburg, 2011, pp. 258, 263, 265–266).

Instead of mastering the shame attached to mental distress, the ending of Limburg's memoir confronts readers with new scenes of shame, for example the shame connected to Limburg's "failure" of "merely" writing "narcissistic" autobiography, the shame or guilt of not having been able to break the silence between herself and her brother, of not having found the courage to fly to the United States to see him (she calls herself a "[s]tupid, selfish woman"), of not having trusted her gut feeling about his withdrawal from her, of not having been able to save him from death as a "proper" sister would have done (Limburg, 2011, p. 317; see Limburg's poem "Sister," which opens *Small Pieces*). The feelings of guilt and shame are transferred and transformed, unfolding their energy in *Small Pieces*, where she traces her brother's life. In this text, Limburg relies on the Jewish tradition of morning *tikkun olam*, a practice of prayers and meditations that aims at an acceptance of shame, guilt, ambivalence, fragmentariness, loss, and (partial) silence and that expresses the hope for a reparation of the world's brokenness (Limburg, 2017, p. 15).

Amanda Green: *My Alien Self: My Journey Back to Me* (2013)

Like Limburg, Amanda Green (born in 1973 into a British working-class family) breaks the silence that surrounds the stigma and shame of mental distress (in her case related to her diagnosis with BPD and OCD). Green's self-published memoir is a collage of readings of fragments from her old diaries, of photos, poems, aphorisms, medical diagnoses, psychiatrists' reports and letters, school reports, short text messages, email conversations, and spoken dialogues. She is a collector of snippets from her own life, an ethnographer of the self. Her act of narrating her life is a practice of reading its fragments (Green, 2013, p. 12).

Green's text contains many passages that depict the shame connected to the display of behavior that is considered inappropriate. The narrating "I" describes a scene in which she masturbated in class at the age of nine. She dwells on the shame the narrated "I" experienced because of her teacher's and her classmates' responses to her behavior:

"Amanda, can I have a word?" said my teacher. "It's about the thing you do in class. It's very wrong and it has to stop." I didn't know it was called masturbation. [. . .] What *was* masturbation? All I knew was that it felt good. [. . .] My legs shook and splayed faster and faster [. . .] and then it would come—[. . .] a wave of pleasure in my parts and throughout my body [. . .]. I would come back to the real world of the school classroom again—friends looking strangely at me, in shock, surprise or a look that implied I was weird. [. . .] I knew something was not quite right with these actions, but I didn't know what, other than the fact that no-one else did it. All I knew was that the comfort it gave was wonderful. I had problems in my head: confusion, loneliness and fear of being bullied at home and in school, and this helped me to deal with them and escape for a few minutes. (Green, 2013, pp. 40–41)

Two years later, her classmates humiliated her because of her actions:

> "*Amanda likes masturbating, Amanda likes masturbating!*" They'd chant as I walked to school. They would crowd around me in a group and enjoy the whole process of humiliation. Smirking, their eyes full of pleasure and faint viciousness; they'd laugh out loud, taking in their power as a group, against little old me who was wiped of pride and life in those moments. (Green, 2013, pp. 40–41)

Although Green was diagnosed with BPD only in 2008, the narrating "I" already links her behavior as a child to the "symptoms" of the disorder (impulsive behavior concerning sex; Green, 2013, pp. 50–51). As her narrative continues, she relates many of her experiences to further "symptoms" (unstable relationships, variable self-image, impulsive behaviors concerning drugs, eating, driving, easily triggered anger). As Janet Wirth-Cauchon has shown, the definition of BPD in the *Diagnostic and Statistical Manual of Mental Disorders* IV (DSM-IV) pathologizes personalities and personal life styles that often simply deviate from social norms and are common among many people (Green, 2013, pp. 50–51; Wirth-Cauchon, 2001, pp. 58, 73, 87–90, 145, 149–150, 177). Is it possible to show that the diagnosis simultaneously trivializes the suffering of the individual through reducing the complex experiences and possible traumas to unidimensional diagnostic criteria? In her memoir, Green addresses and in part challenges this medicalization. She strategically provokes the voyeurism and excitement of her readers, symbolized by the book jacket cover design showing a keyhole. Furthermore, she invokes the mentalist stereotype of the emotionally unstable, irresponsible, promiscuous, sexually adventurous BPD personality on the blurb of her book. *My Alien Self* does not disappoint its readers' expectations: It contains detailed descriptions of mood swings, severe depression, suicidality, drug abuse, verbal and physical fights between Green and her boyfriends, and descriptions of a high number of sexual contacts, including the passages that describe her rape (Green, 2013, pp. 67–78, 299–302). Far from desexualizing, condemning, or pathologizing her own behavior in the masturbation scene quoted above, the narrating "I" adopts the perspective of the narrated "I" and thereby invites readers to empathize with her. Using the technique of interior monologue,[11] the narrating "I" describes her behavior as a source of comfort and relief, as a way in which she dealt with her family's problems that were caused by the hospitalization of her mother (by her mother's experiences of electroconvulsive shocks and ice-cold baths in therapy) and by the lack of social support that her working-class family experienced (Green, 2013, pp. 27, 30, 325, 326, 422).

On the one hand, passages like the one quoted above seem to endorse prevalent stereotypes about BPD. Many readers may simply enjoy the sexual scenes rather than question the stigma of BPD. However, the scenes that depict her "shameful" behavior have an interesting, highly ambivalent effect: Readers find themselves in the productively uncomfortable position of being confronted with what is commonly considered to be "abnormal," "immoral" behavior—and of enjoying the process of reading about it. As Green represents these incidents through the lens of her BPD diagnosis, readers will find themselves oscillating between enjoyment, fascination, interest, and excitement on the one hand and rejection, disgust, and (self-)condemnation on the other. By invoking her readers' interest, excitement, as well as empathy, Green not only challenges stereotypical images of the "immoral" (and mostly female) BPD personality but also unsettles the binary opposition between "normal" and "abnormal" (sexual) behavior.

My Alien Self is less coherent and much more fragmentary in its narrative structure than Limburg's memoir. In many cases, the conspicuous graphic gaps, temporal ellipses, and paralipses in Green's text represent states of dissociation from painful and frightening life experiences (including a rape). At times, the self the narrating "I" encounters when reading her old diaries seems alien to her (Green, 2013, p. 144). Green acknowledges the fragmentariness of her memory that is connected to her mental distress. At the same time, however, she points to the fragmentariness of everybody's memories of childhood: "now it's a haze in my memory. So long ago. But I still remember the feeling of being lost. *We remember only fragments of childhood*" (Green, 2013, pp. 21–22, emphasis in the original). Here, Green subverts the clear distinction between a "reliable" and an "unreliable" narrator and challenges the binary opposition of "mental illness" and "health" that informs mentalist discourse, establishing a speaking position that is so often contested, pathologized, and invalidated in psychiatric literature as well as in public discourse (Guest Pryal, 2010, pp. 479–480). The ellipses and paralipses in Green's memoir activate readers to empathize with the narrated

"I" as well as the narrating "I" to fill the narrative gaps with their imagination of how she might have felt or what might have happened. In the scene that depicts how doctors refused to take Green on as a client when she asked for help and declared that she was suicidal and that describes how Green called the Samaritans (a crisis helpline), she uses this technique of narrative fragmentation through ellipses and paralipses to establish a very intimate relationship with readers:

> I'm not sure what I did next, as I was in a haze, but I do remember calling the *Samaritans* to ask them for help. The call didn't go well, as I couldn't seem to tell them just how suicidal I felt. It was hard to break down like that; to expose my weakness.
>
> *No matter how desperate we feel we hold some of it in.*
>
> Thankfully, I came out of the darkness shortly after, for just long enough to find the strength to walk back into the surgery that I had left years before [. . .] I finally found someone who would listen. (Green, 2013, pp. 226–227; emphasis in original)

Here, the fragmentary communication (visualized by graphic gaps) indicates the narrator's inability to communicate the experiences of suffering and despair to her readers. The aphorism embedded between two graphic gaps points to inexpressible affects, to emotional states that may *always* be held within, that may *always* be beyond verbalization, alerting her envisioned readers (including doctors, psychiatrists, psychotherapists, and medical staff members; see Green, 2014, p. 57) to the experience that persons in mental distress *never* express the full impact of their feelings. The passage in which Green alludes to her inability to communicate her distress when she called the Samaritans demonstrates the complex oscillation between communication, silence, and ineffability that is characteristic of shame as a form of communication. Green admits that she denied her suicidal thoughts in an interview with her psychotherapist and explains that she was too ashamed to tell how desperate she felt (Green, 2013, pp. 431, 450–451). In another passage, she states that she often looked too well to get medical support (Green, 2013, p. 353). In this context, appeals that therapists must create a holding, compassionate environment and should watch closely for implicit and explicit signs of shame in their clients are very important, but as Limburg's and Green's memoirs show, the general practice of therapy is very different from this ideal (Sinha, 2017, pp. 260–263).

Limburg's and Green's memoirs demonstrate that because of the stigma and shame attached to mental illness, it is hard—often impossible—for sufferers to fully express their mental distress in oral conversations with family members and friends as well as with their psychiatrists, psychologists, GPs, and nurses. However, the texts also illustrate that writing about mental distress and the shame and stigma connected with it is an alternative form of expression that can lead to a significant improvement of the authors' mental conditions. Furthermore, reading mental distress autobiographies can enable person-centered care, alerting clinicians to the ambiguous, fragmented form of communication that is typical of narratives infused by shame—that is, to harmful aspects of mental distress (e.g., suicidality and drug abuse) that clients find too painful to share openly and directly.

Conclusion

Limburg's and Green's memoirs show that the predicament of the stigma and shame attached to mental illness can indeed be "air[ed]" by writing about them (Limburg 2011, p. 11). However, both texts also demonstrate that the stigma and shame surrounding mental illness cannot be overcome by individual narrative acts. *The Woman Who Thought Too Much* and *My Alien Self* emphasize that the self is not a transparent, unified entity and that there are limitations to one's capacity to fully control one's affects (see also Tomkins, 1995a, p. 62), especially one's ability to stop oneself from feeling shame about behaviors that are regarded as "abnormal" in medical as well as public discourse. Furthermore, both texts show that memoirs (and especially mental distress memoirs and women's practices of self-representation) are part of a genre tradition that is strongly linked to shame, voyeurism, and self-performance (Green, 2013, p. 292, cover blurb; Limburg, 2011, p. 320; Smith & Watson, 2012, pp. 3–5). The combination of a multiplicity of heterogeneous perspectives on mental distress in Limburg's and Green's memoirs (especially their inclusion of quotations from diagnoses, medical reports, references to the DSM-IV, and the narrating and narrated "I"'s critical responses to them)[12] generates unpredictable, uncontrollable, and highly ambivalent readings as well as intra- and intertextual connections. Not least, Limburg's and Green's memoirs critically address the fact that the shame-inducing social structures are still very much in place.

The Woman Who Thought Too Much and *My Alien Self* exemplify central aspects of shame as a highly ambivalent form of communication that is characterized by narrative discontinuity, fragmentation, and the desire for (re)connection. Limburg's text is marked by a more coherent narrative style, whereas Green's text is highly fragmentary and again and again alerts readers to the ineffability of the suffering and shame that surround mental distress. My analysis shows that the scenes of shame in both texts (related to the embodied "symptoms" of mental distress, sexuality, social interaction, and writing) do not display an overcoming or mastery of shame. Instead, they emit a transformational energy that produces unexpected representations of women in mental distress, becoming-events, startling narrative connections, as well as meditations on the sociocultural sources of shame that challenge the binary opposition between "mental illness" and "mental health." Furthermore, they enable reader responses that are marked by affective plenitude, ranging from (vicarious) shame, disgust, surprise, anger, fear, and distress to interest, excitement, and joy or pleasure, and that oscillate between identification, empathy, and distancing. Because of their capacity to give firsthand testimony about the impact of diagnoses and therapies but also about the needs of users, mental distress memoirs like Green's and Limburg's can be an indispensable contribution to the education of practitioners.

Notes

1. On the role of stigma for shame, see Goffman (1990, pp. 33–36) and Sedgwick (1993, p. 4).
2. "Ableism" is "social stigma and oppression against the physically different" and "mentalism" is the "social stigma and oppression against mental difference." I use the terms in accordance with Lewis (2010, p. 162).
3. On shame-based therapy and its goal to reduce the proneness to pathological shame, see Sinha (2017, pp. 251–275, 262, 265, 269).
4. "Since the experience of shame is all but inevitable in the development of human beings, a critical part of the rewarding socialization of shame and self-contempt must consist in teaching the child the double skills of tolerating his own shame and in overcoming the source of it" (Tomkins, 2008, pp. 451–454; see also p. 456).
5. For similar approaches that highlight the role of shame as a motivator for political and cultural change (especially a change in media representation of mental illness), see Hinshaw (2006).
6. Genette describes a literary character's shameful thought (Octave's thought about his impotence in Stendhal's *Armance*) as an example for paralipsis.

7. In my analysis, I use the terms "women" and "men" as performative, non-essentialist concepts in accordance with Judith Butler (1988).
8. Limburg's condition is very anxiety-related (Limburg, 2010, pp. 176–178, 221, 238) and is related to depression (Limburg 2010, pp. 214–215).
9. Limburg even diagnoses herself with OCD, which is confirmed during her pregnancy.
10. I follow Silvan Tomkins's classification of affects (see Tomkins, 1995a, p. 74). On vicarious shame, see Tomkins (2008, pp. 407–408): "One may feel shame because the other feels shame, but also under circumstances in which the self would feel shame, even if the other does not."
11. I follow the definition by Edouard Dujardin as quoted by Genette (see Genette, 1983, p. 174, n. 18): "a discourse without an auditor and unspoken, by which a character expresses his most intimate thoughts." Genette prefers the notion *immediate speech*, speech "emancipated from all narrative patronage" (Genette, 1983, pp. 173–174).
12. On references to the DSM see Limburg (2010, pp. 315–316) and Green (2013, pp. 49–51, 289, 434, 477–481).

References

Berlant, L. (2015). Crossover/Combover: A Performance Piece. *Berfrois*: 18 April. N. p. Web. Access 28 Decemer 2022. <https://www.berfrois.com/2015/04/vaulting-ambit ion/>.

Bouson, J. B. (2009). *Embodied shame: Uncovering female shame in contemporary women's writings*. State University of New York.

Bouson, J. B. (2016). *Shame and the aging woman: Confronting and resisting ageism in contemporary women's writings*. Palgrave Macmillan.

Brown, B. (2012). *Daring greatly*. Gotham Books.

Butler, J. (1988). Performative acts of gender constitution: An essay in phenomenology and feminist theory. *Theatre Journal*, 40(4), 519–531.

Clare, E. (2015). *Exile and pride: Disability, queerness, and liberation* (3rd ed.). Duke University Press.

Damásio, A. R. (1999). *The feeling of what happens: Body and emotion in the making of consciousness*. Harcourt Brace and Company.

Genette, G. (1983). *Narrative discourse: An essay in method* (trans. J. E. Lewin). Cornell University Press.

Green, A. (2013). *My alien self: My journey back to me* (ed. D. Hobbs-Wyatt). Amanda Green.

Green, A. (2014). *39* (ed. D. Hobbs-Wyatt). Amanda Green.

Guest Pryal, K. R. (2010). The genre of the mood memoir and the ethos of psychiatric disability. *Rhetoric Society Quarterly*, 40(5), 479–501.

Hinshaw, S. P. (2006). *The mark of shame: Stigma of mental illness and an agenda for change*. Oxford University Press.

Hotz-Davies, I. (2007). Scham in den Romanen Jane Austens, oder: Wie die Gender-Studies auf den Affekt gekommen sind. In I. Hotz-Davies & S. Schahardat (Eds.), *Ins Wort gesetzt, ins Bild gesetzt: Gender in der Wissenschaft, Kunst und Literatur* (pp. 181–206). Transcript.

Lelwica, M. M. (2017). *Shameful bodies: Religion and the culture of physical improvement.* Bloomsbury.

Lewis, B. (2010). A mad fight: Psychiatry and disability activism. In L. J. Davis (Ed.), *The disability studies reader* (pp. 160–176). Routledge.

Lewis, H. B. (1971). Shame and guilt in neurosis. *Psychoanalytic Review, 58*(3), 419–438.

Lewis, M. (2011). The self-conscious emotions. *Encyclopedia on early childhood development.* Institute for the Study of Child Development. UMDNJ-Robert Wood Johnson Medical School, Child Health Institute USA.

Limburg, J. (2011). *The woman who thought too much: A memoir of obsession and compulsion.* Atlantic Books.

Limburg, J. (2017). *Small pieces: A book of lamentations.* Atlantic Books.

Lochner, C., Hemmings, S. M. J., & Kinnear, C. J. (2004). Gender in obsessive-compulsive disorder: Clinical and genetic findings. *European Neuropsychopharmacology, 14,* 105–113.

Mantel, H. (2010, May 15). *The woman who thought too much*: A memoir by Joanne Limburg: A clear-eyed exposé of life with a compulsive disorder impresses Hilary Mantel. *The Guardian.* https://www.theguardian.com/books/2010/may/15/woman-who-thought-joanne-limburg

Mental Health Foundation. (2016). *Fundamental facts about mental health 2016.* Mental Health Foundation.

Mitchell, K. (2013). Cleaving to the scene of shame: Stigmatized childhoods in "The End of Alice" and "Two Girls, Fat and Thin." *Contemporary Women's Writing, 7*(3), 309–327.

Munt, S. R. (2008). *Queer attachments: The cultural politics of shame.* Ashgate.

Nosek, M., Kennedy, H. P., & Gudmundsdottir, M. (2010). Silence, stigma, and shame: A postmodern analysis of distress during menopause. *Advances in Nursing Science, 33*(3), E24–E36.

Probyn, E. (2005). *Blush: Faces of shame.* Minnesota University Press.

Sedgwick, E. K. (1993). Queer performativity: Henry James's The Art of the Novel. *GLQ, 1*(1), 1–16.

Sedgwick, E. K. (2003). Shame, theatricality, and queer performativity: Henry James's The Art of the Novel. In E. K. Sedgwick (Ed.), *Touching feeling: Affect, pedagogy, performativity* (pp. 35–66). Duke University Press.

Sedgwick, E. K., & Frank, A. (1995). Shame in the cybernetic fold: Reading Silvan Tomkins. In E. K. Sedgwick & A. Frank (Eds.), *Shame and its sisters: A Silvan Tomkins reader* (pp. 1–28). Duke University Press.

Sinha, M. (2017). Shame in psychotherapy: Theory, method and practice. In E. Vanderheiden & C. Mayer (Eds.), *The value of shame exploring a health resource in cultural contexts* (pp. 251–275). Springer.

Smith, S., & Watson, J. (2010). *Reading autobiography: A guide for interpreting life narratives* (2nd ed.). University of Minnesota Press.

Smith, S., & Watson, J. (Eds.). (2012). *Interfaces: Women, autobiography, image, performance.* University of Michigan Press.

Tangney, J. P., & Dearing, R. L. (2002). *Shame and guilt.* Guilford Press.

Tomkins, S. S. (1995a). What are affects? In E. K. Sedgwick & A. Frank (Eds.), *Shame and its sisters: A Silvan Tomkins Reader* (pp. 33–74). Duke University Press.

Tomkins, S. S. (1995b). Shame-humiliation and contempt-disgust. In E. K. Sedgwick & A. Frank (Eds.), *Shame and its sisters: A Silvan Tomkins reader* (pp. 133–178). Duke University Press.

Tomkins, S. S. (2008). *Affect imagery consciousness: The complete edition.* Springer Publications.

Ussher, J. M. (2013). Diagnosing difficult women and pathologizing femininity: Gender bias in psychiatric nosology. *Feminism & Psychology, 23*(1), 63–69.

Vanderheiden, E., & Mayer, C. (2017). An introduction to the value of shame: Exploring a health resource in cultural contexts. In E. Vanderheiden & C. Mayer (Eds.), *The value of shame: Exploring a health resource in cultural contexts* (pp. 1–40). Springer.

Wirth-Cauchon, J. (2001). *Woman and borderline personality disorder: Symptoms and stories.* Rutgers University Press.

World Health Organization. (2019). *Mental health.* https://www.who.int/features/factfiles/mental_health/en/

13

Psychic Relief and Nonnarrative
Configurations in Graphic Memoirs
About Mental Health

Lasse R. Gammelgaard

This chapter contributes to scholarly discussions within the health humanities concerning illness narratives and graphic memoirs as two proliferating genres. More specifically, I examine how graphic memoirs about mental illness encompass nonnarrative features that engage in complex ways with the illness narratives being told. Narrative medicine holds the conviction "that narrative competence can widen the clinical gaze to include personal and social elements of patients' lives vital to the tasks of healing" (Charon et al., 2017, p. 1). A cornerstone of narrative medicine is that telling one's story and organizing it into a coherent narrative can help reconfigure the ill person's identity and self-perception in a way that provides comfort and possibly recovery (Williams, 2011, p. 359). It has also been posited that graphic memoirs about illnesses are flourishing because they afford some measure of catharsis for the artist (Williams, 2011). My aim in this chapter is not to try to repudiate those positions. In fact, I do support these positions. Rather, I am claiming that this focus on narrative aspects of illness representations in graphic memoirs has led to an oversight of a number of strategies in graphic memoirs that are not narrative in nature and that are, in some cases, even more central to artists' experiences of auto-therapeutic benefits. I introduce the concept of *nonnarrative configurations* as a catch-all for such abstract, nonnarrative poetic devices, and I explore how they interact with the narrative strategies in a selection of graphic memoirs about mental illness. I analyze passages from three graphic memoirs—Art Spiegelman's *In the Shadow of No Towers* (2004), Terian Koscik's *When Anxiety Attacks* (2016), and Ellen Forney's *Marbles: Mania, Depression, Michelangelo, & Me* (2012)—to make this case, but before I turn to my close readings, I will (1) say something

Lasse R. Gammelgaard, *Psychic Relief and Nonnarrative Configurations in Graphic Memoirs About Mental Health*
In: *Narrative and Mental Health*. Edited by: Jarmila Mildorf, Elisabeth Punzi, and Christoph Singer, Oxford University Press.
© Oxford University Press 2023. DOI: 10.1093/oso/9780197620540.003.0014

general about illness in relation to time and narrative, (2) account for graphic memoirs' propensity to play with the experiencing "I" and the narrating "I" and for catharsis in graphic memoirs, and (3) claim that comics and graphic memoirs have affinities with poetry, and that this generic kinship has been neglected due to the tendency for definitions of comics to align it with narrative in literature and film.

Illness, Narrative, and Graphic Memoir

Attempts at defining what makes something a narrative or makes it possess the quality of narrativity have traditionally been centered on time and more specifically time in relation to plot, which might be defined as events unfolding or progressing over time. It is noteworthy that Gerard Genette's seminal work of structuralist narratology, *Narrative Discourse*, contains three chapters on time and none on, for example, space. Likewise, Paul Ricoeur wrote no less than three books titled *Time and Narrative*. Illness, however, impedes teleology and introduces a rupture in time. Given that "[d]isruption is the rule rather than the exception" (Rimmon-Kenan, 2006, p. 243), Shlomith Rimmon-Kenan asks if illness narratives then "are non-narrative," or if narrative theory should be "rethought in terms of contingency, randomness, and chaos rather than order and regularity?" (2006, p. 243). She appositely describes the battle between order and chaos in illness in the following way:

> The ill person has limited control over both the dictated order and the overwhelming inner disorder. Autobiographical writing about illness may be an attempt to control the uncontrollable, and hence it can become a battleground between the two competing principles. But beyond illness narratives, it also suggests a coexistence of or, better, a collision between regularity and contingency in all narrative. (p. 244)

The same observation is fundamental to Arthur Frank in *The Wounded Storyteller* from 1995. Ill people are presented as wounded storytellers, and Frank then designates three frequently recurring illness narratives: the restitution narrative, in which medicine triumphs over the illness and health is restored; the quest narrative, where the illness is seen as a journey through which something is to be gained; and finally, the chaos narrative, in which chaos prevails and no positive or coherent narrative is constructed. Both Rimmon-Kenan and Frank discuss ill people's attempts at mastery over their illness through narrative means, and they both address the impact of the ill body on the mind's cognitive and emotional faculties. That is, they draw attention to the fact that physical illness has implications for one's mental health. However, to be in ill mental health frustrates narrative comprehension of selfhood just as it affects one's bodily perception. Or vice versa: Ill mental health can develop from a troubled selfhood.

While for the past 20 years or so graphic memoirs (i.e., comics autobiographies) have proliferated, the trend dates all the way back to the 1970s (cf. Gardner, 2008). Many of these graphic memoirs are illness narratives. This has given rise to the interdisciplinary network and research field of graphic medicine, which investigates how comics and graphic pathographies can have an impact on our medical practices and view on health. Numerous graphic memoirs about illnesses are specifically about mental illnesses. Though not at any rate a complete list, graphic memoirs about mental illness comprise Justin Green's *Binky Brown Meets the Holy Virgin Mary* (1972), Art Spiegelman's *Maus I and II* (1973–1991), *Breakdowns: Portrait of the Artist as a Young %@&*!* (2008; a version with less material was published in 1977 under a different title), and *In the Shadow of No Towers* (2004), as well as Alison Bechdel's *Fun Home: A Family Tragicomic* (2006), Allie Brosh's blog/webcomics *Hyperbole and a Half* (2009–), Willy Linthout's *Years of the Elephant* (2009), Darryl Cunningham's *Psychiatric Tales* (2010), Ellen Forney's *Marbles: Mania, Depression, Michelangelo, & Me* (2012), Katie Green's *Lighter Than My Shadow* (2013), Tyler Page's *Raised on Ritalin: A Personal Story of ADHD, Medication and Modern Psychiatry* (2016), Terian Koscik's *When Anxiety Attacks* (2016), and Rachel Lindsay's *RX: A Graphic Memoir* (2018).

The graphic memoir is a genre well suited to depict mental illness (and illness in general) autobiographically due to its multimodality—that is, the visual track and the verbal track create a number of unique affordances that can be employed creatively. I want to highlight two aspects that are foregrounded particularly often in graphic memoirs about mental illness: the narrative situation and psychic catharsis.

First, from a narratological standpoint, graphic narratives productively foreground the split between the narrating "I" and the experiencing "I." As Jared Gardner has theorized, this allows "the autographer to be both victim of the trauma and detached observer" (2008, p. 12). In the standard graphic narrative situation, the experiencing "I" inhabits the visual track (including verbalization through speech and thought bubbles), whereas the narrating "I," who narrates from an experienced position later in time, is represented as text in the captions. Hence, one way to represent the chaos and order that—according to Rimmon-Kenan—characterizes illness narratives is to let the chaos of the experience play out in the visual track, and represent the attempt at mastery and control in the captions. As I have argued elsewhere (Gammelgaard, 2019), comics artists can then limit or delete the captions if they want to try to find expression for something approximating Frank's chaos narrative.

The second aspect, which is often foregrounded in graphic memoirs about mental illness, is the notion of psychic relief. Forney explicitly entertains the idea that drawing is cathartic. In addition to the comics style in *Marbles*, Forney has inserted photographs of a number of sketch-book drawings, of which she states that "it was really my sketchbook where I could face my emotional demons in a wholly personal way" (2012, p. 92), and, furthermore, that "I soon learned to keep drawing until I really nailed my feelings down. I didn't get nearly the same relief if I only came close" (2012, p. 96).

This notion of psychic relief through drawing is not unique to Forney. In "Autography as Auto-Therapy: Psychic Pain and the Graphic Memoir," Ian Williams interviews a number of prominent graphic memoir artists (Katie Green, Phoebe Gloeckner, Willy Linthout, Nicola Streeten, and Darryl Cunningham) and asks them if they experience some kind of catharsis in the working through of their stories in the comics format. Williams's article is also based on scientific scholarship (and not just interviews). Williams comes to the following conclusion:

> It seems likely that, among the multiple and complex reasons for publishing a graphic memoir of suffering, some artists hope that the process will afford some measure of healing and some artists find some therapeutic effect, whether expected or not. (Williams, 2011, p. 365)

Besides the auto-therapeutic effect, the graphic memoir is believed to help others face their demons—in other words, that it has the potential to trigger a common catharsis among artist and audience. Jared Gardner has formulated this point succinctly:

This was perhaps the greatest surprise of the first comics autobiographers: that the most personal stories became the ones that forged the most meaningful connections with others, opening up a dialogue with audiences and a sense of communal experience and release. (Gardner, 2008, p. 13)

The autobiography is most often conceived of as telling someone's life story. Hence, it is arguably always characterized by being narrative in nature. As such, it is a nonfiction equivalent of the novel, in being a narrative of some length (although, of course, the relationship between fiction and nonfiction in discussions of novels vs. autobiographies is much more complex than that). One could argue that the graphic memoir is to the graphic novel what the autobiography is to the novel in being an extensive narrative about someone's life. With reference to trauma scholar Dori Laub, Williams also highlights the process of making a narrative as being essential to the healing process. The idea is that "the narration of events can help to reconfigure a self whose integrity has been threatened," and that the memory must be "organized into a coherent narrative sequence" for the healing to work, which is "a central idea of Narrative Medicine" (Williams, 2011, p. 359). I am not in disagreement with this position, but I want to supplement it by drawing attention to the fact that the therapeutic effects of composing and/or reading a graphic memoir about mental illness are not only limited to the works of narrative reconfiguration. In what follows, I would like to highlight how nonnarrative configurations are at work within graphic memoirs that tell a story. This requires a minor theoretical detour, before I can turn to close readings of such configurations.

Nonnarrative Configurations

Attempts at defining what makes something a narrative center on the essential aspects of a narrative like time, plot, causality, world disruption, and more, but all narratives of some length encompass a number of features that do not essentially constitute core aspects of narrativity. When nonnarrative features are elevated to a more prominent role in a narrative, they can even threaten the narrative impetus. Georg Lukács discussed this dilemma in relation to nineteenth-century realism and more specifically to the naturalistic novel's propensity to indulge in extended descriptions that are not essential to the plot. Despite the verbal virtuosity of, for example, Émile Zola, his comprehensive descriptions function as a "mere filler in the novel [i.e., *Nana*]" (Lukács, 1971, p. 110). Hence, descriptions that are not narrativized or otherwise integrated thematically seem to impede narrative progression. The conflict between narrative and nonnarrative features is even more conspicuous in narrative poetry due to the materiality of poetry. In my work on narrative poetry, I have made the following claim concerning this:

> [T]he reader responds to a poetic trajectory in addition to a narrative trajectory. I see readerly dynamics in narrative poetry as a response to or an engagement with the textual dynamics of the two trajectories. [. . .] The poetic trajectory designates the reader's interpretation or processing of the poeticity. By poeticity [. . .] I mean two things. On the one hand, as that which is unique to poetry: versification and stanza form [. . .]. On the other hand, I take it to mean that which is not exclusively found in poetry, but which is often highly *foregrounded* in poetry: the artificiality of language, accentuated by flaunting the acoustic or visual materiality of language. This includes, for example, puns, alliteration, rhymes, and metaphors. In reading a narrative poem, this poetic trajectory has a significant impact on the readerly dynamics. (Gammelgaard, 2014, p. 204)

The poetic trajectory can have an impact on readers at a very local level (say, in a pun or a rhyme), but it can also unfold over the course of the entire narrative (e.g., through developing a symbol). The main crux of this discussion is transferable to the comics genre. Two of the most prominent definitions of comics perceive of comics in terms of time sequence and, hence, in narrative terms. The first one, Will Eisner's, states that comics is "sequential art" (quoted in Bennett, 2012, p. 16). The second one is Scott McCloud's definition in *Understanding Comics: The Invisible Art*: "Juxtaposed pictorial and other images in deliberate sequence, intended to convey information and/ or to produce an aesthetic response in the viewer" (1993, p. 9). In her dissertation *Comics Poetry: Beyond Sequential Boundaries*, Tamryn Bennett takes issue with the inherently narrative understanding of comics: "Comics critics like Scott McCloud, Charles Hatfield, David Kunzle, David Beroä and Douglas Wolk, among others, view comics as narrative constructs, preferencing images in sequence over all other elements in the visual-verbal comics vocabulary" (Bennett, 2012, p. 11). In opposition to this, she argues that "a new model for comics analysis is needed to address narrative, non-narrative, multi-linear, abstract and experimental developments within the form" (Bennett, 2012, p. 10). She then theorizes the genre of comics poetry to account for works that "experiment with the combination of comics and poetic devices" (2012, p. 23). The poetry connection is more appropriate than the narrative connection "because of both the condensing of words and the emphasis on rhythm" (Seth, quoted in Bennett, 2012, p. 10). My cases in this chapter do not strictly speaking qualify as comics poetry, but I see many similarities between Bennett's work on comics poetry and my own work on narrative poetry, and I want to make the claim that the poetic or nonnarrative configurations at work in graphic narratives about mental illnesses are essential to the purposes of these illness narratives, not least to the aim of achieving psychic relief. Or, put differently, I do not suggest that we should conceive of graphic memoirs *as* poetry. Rather, I want to show how nonnarrative (among them poetic) configurations are at work within the narrative composition. Jan Baetens has touched on this in his 2011 article "Abstraction in Comics," in which he writes that "[a]bstraction seems to be what resists narrativization, and conversely narrativization seems to be what dissolves abstraction. Abstract comics melt in the air when narrative walks in—and vice versa" (quoted in Bennett, 2012, p. 48). However, whereas he suggests that they replace each other, I will suggest that they often coexist, that both modes may be applied simultaneously.

In an article about metaphors in graphic medicine in relation to depictions of anorexia, Venkatesan and Peter (2019) write: "Comics can help sufferers to externalize cognitive and corporeal memories of suffering/illness through symbolization using visual metaphors, verbo-visual metaphors, method-ical use of imagination, and a wide range of drawing techniques" (p. 1). They furthermore argue that "[m]etaphors help individuals in revisiting, confronting, and externalizing the experience of physical or psychological trauma" (p. 12). By externalizing an experience through comics, it is argued, the artist is enabled to mix what is deeply personal and subjective with a concomitant objectifying stance (p. 2). The narrative components and the nonnarrative configurations in graphic memoirs about mental health there-fore share the aim of attaining a kind of mental catharsis by reconfiguring the self, but the means to that end differ. The nonnarrative configurations investigate and analyze mental states by creative means and in a condensed verbal-visual language, which supplements and interacts with the narrative aspects of graphic memoirs.

Before an extended interpretation of a case, I will give two examples of how these nonnarrative, poetic devices are employed productively in graphic memoirs about mental illness. The first example is from the third page (out of 10 original pages) by Art Spiegelman in his broadsheet-size board book *In the Shadow of No Towers* (which, in addition to the 10 original pages, contains reprints of early American comic strips). The 10 pages are single-page units about Spiegelman's reaction to 9/11. The second page in the series suggests that he suffered from post-traumatic stress disorder (PTSD) in the aftermath of the terrorist attack in New York. Hence, Spiegelman's autobiographical avatar states the following: "I insist the sky is falling; they roll their eyes and tell me it's only my Post-Traumatic Stress Disorder" (Spiegelman, 2004, p. 2). In the preface to the book, Spiegelman suggests that one reason for creating the pages was for auto-therapeutic purposes: "I had anticipated that the shadows of the towers might fade while I was slowly sorting through my grief and putting it into boxes" (unpaginated). Additionally, he describes the book as "a slow-motion diary of what I experienced while seeking some provisional equanimity" (unpaginated). The third page gives an account of how Spiegelman and his wife raced to their daughter's school, which was close to the twin towers, to make sure she was safe. The page is highly condensed, intermingling his concerns for the air quality in the school after the collapse of the towers with a memory of his father describing the smell of the smoke in Auschwitz as "indescribable" and additionally with his own smoking habit (he initially states that he smokes two packs of cigarettes a day).

The central poetic device of the page consists of a kind of visual simile between the burning, collapsing tower and a cigarette. The tower is placed on the left side of the page and extends from the top to the bottom. The cigarette is in a similarly vertical position on the right-hand side of the page and is also burning down. It extends from the top to the bottom of the page as well. The comics panels are placed in between the tower and the cigarette. The logic functions like many verbal metaphors: Spiegelman compares two entities that have some similar features even though they are also extremely different. Firstly, the tower and the cigarette have a similar physical shape, but, of course, the tower is much, much bigger in reality. On this page, however, they are equal in size. Secondly, they are both burning down from the top of the page towards its bottom. Comics, of course, only have "frozen," non-moving images. The tower and the cigarette have approximately burned equally far down, but in real life, once the tower starts collapsing, it reaches the ground much more quickly than the cigarette will reach its bud, paradoxically despite the great difference in size. Thirdly, both the chemicals from the building and in the cigarette are detrimental to your health. This intermingling of the collective trauma and disaster of 9/11 and personal issues is epitomized by the comparison between the crashing tower and the vertically burning cigarette. Spiegelman's avatar is frustrated by the potentially dangerous air pollution, and the page concludes with the following two speech balloons (quoted in succession): "all this has gotten me so anxious I smoke more than ever now"; "I'm not even sure I'll live long enough for cigarettes to kill me. 'cof! cof!'" (Spiegelman, 2004, p. 3). The visual metaphor, comparing the building to the cigarette, surrounds (and literally frames) the narrative told in the panels, in which Spiegelman and his wife run toward the school to retrieve their daughter on 9/11. Hence, the narrative and nonnarrative aspects of the page interact to create meaning in complex ways.

My second small-scale example is from Koscik's *When Anxiety Attacks*. It is a short graphic memoir about the artist's struggle with anxiety. When Koscik's avatar experiences anxiety, the background and the avatar are drawn in a red color, but despite that, the graphic memoir experiments less with the comics genre within the book than Spiegelman did in *In the Shadow of No Towers*. The message conveyed on the front page, however, is condensed and experimental (Figure 13.1).

The title of the book is an obvious pun in which the compound noun "anxiety attack" is employed as a verb. The brilliance of this is that "anxiety" then becomes the grammatical subject for the verb "attack," which puts the onus of agency on anxiety itself. The visual track attempts to visualize this grammatical subject. Hence, a complex and abstract concept like anxiety, which from a medical perspective is described through a list of symptom clusters, is endowed with an actual, physical shape. The attack takes place on a foreign planet in outer space, and anxiety is personified as an alien-like robot. The robot attacks her from behind. It finds her and illuminates her with a light beam. The attack itself, however, consists of an accusation framed as a question, which causes guilt: "When was the last time you called your grandmother?!" In a humorous way, it communicates how something that would not entail so much concern for most people elicits such a vehement emotional response in a person who suffers from anxiety. The front page appears to be quite narrative—a robot chasing and attacking the protagonist on a foreign planet—but actually this small narrative scenario is at the service of the verbal-visual interaction of the poetic personification that describes an abstract illness. Through this maneuver, Koscik achieves

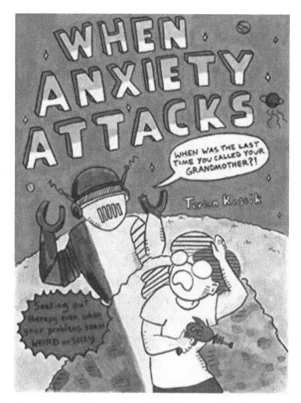

Figure 13.1. Front page of Terian Koscik's *When Anxiety Attacks*.
Used with permission from the artist.

multiple goals. The person on the front page, in fact, finds herself in a dangerous situation, if the scenario were to be processed as an actual situation: Most people would be fearful if they were put in a war-like or battle-like situation. Employing the scenario to describe anxiety, Koscik conveys the notion that people experiencing anxiety actually do fear that some catastrophe is imminent and consequently operate as a radar scanning for danger. The felt imminence of danger is real. At the same time, the comics style and humor—not least achieved through the visual intertextual reference to the science fiction comics magazine *Weird Science*—deflate any straightforward, serious reading of the front page. It contributes to a self-deprecating humor, in which Koscik communicates that the anxiety is sincerely and severely felt even though there is an awareness of not actually being in danger (this awareness is inherent in anxiety). The danger is not *out there* (in outer space or on Earth). Rather, it originates or emanates from within, and, despite the self-mocking stance, readers can infer the serious, non-ironic statement that taking on anxiety is heroic.

Readerly Dynamics in Ellen Forney's *Marbles*

In the Shadow of No Towers works in single-page units. *When Anxiety Attacks* is relatively short, and my interpretation of it focused solely on the front page. The final case—Ellen Forney's *Marbles: Mania, Depression, Michelangelo, & Me*—is a full-length graphic memoir of 256 pages. I will highlight what to my mind is the book's central nonnarrative configuration, how its trajectory reflects or intermingles with the narrative trajectory, and, finally, how the reader responds to the two trajectories.

I have already described how it is a book with auto-therapeutic purposes. As a pathography, it resonates well with Arthur Frank's restitution narrative. Readers are invited along Forney's journey. Readers are told about the onset of a manic episode. We see Forney receive the diagnosis. We gain insight into her subjective experience with depressive and manic episodes. We witness her struggle to strike a balance with the right combination of therapy, sleep, yoga, and biomedical treatment. The book even ends with a staged, fictionalized conversation between her older and younger self, in which she reassures her younger self that she will be okay—that is, even though she will not recover from bipolar disorder, she will learn to cope with the illness.

As with *When Anxiety Attacks*, I will argue that there is great analytical dividend in paying special attention to the front page. I have had the good fortune to be able to teach this book with approximately 10 different classes, which has given me the opportunity to collect responses from a diversity of university students. In relation to reader response (whether based on speculative readers or actual readers), the response begins with the front page; it is the first element one encounters, and it shapes one's perception of the book. Each time I teach the book, students are asked to do a close reading of the front page, paying attention to both the visual track and the verbal track, and the interaction between the two. I prompt them to extrapolate as much information as possible from the front page alone. At the top of *Marbles*'s front page, one sees four circles in different colors. All four circles extend beyond the actual page (thus one must imagine their completion). The title, subtitle, genre designation, and name of the author are placed below the circles. At the bottom, one sees the upper half of the head of the protagonist (Figure 13.2).

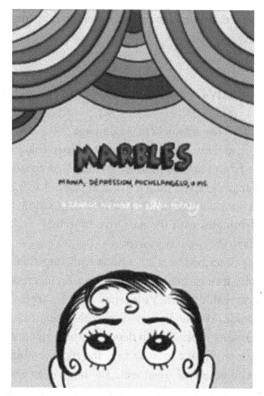

Figure 13.2. Front page of Ellen Forney's *Marbles: Mania, Depression, Michelangelo, & Me.*
Used with permission from the artist.

With respect to the verbal track, the students note that it is a graphic memoir by Ellen Forney, so they expect what they are about to encounter to have some referential truth value. They note that it is about mania and depression. They mention the salient use of m-alliteration (marbles, mania, Michelangelo, me, memoir). They highlight that the word "Marbles" is equivocal. It plays on the idiom "to lose one's marbles," which means to go crazy. At the same time, it establishes a connection with Michelangelo or the creation of art and with Forney as an artist (with the not-so-humble juxtaposition of "Michelangelo & Me"), and, of course, there is an entire chapter devoted to the notion of the mad genius, which Forney refers to as the "Van Gogh Club."

The students always immediately establish that the abstract shapes (we assume they are circular) at the top resemble actual marbles and that the bright colors opposed to the dark ones are affiliated with mania and depression respectively. Some students remark that the colors remind them of the flag for the LGBT movement (and, in fact, being bisexual is a significant topic of the memoir). We cannot see the entire head of Forney's avatar, but enough is visible so that when I ask students if the face reminds them of a well-known character, there is always at least one student suggesting she resembles Betty Boop, the performing cartoon character from the 1930s. This prompts some students to suggest that the circular shapes are reminiscent of stage curtains, a point that resonates well with the graphic memoir's proclivity for performance and self-exhibition. The genre mixes the private and the public. In *Marbles*, it also feeds into the overall message that you should perform and flaunt your mental illness instead of being subdued or ashamed by society's stigmatization thereof.

Hence, the front page is characterized by condensation and overdetermination, and all this information shapes our understanding of the rest of the book. Midway through the book, readers encounter abstract circles that are reminiscent of those on the front page. On page 124, readers see a photocopy of one of the depression drawings from Forney's sketchbook. In this sketch, big round shapes are ominously close to a little, fragile figure. The caption reads: "I wanted to depict floating, rumbling anxieties." The sketchbook drawings have up until this point only been inserted as individual pages. It is therefore significant that this particular drawing is the only one that Forney actually transposes into the comics panels. On the right-hand page (p. 125), you see the dark, round, "rumbling anxieties" interfere with her attempt at a yoga plank pose.

If the interpretation of the front page has an impact on readerly expectations going forward, the encounter with the sketchbook drawing, which is similar to the front page in its composition with the circular shapes above a person's head, establishes grounds for a comparison with the front page. In the sketchbook, the shapes are many times larger than the fragile person that they seem to threaten to crush. On the front page, however, the avatar's head is of about the same size as the round shapes (perhaps even a bit larger), and the circles are further removed from the head, which along with the bright blue background color gives the impression of more hopeful prospects. Since you only see the upper half of the head, it is difficult to decipher the emotional state, but she seems to be glancing at the circles, and based on what we can see (the eyes and the eyebrows), she does not appear to be anxious.

Forney's use of these nonnarrative configurations helps shape readers' expectations for and responses to her illness narrative. Whether they represent the two moods of bipolar disorder, marbles that kids play with, marbles that you use to make art, stage curtains, "floating, rumbling anxieties," or all of those, they support the narrative trajectory of *Marbles* as a restitution narrative. The differences between the front page and the sketchbook drawing suggest that this is a story about someone who has learned to manage her bipolar disorder and regain balance.

Conclusion

Graphic memoirs about mental illness have proliferated in the past 20 years concurrently with a turn within humanities and health sciences to collaborate extensively. In this chapter, I have highlighted that illness narratives may pose a challenge to our received understanding of narratives in that they introduce a rupture in time and teleological progression. Research on the genre of pathography has accounted for specific types of illness narratives, but insufficient attention has been paid to nonnarrative configurations within illness narratives. The same could be said of research on comics. Definitions of comics most often highlight its narrative qualities by accommodating theory from literary fiction and fiction film. This has led to a relative neglect of nonnarrative configurations in comics in general, and, in relation to my empirical material, to a neglect of nonnarrative configurations (among them abstract and poetic) in research on graphic memoirs about mental illness.

Furthermore, I have argued that graphic memoirs about mental illness often fulfill cathartic purposes. These entail auto-therapeutic relief in formulating a feeling as well as relief in sharing this within one's community of peers (or "co-sufferers") and with the public. Research on catharsis in illness narratives and in graphic memoirs has predominantly explained this through narrativization strategies, but I have claimed that it may also be a result of nonnarrative configurations.

In three case studies, I have explored the multifarious ways in which such nonnarrative configurations supplement and interact with the overall trajectory of their respective illness narratives. In one of the single-unit pages in Spiegelman's *In the Shadow of No Towers*, the artist tells a brief story about his experience on September 11, 2001, and to sum up the chaos and intermingling of his own traumas and the collective trauma imposed on New Yorkers by the terrorist attack he creates a complex visual metaphor that dominates the page and, hence, the story that he is telling. In Koscik's

When Anxiety Attacks, the implication of an action-filled narrative event on the front page is employed to create a personification of an abstract condition. The narrative is at the service of explaining this condition. Finally, in an extensive interpretation of reader response to abstract, nonnarrative configurations in Forney's *Marbles: Mania, Depression, Michelangelo, & Me*, I have highlighted how the creation of condensed, overdetermined, and abstract geometrical shapes supports the overall purpose of the illness narrative as a restitution narrative.

The nonnarrative, poetic features foregrounded in this chapter are by no means an exhaustive list. Future work on illness narratives and more specifically on representations of mental illness in graphic memoirs might profitably explore further how both graphic memoir and poetry flaunt the acoustic and visual materiality of language (in the case of comics also its visual materiality) and examine how graphic memoirs employ poetic strategies (like, for example, play with the verbal-visual vocabulary, puns, enjambment, metaphors, similes, hyperboles, condensation, and more). Additionally, more research is needed on the ways in which such nonnarrative configurations relate to narrative trajectories in graphic memoirs about mental illness.

References

Bechdel, A. (2006). *Fun home: A family tragicomic*. Jonathan Cape.

Bennett, T. (2012). *Comics poetry: Beyond sequential boundaries*. Doctoral dissertation, University of New South Wales.

Brosh, A. (2009–). *Hyperbole and a half.* http://hyperboleandahalf.blogspot.com/

Charon, R., DasGupta, S., Hermann, N., Irvine, C., Marcus, E. R., Rivera, Colón, E., Spencer, D., & Spiegel, M. (2017). *The principles and practice of narrative medicine.* Oxford University Press.

Cunningham, D. (2010). *Psychiatric tales*. Blank Slate.

Forney, E. (2012). *Marbles: Mania, depression, Michelangelo, & me*. Gotham Books.

Frank, A. (1995). *The wounded storyteller: Body, illness, and ethics*. University of Chicago Press.

Gammelgaard, L. (2014). Two trajectories of reader response in narrative poetry: Roses and risings in Keats's "The Eve of St. Agnes." *Narrative, 22*(2), 203–218.

Gammelgaard, L. (2019). Chaos narrative and experientiality in the graphic memoir: The case of Thomas H. Nøhr's "Cirkus." *Journal of Research in Sickness and Society, 16*(31), 89–105.

Gardner, J. (2008). Autography's biography, 1972–2007. *Biography, 31*(1), 1–26.

Green, J. (1995). *Binky Brown: Samplerincluding the unexpurgated 1972 Classic "Binky Brown Meets the Holy Virgin Mary"*. Last Gasp.

Green, K. (2013). *Lighter than my shadow*. Jonathan Cape.

Koscik, T. (2016). *When anxiety attacks.* Singing Dragon.

Lindsay, R. (2018). *RX: A graphic memoir.* Grand Central Publishing.

Linthout, W. (2009). *Years of the elephant.* Fanfare/Ponent Mon.

Lukács, G. (1971). Narrate or describe? In *Writer and critic and other essays* (pp. 110–149). Grosset & Dunlap.

McCloud, S. (1993). *Understanding comics: The invisible art.* Harper Collins.

Page, T. (2016). *Raised on Ritalin: A personal story of ADHD, medication, and modern psychiatry.* Dementian Comics.

Rimmon-Kenan, S. (2006). What can narrative theory learn from illness narratives? *Literature and Medicine, 25*(2), 241–254.

Spiegelman, A. (1997). *Maus: A survivor's tale.* Pantheon.

Spiegelman, A. (2004). *In the shadow of no towers.* Pantheon.

Spiegelman, A. (2008). *Breakdowns: Portrait of the artist as a young %@&*!* Pantheon.

Venkatesan, S., & Peter, A. M. (2019). Anorexia through creative metaphors: Women pathographers and graphic medicine. *Journal of Graphic Novels and Comics, 12*(5), 429–442. doi:10.1080/21504857.2019.1657158

Williams, I. (2011). Autography as auto-therapy: Psychic pain and the graphic memoir. *Journal of Medical Humanities, 32,* 353–366.

14

Memory Is a Strange Thing

Science Fiction, Trauma, and Time in *Arrival*

Christoph Singer

Introduction

"Memory is a strange thing," we are told in Denis Villeneuve's (2016) science-fiction film *Arrival*, which is based on Ted Chiang's short story "Story of Your Life" (2002). In the following discussion, I will read the time-bending film as a trauma narrative at the heart of which we observe the protagonist Louise Banks coming to terms with the death of her child. As a consequence of her traumatic experience, (1) chronological temporalities are upended for Louise, (2) the experience of loss is presented as highly difficult to transform into a coherent narrative, and (3) most importantly, the film complicates and deconstructs the audience's sense of temporality and possibility of emplotment. By shifting the focus from the *story*, what is being told, to *discourse*, how the narrative is being told, the film foregrounds the pitfalls in telling and listening to trauma narratives. Regarding the relationship of narrative and mental health, I will argue that this specific shift of focus subverts normative notions of what a narrative actually is and can be. More importantly, a discourse-based reading of trauma narratives highlights the various implicit readerly expectations when it comes to approaching narrative texts.

In the following discussion, I will address how *Arrival*, as well as Chiang's short story, attempt to represent and communicate the trauma of child loss by creating a sense of nonlinearity in a linear medium. To do so, the film defamiliarizes a range of narrative markers from genre to causality, to chronology, to the film's soundtrack. I am especially interested in the connection of temporality and trauma. After a short introduction to and summary of the film (which, given its time-bending structure, is a paradoxical undertaking in and of itself), I will discuss the film's attempts at deconstructing any narrative closure while foregrounding various processes of reading narratives.

Christoph Singer, *Memory Is a Strange Thing* In: *Narrative and Mental Health*. Edited by: Jarmila Mildorf, Elisabeth Punzi, and Christoph Singer, Oxford University Press. © Oxford University Press 2023.
DOI: 10.1093/oso/9780197620540.003.0015

Narratives are, after all, highly connected to normative perceptions of what a narrative's structure and temporality should ideally look like. At the end, time-bending trauma narratives, as seen in *Arrival*, may not be a presentation of what it feels like to be out of time. But what these narratives may achieve is to keep the narrative's addressees in a state where they constantly question whether their own emplotment and interpretations are actually correct. Such narratives may also create empathy with a traumatized person struggling to transform the traumatic events into a coherent and chronological narrative.

Temporality and Trauma Narratives

A summary of time-travel plots is often a rather futile attempt; since the plot continually deconstructs itself in the time-looping logic of warped temporalities. So rather than offering a summary of *Arrival*, I will, for now, quickly introduce the film by means of its premise and by outlining some of its central narrative events, whose narrative order will be discussed in detail below. *Arrival* only superficially comes in the disguise of an alien-invasion film: 12 ovoid spaceships appear in random places scattered over the globe. Their appearance is reminiscent of Douglas Adams's *The Hitchhiker's Guide to the Galaxy* (1979): "The ships hung in the sky in much the same way that bricks don't." In *Arrival* the fear of what will appear from the egg-like spaceships results in mass hysteria and military mobilization. While an invasion film like Roland Emmerich's *Independence Day* grounds its terror in weaponry, *Arrival*'s anxiety stems from uncertainty. The film's protagonist, Louise Banks, is a linguist who is asked by the U.S. military to decipher and translate the written and spoken languages of a race of aliens that suddenly arrived in these spacecraft. The effect of learning these languages is such that Louise's sense of temporality and perception of linear time collapses. Her altered state of time allows her to perceive events past, present, and future in perfect synchronicity. One of the film's central events is the traumatic death of Louise's daughter, Hannah, whose terminal illness leads to a sudden death.

Yet, herein lies *Arrival*'s premise: As said, the military asks Louise to translate the extraterrestrials' languages—that is. their spoken and their written, inky, nonlinear languages. These written logograms lack beginning, end, and temporal markers of any kind. This makes Ian, Louise's colleague and husband-to-be, wonder: "Like their ship or their bodies, their written language has no forward or backward direction. Linguists call this 'nonlinear orthography,' which raises the question, 'Is this how they think?'" The answer is a time-bending "yes." By internalizing this language, Louise's perception of time changes, allowing her to perceive future events. This results in two painful epiphanies shared by the audience: What we perceive as the plot's past is actually the future. And it is in the future that Louise's daughter will be born, become sick, and die. Yet, viewers unknowingly judge every event as if the daughter has already died. We perceive Louise as a grieving mother when actually she is not. And the film forces the audience to create a seemingly cohesive plot and filmic memories based on a misconceived temporal order of events. In that sense, *Arrival* is reminiscent of what psychologist Jens Brockmeier calls retrospective teleology: "In the process of being narrated the flux of life seems to be transformed into a flux of necessity" (2001, p. 253). Polychronic plots and trauma narratives like *Arrival* play with the idea that time is nonlinear in the first place. From a narrative point of view, this leads to a seemingly anti-teleological worldview, which raises a number of problems, such as: How do we relate the time-disrupting experience of trauma in a medium that is mostly a temporal one?

In the logic of *Arrival*, the eventual pregnancy and Hannah's death are "not yet" and simultaneously an event of the past, a dual structure that is replicated by the film's dual plot. We observe an almost biblical annunciation scene of sorts, which leaves not only the plot but also Louise as a double. In the words of Iris Marion Young, the pregnant subject is "decentred, split, or doubled" (2005, p. 46).

In hindsight, the film attempts to transform narrative linearity into a mimicry of synchronicity. Louise's ability to suddenly "remember" the future is reminiscent of a central statement found in *Alice's Adventures in Wonderland* (1865): "It's a poor sort of memory that only works backwards." This experience leads Louise and the audience to ask: "If you could see your whole life from start to finish, would you change things?" Consequently, *Arrival* is less interested in the logic of time travel than in how traumatic experiences can be integrated in a narrative sense of self.

Trauma and Temporality

How are temporality and narrative related? Are they reciprocal, or is one the precondition for the other? If they are conditional, who comes first: narrative or temporality? Philosopher Eric Levy argues that "the need thus to achieve cohesion through time presupposes a construction of time. Hence the most fundamental ground of self-awareness is not narrative, which binds together the moments or phases of personal unfolding, but the sense of time itself" (2016, p. 215). And Brockmeier argues in a similar vein: "I believe that human identity construction can essentially be viewed as the construction of a particular mode of time" (2001, p. 248). Yet, narrative is a major mode of giving a semblance of time and orienting oneself in time. And exactly this sense of temporal orientation by means of narrative is often afflicted due to the experience of trauma. Psychology and literary representations show that subjects in crisis may perceive themselves as being catapulted outside of chronological and social time. This is confirmed by literary scholar Elizabeth Larsen, who argues: "[In] instances of catastrophe or events that restructure life, time is released from the typical routines of everyday life. Everyday notions of time are overturned or unhinged" (2004, p. 27). As a result, the experience of trauma may be perceived as being plotless. Robert Stolorow also argues:

> In the region of trauma all duration or stretching along collapses, the traumatic past becomes present, and future loses all meaning other than endless repetition. Because trauma so profoundly modifies the universal or shared structure of temporality, I claimed, the traumatized person quite literally lives in another kind of reality, an experiential world felt to be incommensurable with those of others. This felt incommensurability, in turn, contributes to the sense of alienation and estrangement from other human beings that typically haunts the traumatized person. (2018, p. 21)

Stolorow then concludes that "Trauma destroys time: the traumatized person lives in an alien reality" (2015, n.p.). In the case of Louise Banks and *Arrival*, this alien reality holds true in both the literal and figural sense of the word. As said, Louise encounters alien creatures in a UFO, an experience whose impact renders her an outsider among her peers. Due to her experiences she is placed, in the logic of the film, quite literally outside of chronological time. This is reminiscent of Peter Brooks's argument that firstly, narrative is the "organizing dynamic of a specific mode of human understanding" (1984, p. 7). Secondly, and more importantly, Brooks argues that "Until such a time, as we cease to exchange understandings in the form of stories, we will need to remain dependent on the logic we use to shape and to understand stories, which is to say, dependent on plot" (1984, pp. 6–7). Yet, what happens if trauma complicates the possibility to create a coherent and chronological plot on the side of the traumatized subject?

Time-Loop Narratives

Regarding trauma's effect on the perception of time, *Arrival* and Ted Chiang's short story recall various literary predecessors and trauma narratives. In Chiang's short story Louise claims that "I perceive—during those glimpses—that entire epoch as a simultaneity" (2002, p. 141). In W. G. Sebald's novel *Austerlitz*, for instance, the protagonist claims that "a certain degree of personal misfortune is enough to cut us off from the past and the future" (2001, p. 143). He also states that in a moment of crisis "I shall find that all moments of time have co-existed simultaneously" (2001, p. 144). One is also reminded of French-American author Raymond Federman and his postmodern science-fiction memoir *The Twofold Vibration*. The protagonist—a Holocaust survivor called the Old Man—is confronted with a "barrage of unresolved events" (Federman, 1982, p. 326). He perceives his existence as "plotless." The way the resulting silences are being broken, especially in the case of Federman, directly links in a postmodern fashion the extra-textual and the intra-textual level. It is at the same time an act of memorization and an attempt at avoiding sentimentality. Sentimentalism is what the Old Man in Federman's novel detests the most. Upon finishing his 20-page memoir (presented in a novel of 400 pages) the Old Man is disappointed by his friend's lukewarm reaction. He stresses the fact that he "had to do it this way, it's a demanding subject for which a demanding form had to be invented" (Federman, 1982, p. 223). This comment relates directly to the novel at large and by extension to Sebald's *Austerlitz*, as earlier in the novel the Old Man claims that "it's not the story that counts, it's the way you tell it" (Federman, 1982, p. 109) This statement is a direct literal translation of Federman's argument made in his essay on *surfiction*:

> If life and fiction are no longer distinguishable one from the other, nor complementary to one another, and if we agree that life is never linear, that in fact life is always discontinuous and chaotic because it is never experienced in a straight line or an orderly fashion, then similarly linear, chronological and sequential narration is no longer possible. (1993, p. 42)

The characters in Federman's and Sebald's texts and in the film *Arrival* more or less successfully try to regain a sense of order and chronology. On the one hand, they need to re-establish a sense of self. On the other hand, they are forced to relearn to communicate their experiences with those around them. And here is yet another similarity that connects all of these texts: They represent characters who lost their narrative sense of self, but would be able to partially regain it with the help of patient listeners. Since they lack such listeners, however, the cyclical nature of the respective plot is doubled down by the cyclical narrative situation. Most of these tales are in a sense autotelic: Narrator and narratee are the same. In *Arrival*, Louise basically tells her story to herself. So do Federman's Old Man or Samuel Beckett's Molloy. Sebald's Austerlitz and James Joyce's Leopold Bloom—who also lost a child— chose younger versions of themselves to do so. This leaves the respective audiences and readers with the task of creating a seemingly logical, chronological, and causal plot. As argued, subjects who experience a crisis of sorts may perceive themselves as being catapulted outside quotidian time. Is the experience of crisis and trauma consequently a plotless one?

This connection of themes and approaches appears to be a current trend in cinema, a trend that is based less on classic time-travel plots in the vein of H. G. Wells's *The Time Machine* (1895), in which a protagonist travels along linear time tracks into the future or the past. The combination of time-bending science-fiction films whose cerebral musings on physics are humanized by protagonists who suffered the loss of a child is quite popular. Christopher Nolan's film *Interstellar* (2014) depicts a father who, through the physics of space travel, retains his young self only to return to his daughter dying of old age on her deathbed. The Marvel blockbuster *Endgame* (2019) presents a more conventional superhero plot, which is made more humane and is motivated by two of the heroes who lost their children due to time travel. And Alex Garland's film *Annihilation* (2018) depicts a heroine who, while grieving the death of her partner, encounters an alien form called "the Shimmer" that slowly reconstructs her sense of self and her identity. Especially in light of the trope of the dead child, *Arrival* can be recategorized as a "puzzle film" that requires viewers to piece together various events and narrative clues to create a sense of narrative coherence. Especially this sense of narrative fragmentation and the need to create a sense of causality and sequentiality is an important foundation of this genre for its trauma narratives. According to Warren Buckland, puzzle films "represent radically new experiences and identities, which are usually coded as disturbing and traumatic" (2009, p. 1). And here, as exemplified by a film like *Memento*, the disruption of time and memory are central elements, which lead us to various psychological considerations.

Trauma, Time, and Puzzle Films

One peculiarity of *Arrival* is the fact that the audience only realizes at the very end that it has observed a puzzle film. As such, the film and its source text confront the audience with a narrative conundrum: *Arrival* highlights the fact that viewers cannot stop themselves from transforming the depicted events into a narrative of their own making. It is literally impossible to observe the events without coming up with interpretations and conclusions. Consequently, the film forces viewers to acknowledge that their constant and automatic emplotment and the resulting empathy with the traumatized protagonist is the result of a misunderstood narrative. The main protagonist, whom one perceives as being guided by her traumatic experiences, is anything but. Importantly, *Arrival* invites the audience's empathy not by making the event that triggered the trauma relatable. Rather, the extra-textual audience and the intra-textual character Louise are aligned in their respective acts of constructing the story of Louise's life. And for both Louise and the audience narrative closure becomes impossible due to the temporal disruptions of trauma and the film's nonchronological sequencing of events. Consequently, *Arrival* defamiliarizes the audience's preconceived ideas of genre, chronology, causality, and closure and the resulting representation of memory and (narrative) identity. This matters especially when regarding mental health issues in relation to narrative, as this approach foregrounds how certain genres and the related narrative expectations shape our (mis-) reading of the events related to us.

As argued, *Arrival* addresses an essential paradox: If trauma has the effect of deconstructing the traumatized subject's sense of linear time and chronology, how can such an experience be expressed in media, be they literary or filmic? After all, does the textuality of these media render them inherently linear and chronological? The codes we are presented with, be they words or moving images, cannot but appear in a linear and consecutive fashion. Hence, every attempt at subverting the temporalities at hand is necessarily metaphorical, stylistic devices that make the addressee understand how events relate to the chronological timeline. One can find, of course, a variety of stylistic devices in storytelling that allow for the perceived alteration of the flow of time. Either chronology is affected by flashbacks, flash-forwards, ellipsis, and so forth, or the sense of duration is altered by means of summaries, excessive descriptions, repetitions, slow-motion, speed-ups, cutting, and so forth. Importantly, however, these temporal devices only become effective relative to an understanding of the narrative's sense of normative, chronological time. Surely, the audience's perception whether a narrative in film or literature is perceived as slow or fast may vary depending on the cultural or historical context. Ridley Scott's *Alien* may "feel" relatively slow compared to the later *Prometheus*.

What these examples are intended to highlight is a central issue inherent in judging what is called trauma narratives. Very often one will find arguments like Anne Whitehead's, who states that "the impact of trauma can only adequately be represented by mimicking its forms and symptoms, so that temporality and chronology collapse, and narratives are characterized by repetition and indirection" (2004, p. 3). If linear time falters for the traumatized subject, how can narrative identities remain intact? This quotation I would, firstly, like to relate to my argument above: Narratives cannot represent the alteration of chronological time. They can only—to borrow Whitehead's words—mimic such temporal disruption. Secondly, Whitehead implies that trauma is nonrepresentable. One way to represent trauma is by means of second-order signification. This second-order signification, however, will be judged against a normative understanding of how chronology and narrative are supposed to interact. Hence, various claims about the nonchronological experience of time by traumatized persons carry within them an implicit presupposition of what time supposedly is like, how it should be perceived, and how it can be communicated. Time, after all, is a symbolic construct, as Norbert Elias (1992) argues.

How does *Arrival* mimic Louise's perception of a nonchronological experience of time? How can a linear medium such as film or literature undermine its own constitutive temporalities? To illustrate how the film's director, Denis Villeneuve, manages to give a semblance of nonlinearity, I will look at three elements: the film's soundtrack, its use of space, and, most importantly for my discussion of the plotless structure of trauma and the audience's conception of narrative, its memory-subverting sequencing of events. Whereas the former two can be regarded as stylistic devices that merely play with filmic conventions, the latter tells us a lot about linear sequencing and time in storytelling.

Music, Soundtrack, and Nonlinear Time

Arrival's soundtrack was composed by Icelandic composer Johann Johannson. Johannson's ambient music is closer to the "time-less" music of Brian Eno's "Music for Airports" rather than Hans Zimmer's swelling score for *Interstellar*. *Arrival*'s score is remarkable for its unpredictable repetition of themes and patterns. Listeners will certainly recognize combinations of sounds, themes, or short musical phrases they may have heard before, but it is hard, if not impossible, to predict the occurrence of specific patterns. When Anne Whitehead, as quoted above, attests to trauma narrative's overt use of "repetitions" and "indirections," then Johannson's score may even be called trauma music. As a consequence of its use of these "indirections" and a refusal to follow the musical patterns and structures of (popular) music, viewers have a hard time at predicting and foreshadowing the musical score's development, leaving them slightly unsettled. In the words of Anthony Lane, the *New Yorker*'s film critic, the music is "rife with choral chanting, swelling brass, skitterings, and booms. [. . .] Should we be threatened or thrilled?" (2016, n.p.). Just as readers, based on their understanding of genre conventions, are able to predict the narrative's flow of events, listeners are likely to anticipate the progress of a musical piece. This ability to foreshadow the immediate future—albeit with some variations—is one of the reasons why particularly conventional narratives and popular music produce a sense of security. This observation evokes Edmund Husserl's phenomenology of time (1960/2002). Husserl structures the perception of time into *retention*, which can be loosely translated as memory, and *protention*, which can be understood as a sense of anticipation. Using music as an example for the human mind's ability to retain the (immediate) past and predict the (immediate) future, Husserl proposes the following argument: In our mind as listeners, the sounds we just heard, the sound we are hearing at the moment, and the sound we anticipate hearing are connected in a linear perception of time. By means of tropes and a conventional architecture of the composition, a well-structured piece of music allows us to anticipate a song's progression—a glimpse into the future, giving listeners a sense of order and control.

Additionally, if retention, immediate perception, and protention fulfill our expectations, we are left with a sense of ordered and structured time. Past, present, and future appear to move forward in a chronological fashion. The individual parts form a larger whole. If this linear perception of time, however, is disrupted, we are left with a sense of unease and disorientation—and this is exactly the time-bending effect of Johannson's music. To support my argument, it is important to mention that the soundtrack at the film's beginning is provided by a different composer, the German Max Richter. The first minutes of the film that tell us in linear fashion about the birth, illness, and death of Hannah are underscored by a musical piece that may be regarded as more classical in its composition. Reminiscent of Gustav Mahler's music, the piece with the title "On the Nature of Daylight" serves as a separate score that particularly accompanies the traumatic event that is Hannah's death. In doing so, Richter's more ethereal score stands in direct contrast to Johannson's ambient jitters and unpredictable repetitions.

In a sense, protention may also be connected to imagination. A possible or desired future that is imagined based on past experiences may or may not materialize. But what happens to a traumatized subject who may feel unable to imagine any future at all, due to the disruptive effects of the traumatizing event? As a result of being stuck in such an existential situation, in which the hoped-for future remains uncertain and the perception of time and chronology becomes warped, the importance of the imagination for escaping a present perceived as oppressive would be all the more important. Hence, to argue with Gail Womersley, who discusses projections of the future by refugee victims, imagination not only is a process of re-establishing a sense of temporality but more importantly

> emphasizes the importance of non-linear temporality in the context of migrants' changing subjective current realities—as individuals weave together images of the past, present and future to cope with situations of trauma, confer meaning to their current situation and redefine-reposition themselves toward the future. This includes tracking the processes of change in imagining alternative possible lives. (2020, pp. 715–716)

Interestingly, Womersley, intentionally or not, avoids the term *narrative*, despite the fact that her description of how imaginative work helps an individual to connect past, present, and future from a subjective point of view is actually a very good definition of narrative. Additionally, Womerley's use of the metaphor "weaving" is also very helpful in this context. Firstly, she implicitly alludes to one of Western literature's foundational, narrative works: Homer's *Odyssey*. Here we find Penelope, waiting for her refugee husband and literally and metaphorically weaving and unraveling her own future, as represented by the funeral shroud she creates for her father-in-law, who himself is waiting to die. From a more conceptual point of view, this famous metaphor of the woven textile as text, a text woven by connecting various strands, is also quite apt in the context of refugees and trauma: Without an immediate future in sight, one's biographical text has to be "unwoven" again and again, thus complicating the writing and telling of a future-oriented narrative. Thirdly, this metaphor stresses that the work of narrative imagination and narrative as imagination is not solely the result of a subjective and self-centered process. Every narrative requires a listener able to make sense of such a text. Yet, especially traumatic experiences are likely to subvert not only the communicative aspect of narrative but also the very ability to form a narrative: Exposure to trauma "risks the individual being caught up in a vicious cycle where no addressee may be found, no language exists to form a coherent narrative whereby trauma may itself be collectively represented and made sense of" (Womersley, 2020, p. 718).

Metaphorical Space, Trauma, and Time

Next to *Arrival*'s music, the film's use of space is equally intended to undermine the audience's perception of chronological time. This alignment of time and space is not surprising, given that in language also, time is often communicated in terms of spatial metaphors such as "the past is behind me," "the future lies before us," or "time is running its course." While the directionality of time as metaphorical space may differ given the specific cultural context, the combination of time and space in language appears to be fairly universal. *Arrival* uses this metaphorical connection of time as space to deconstruct a sense of the former.

Firstly, most spaces in the film are *non-spaces* whose warped temporalities Marc Augé has described in detail (1995). These are uniform spaces such as lecture halls, offices, and military interiors that seem rather interchangeable. Since the film is set mostly inside these spaces, which are lit by artificial light, the respective time of day remains unclear. In the words of Max Richter's soundtrack, "The Nature of Daylight" does not allow the audience to temporally locate the narrative's events. As with the soundtrack, one big exception is the aforementioned depiction of Hannah's short life, which mostly plays out on the outside or inside Louise's house, whose walls are mostly made of glass windows, thus allowing a clear understanding of "when" we are.

Additionally, *Arrival* undermines the conventions concerning spatial mobility found in Western cinema. In Western cinema, the preferred movement is akin to reading a sentence, namely from left to right, whereas right-to-left movement is perceived as unsettling. When a director subverts this direction, the effects are immediate. *Arrival* uses this sense of temporal disruption, for example when Louise enters the ovoid UFO's perfectly symmetrical chamber, a gray, dark contact zone. Due to the craft's subverted internal gravity, she is depicted as entering the chamber from right to left, and upside down. This already foreshadows the time-bending abilities Louise will acquire in that very room.

The Dangers of Emplotment

As argued above, a central narrative trick to play with the perception of time is the film's employment of emplotment and the so-called Kuleshov effect. (Puschak 2017, n.p.) By being made aware only at the end of the film that the events were presented in nonchronological fashion, the audience cannot help but create a sequential narrative based on what they see. As argued above, emplotment is partially a retroactive process. One looks at the past and turns different episodes and events into a meaningful plot by asking for their causal and chronological relationship. Yet, exactly this construction is problematized in trauma narratives. In Federman's novel *The Twofold Vibration*, the Old Man is not too concerned about such retroactive reading; rather, he claims to be "inventing and twisting my life into premembrances, distorting myself, my many selves into a strange time loop" (1982, p. 281).

The short story by Ted Chiang subverts temporality by means of grammatical tense as expressed in the following example: "I remember once when we'll be driving to the mall to buy some new clothes for you. You'll be thirteen" (Chiang, 2002, p. 114). The film *Arrival* attempts to present such a time loop in the form of its sequencing. *Arrival's* trauma narrative consists of two plots rather than one. Here is a summary of what we see, *Arrival's* discourse. The film begins with Louise's voice-over. She addresses her daughter, whom we observe in a montage of slow-motion scenes covering Hannah's happy childhood and terminal illness. After a cut, we then follow the seemingly grief-stricken Louise entering her university, only to find the seminar room almost empty. Louise is tasked by the military to communicate with the aliens, to learn their language. After a dramatic climax—to give Hollywood its due—the aliens leave befriended rather than conquered. Louise and her co-worker Ian, a physicist, marry. The conventionality of this ending seems to be at odds with the film's refusal to recycle time-honored tropes—if not for the film's eventual revelation. As mentioned before, the film plays with our perceptions of story and discourse, which are subverted by the final outcome. This is more than just a play: The chosen order of events subverts the viewer's expectations, memory, and reasoning.

What is essential to achieving that ending is *Arrival's* use of the Kuleshov effect. According to Sermin Ildirar and Louise Ewing:

> The Kuleshov effect is a film-editing effect that was demonstrated during the late 1910s and early 1920s by the pioneering Russian filmmaker and theorist Lev Kuleshov (1899–1970). Famously, Kuleshov is reported to have intercut a close-up of the Russian actor Ivan Mozhukhin's neutral, expressionless face with various other camera shots, including a bowl of soup, a woman in a coffin, and a child playing with a toy bear. He observed that these additional shots interacted with the original, leading viewers to perceive the (objectively neutral) face as expressing happiness, sadness, and hunger/thoughtfulness, respectively ... (2018, p. 19)

Alfred Hitchcock's famous example uses two linear sequences of three images each. The first and third image always remain the same: an old man—Hitchcock himself—firstly, observing something and, secondly, reacting with a smile to what he sees. The center image is changed in each sequence. In sequence one, it is a mother with a young child. The total sequence of images, which already imply a temporality and a causal reaction, likely prompt us to perceive an old man observing mother and child, which in turn results in a benevolent smile. Sequence two, however, presents us with a central image of a woman sunbathing in a bikini. While the reaction shot is identical, the audience will read the smile as that of a leering, male gaze—a radically different perception and interpretation of the text.

Arrival uses this effect to guide the audience's perception of Louise in a similar way. Upon viewing the film for the first time, Louise is perceived as somebody who merely reacts and whose reactions seem mostly motivated by her grief. The audience observes Louise sitting at her daughter's deathbed and then cuts to Louise entering her university. Her somber expression and slow walk naturally invite the interpretation that she is grieving. And it is likely that all of her actions are being read as a response to the loss of her daughter.

Upon entering the UFO for the first time, she is confronted with an unconscious scientist being taken out of the spacecraft. Her decision to continue and enter a potentially life-threatening situation could also be interpreted in this light. Yet, once the audience understands that the supposed past—Hannah's death—is actually the future, Louise turns into a protagonist whose life is guided by her own informed decisions. She is the one writing and narrating her story by accepting the grief the future holds for her. Suddenly, the audience simultaneously perceives two versions of one plot. This matters for narratives and for dealing with grief. Barney Downs argues: "Each time I tell my story it occupies less space and grief in my soul" (1993, p. 303).

Normative Narratives and Time

All of these films are firmly embedded in a cultural system that is more interested in revenue than artistic experimentation. How does that matter? I would argue that all of these films are, by means of their intended audience, required to present unconventional science fiction in narrative forms that remain understandable, palpable, and marketable to a wider audience. This also means that as viewers—and this will become important regarding the reading of other people's narrative accounts—our interpretation of and response to the narrative at hand is of course framed by our expectations. And genres are, after all, normative cultural constructions. Genre conceptions tell readers and audiences not only what to expect, but also how to react to the narrative. Depending on the respective sociocultural context, most people are (self-)educated enough to understand the basic elements of different genres, be they a Shakespearean comedy or a romantic Bollywood film. Put simply, our understanding of genre not only helps us in the readerly construction of a narrative, but we are also made to understand how to emotionally respond to given narratives. *King Lear* is no laughing matter, comic relief notwithstanding; *Pretty Woman* is not intended as a social documentary but a romantic love story. In short, specific genres trigger specific expectations and expected reactions.

This may be an obvious insight. But how then does this relate to narratives of mental health and an addressee's or listener's response to such narratives? The expectation of genre conventions and narrative conventions such as chronology, causality, and a tripartite structure with beginning, middle, and end raises a number of concerns:

1. How do implicit and explicit notions of genre conventions guide our perception and reaction to trauma narratives? Can readers and listeners take in nonchronological and noncausal narratives without attempting to create a sense of chronology and coherence, and rather accept the seemingly disjointed narrative for what it is, an expression of a traumatic self?

2. If traumatic experiences undermine a sense of chronology and causal coherence, how can one expect a traumatized subject to communicate in narrative form in the first place?

3. Most importantly, if a trauma narrative is told in a seemingly incoherent, noncausal, nonchronological way, how can we as readers avoid superimposing a sense of order and chronology, where, for the traumatized subject, none exists?

Herein lies the beauty of *Arrival*, as this film juxtaposes exactly these two sides: (1) the audience's expectations of an alien-invasion film and the related expected plot elements and (2) the protagonist's sense of being out of time due to her traumatic experience. Already the film's marketing campaign and trailer, probably for different reasons, were misleading in the generic framing of *Arrival*. The trailer marketed *Arrival* as a film that mostly seems to be about fending off an alien invasion, a narrative premise presented over and over again.

Conclusion

In the end, the grief and sadness we feel by empathizing with Louise is replaced by a strong sense of acceptance and cathartic closure. The anagnorisis—the insight that "there is no time," as the aliens would have it—affects Louise and the viewers simultaneously, and confers, according to Hannah Wojciehowski, "a quasi-metaphysical consolation" (2018, p. 68). In *Arrival* the past turns into future, beginning turns into end, flashbacks turn into flash-forwards. Hannah holds a stretched—read linear—black caterpillar that partially echoes/foreshadows the aliens' cyclical language. The caterpillar also illustrates how Louise herself is unmade by the traumatic experience she faces, only to re-emerge with a rewritten, linear, sense of self. Ultimately, the unease caused by the music, the various visual devices, and an increasing cognitive dissonance concerning the plot's chronology are transformed into a cathartic experience of closure.

To conclude, I would like to complete Louise's statement that I quoted in my title incompletely: "Memory is a strange thing indeed. It doesn't work like I thought it did. We are so bound by time, by its order."

References

Augé, M. (1995). *Non-places: An introduction to supermodernity* (trans. J. Howe). Verso.

Brockmeier, J. (2001). From the end to the beginning: Retrospective teleology in autobiography. In J. Brockmeier & D. Carbough (Eds.), *Narrative and identity: Studies in autobiography, self and culture* (pp. 247–282). John Benjamins Publishing.

Brooks, P. (1984). *Reading for the plot: Design and intention in narrative.* Harvard University Press.

Buckland, W. (2009). Introduction. In *Puzzle films: Complex storytelling in contemporary cinema* (pp. 1–12). Blackwell.

Chiang, T. (2002). Story of your life. In *Stories of your life and others* (pp. 91–145). Vintage.

Downs, B. (1993). Lessons in loss and grief. *Communication Education, 42*(4), 300–303.

Elias, N. (1992). An essay on time. In S. Loyal & S. Mennell (Eds.), *The collected works of Norbert Elias* (Vol. 9, pp. 31–162). University College Dublin Press.

Federman, R. (1982). *The twofold vibration.* Green Integer.

Federman, R. (1993). Surfiction: A postmodern position. In *Critifiction: Postmodern essays* (pp. 35–47). State University of New York Press.

Husserl, E. (1960/2002). The phenomenology of internal time consciousness. In D. Moran & T. Mooney (Eds.), *The phenomenology reader* (p. 110). Routledge.

Ildirar, S., & Ewing, L. (2018). Revisiting the Kuleshov effect with first-time viewers. *Projections, 12*(1), 19–38.

Lane, A. (2016, November 14). The consuming fervor of *Arrival. The New Yorker.* https://www.newyorker.com/magazine/2016/11/14/the-consuming-fervor-of-arrival

Larsen, E. (2004). The time of our lives: The experience of temporality in occupation. *Canadian Journal of Occupational Therapy, 71*(1), 24–35.

Levy, E. (2016). *Detaining time: Temporal resistance in literature from Shakespeare to McEwan.* Bloomsbury.

Puschak, E. (2017). *Arrival: A response to bad movies.* https://www.youtube.com/watch?v=z18LY6NME1s

Sebald, W. G. (2001). *Austerlitz* (trans. A. Bell). Penguin.

Stolorow, R. D. (2015). Trauma destroys time: The traumatized person lives in an alien reality. *Psychology Today.* https://www.psychologytoday.com/us/blog/feeling-relating-existing/201510/trauma-destroys-time

Stolorow, R. D. (2018). Emotional disturbance, trauma, and authenticity: A phenomenological-contextualist psychoanalytic perspective. In K. Aho (Ed.), *Existential medicine: Essays on health and illness* (pp. 17–26). Rowman and Littlefield.

Villeneuve, D. (Producer), & Heisserer, E. (Screenplay). (2016). *Arrival.* Paramount Pictures.

Whitehead, A. (2004). *Trauma fiction.* Edinburgh University Press.

Wojciehowski, H. C. (2018). When the future is hard to recall: Episodic memory and mnemonic aids in Denis Villeneuve's *Arrival. Projections, 12*(1), 55–70.

289

Womerlsey, G. (2020). (Un)imagination and (im)mobility: Exploring the past and constructing possible futures among refugee victims of torture in Greece. *Culture & Psychology*, 26(4), 713–731.

Young, I. M. (2005). Pregnant embodiment: Subjectivity and alienation. In *On female body experience: "Throwing like a girl" and other essays* (pp. 46–61). Oxford University Press.

Index

For the benefit of digital users, indexed terms that span two pages (e.g., 52–53) may, on occasion, appear on only one of those pages.
Tables and figures are indicated by t and f following the page number

"Abstractions in Comics"
  (Baetens), 262–63
addiction/addiction recovery
  analysis/proposals, of McConnell and
    Snoek, 45, 46, 47–53
  Australian-based narrative therapy
    study, findings, 46, 48, 50–51
  DSM-5 and, 142–43
  influence/role of self-narratives,
    45, 48–54
  need for special narrative strategies,
    tactics, 51
Ahrens, Courtney E., 87
alcoholism/alcohol abuse, 35–36, 37, 108,
  138, 170–71
Alexander, June, 107–8
Alice's Adventures in Wonderland
  (Carroll), 279–80
Alien film (Scott), 279–80
Alpert, Judith, 89, 100–1
Alzheimer's disease
  Alzheimer's Society warning against
    categorization, 193, 195
  characteristics/symptoms of, 179, 190–
    91, 192–93, 199–200
  consequences for affected
    person, 190–91
  construction of a person identity
    with, 174
  descriptions of caring for parents with,
    179, 186–87
  normative assessment/categorization
    of, 192–93
  vascular dementia comparison, 195
Alzheimer's Society, 190–91, 193, 195
American Psychological Association

number of divisions, 2–3
anorexia, 46, 263
Armstadter, Ananda B., 86–87
Arrival (film), 9–10, 273–88
  trauma and temporality, 275–77
artistic expression, 3–4, 9
Aubourg, Jarrah, 155
Augé, Marc, 283
Australian-based Narrative Therapy, 7
autobiographical narratives. See also
    first-person delusions; first-person
    narratives; life stories (life storying);
    My Alien Self: My Journey Back to Me
    (Green); The Woman Who Thought
    Too Much (Limburg)
  autobiographical "truth" and, 119–20
  benefits of, 171, 191
  Bruner on, 154
  fictive bracketing and, 61
  graphic memoir genre and, 259
  relation to novels, 261
  Rimmon-Kenan on, 258
  shame-based, 61, 237–38, 240–52
  use for neurodegenerative diseases, 191
"Autography as Auto-Therapy:
    Psychic Pain and the
    Graphic Memoir"
    (Williams), 260
auto-therapeutic
  effect, 257–58, 260, 264, 267, 270

Baetens, Jan, 262–63
Bamberg, Michael, 156–57.
  See also narrative positioning
  theory
Barthes, Roland, 104, 109–11, 154

Basic Elements of Narrative (Herman), 5–6
Bechdel, Alison, 259. See also
    Fun Home: A Family
    Tragicomic (Bechdel)
Becoming Myself: A Psychiatrist's
    Memoir (Yalom), 108–9
Bennett, Tamryn, 262–63.
    See also *Comics Poetry: Beyond*
    Sequenetial Boundaries (Bennett)
Beroä, David, 262–63
Binky Brown Meets the Holy Virgin Mary
    (Green), 259
biopsychosocial (BPS) model of
    psychiatry, 125–26, 135–37, 139–
    40, 144–45
blogs/blogging, 110–11, 119–20, 259
Blustein, Jeffrey, 174, 178–79, 181–
    10, 186–87
Bohlmeijer, Ernst T., 155, 158–59
borderline personality disorder (BPD), 46,
    238–39, 248, 249–50
Bourdieu, Pierre, 86–87
BPS (biopsychosocial) model, 125–26,
    135–37, 139–40, 144–45
Brancazio, Nicolle Marissa, 155
Breakdowns: Portrait of the Artist as a
    Young %$@&!* (Spiegelman), 259
British Psychological Society, 1–2
Brooks, Peter, 276–77
Brosh, Allie. *See also Hyperbole and a Half*
    (Brosh)
Bruner, Jerome, 154
Buckland, Warren, 278–79
bulimia, 46, 108

Carroll, Lewis, 279–80
Chamberlain, Judith, 235
Charon, Rita, 33–34, 39
Chiang, Ted, 273–74, 277,
    284–85. *See also* "Story of Your Life"
    (Chiang)
clinicians/practitioners
    belief in the efficacy of narrative
        practices, 46
    challenges, 142–43
    control limitations of, 78–79
    demential classification challenges
        of, 199

focus on trauma-induced
    tinnitus, 95–96
patience required by, 79
protocol with clients, 23, 69–70, 75, 76,
    80–81, 91–92, 100, 204
role of trust with clients, 80
skepticism about open form of a
    diary, 108
cognitive-behavioral therapy (CBT), 107–
    8, 117
Comics Poetry: Beyond Sequential
    Boundaries (Bennett), 262–63
Compagnon, Antoine, 109–10
conceptual metaphor theory (CMT), 211–
    13, 214–15
conversational narrative analysis, 210
Conway, Kathlyn, 200
Couser, G. Thomas, 183
COVID-19 global pandemic, 2–3
cross-fictionality theory, 156, 169
Cullberg, Johan, 138–39
Cunningham, Darryl, 259, 260. See also
    Psychiatric Tales (Cunningham)

Dean, Sandra M. (alias Amanda Green).
    See Green, Amanda
de Beauvoir, Simone, 241–42, 244–45
Deignan, Alice, 212–13
delusions/delusional episodes. *See also*
    first-person delusions
    delusional variables, 18–21
    first-person delusions, 21–28
    of grandeur, 25–26
    narrative beginnings of, 24–26
    persecutory delusions, 18–22
    of reference, 25–26
dementia/dementia patients, 8–9. *See also*
    external narratives, for dementia
    patients; *House Mother Normal*
    (Johnson), individual experiences/
    normative categorizations of mental
    health, pathology
    challenges of expressing in literature,
        191–92, 200
    characteristics/symptoms of, 185, 190–
        91, 192–93, 198–201
    confusion caused by normative
        categorization, 192–93

consequences for affected person, 190–91, 198–99
criticisms of external narratives for, 174–75, 181, 183–85
difficulties in diagnosing progression of, 199
importance of considering first-person experiences of, 175, 183–84, 186–87
importance of diminishing the diachronic unity perspective, 185–86
Kane/Thomas, on classificatory norms, 199
Lewy body dementia, 195
narrative identity, ethics, and, 180–85
need for modifications of external narratives for, 185–87
normative assessment/categorization of, 192–93
person-to-person variations in symptoms, 193
points made by proponents of external narratives for, 178–79, 180–82
positive contribution of narrative fiction, 191
psychoses related to, 132–33
qualitative identity and, 175–76
related DSM-III disorders, 132–33
risk of disregarding first-person expressions by, 184
role of external narratives in construction of a person's identity, 174–75, 178–79
transfer of narrative approaches to, 178–256
use of fictional texts/autobiographical narratives with, 191
vascular dementia, 195
depression. *See also* depression, representations in German mass media
diary writing and, 104, 105–6, 107–8
Klein on normalcy of, 98–99
mood treatment protocols, 107–8
narrative practices and, 45
rape/sexual violence and, 88–89, 94–95
re-authoring techniques and, 46
SORC scheme analysis of client behavior, 107–8

term derivation, 214
WHO data on, 207
depression, representations in German mass media, 213–24. *See also* linguistic discourse analysis
depression is a fall (metaphor), 218–20, 221
depression is a heavy burden (metaphor), 215–18, 219
depression is a journey (metaphor), 221
depression is a loss of control (metaphor), 219
depression is darkness (metaphor), 220–21
metaphor and narrative in the examples, 221–23
diachronic holism, 180–81, 184, 185
Diagnostic and Statistical Manual of Mental Disorders (DSM-5), 3, 141, 142–43, 214
Diagnostic and Statistical Manual of Mental Disorders (DSM-I), 132, 135–36
Diagnostic and Statistical Manual of Mental Disorders (DSM-II), 132, 135–36
Diagnostic and Statistical Manual of Mental Disorders (DSM-III), 126–27
behavioral categories (1832-1980), 134*t*
BPS model, 135–36
changes in behavioral diagnostic categories (1832-1980), 133–34
changes in the grand narrative of mental disorder (1832-1980), 134–35
diagnostic description of mental disorder and, 132–36
differences with Engström's diagnoses categories, 133–35, 138–39
influence on use of diagnosis, 127–28
Melancholy/mania category, 132–34
nosological character of, 147–48
Psychosis category, 132–33
Specific extreme behaviors category, 133–34
use of biological *vs.* psychodynamic emphasis, 127–28, 135–36
Withdrawal category, 133–34

Diagnostic and Statistical Manual of Mental Disorders (DSM-IV), 249–50
diaries/diary writing, 3–4, 8. *See also* diaries/diary writing, case study (Client S.)
  benefits for depression, 107–8
  as complementary to traditional psychotherapy, 3–4
  Lejeune's research on, 106–7
  literary diaries, 109–12
  research and practice overview, 106–9
  Seiffge-Krenke's research/findings, 108
  sociolinguistic/psychological perspectives, 106–7
  Suhr's research/findings, 107–8
  types of, 104
  usefulness in psychotherapy, 3–4, 8, 105, 107–8, 119–20
diaries/diary writing, case study (Client S.), 112
  orientation toward the future, 117–18
  quasi-philosophical introspection, 118–19
  reflection, implied audience, daily life, 113–14
  work and relationships, 114–17
Dilthey, Wilhelm, 136–37
disassociation theory (Janet), 95–96
discourse analysis. *See* linguistic discourse analysis
discourse narratology, 153–58, 169
Divina Commedia (Dante), 241–42
Dolto, Françoise, 89
La domination masculine thesis (Bourdieu), 86–87
Downs, Barney, 285–86
dreams
  dream narratives, 36–37
  Freud's study/findings, 96–97

eating disorders, 46, 108, 263
Eisner, William, 262–63
elderly people, life narratives (Vitality 90+ research project), 8, 157–72
  Oskari: a life unfolding, 159–60, 164–69
  Simo: retrospective life story, 158–59, 160–64

  uses of level-one (story-level) positioning, 160–61, 164–65, 166, 167, 168–69
  uses of level-three positioning, 160–62, 163–65, 167, 169
  uses of level-two (interview-level) positioning, 163–64, 165, 166, 167, 168–69
  uses of narrative discourse modes, 169–70
  victim plot identification, 168
  ways of narrating, 169–72
Engström, Georg, 128–32, 131*t*, 134–36, *See also under* psychiatry
Eno, Brian, 281
Epstein, Seymour, 89
Erikson, Malgorzata, 73, 74
Ette, Ottmar, 109–10
Ewing, Louise, 285
existential philosophy, 118
existential psychiatry, 125–26
existential psychotherapy, 108–9
experientiality, 5–6
Explanatory Challenge, 53–56
external narratives, for dementia patients
  advantages of, 180, 181
  Blustein's advocacy for, 174
  Boetzkes's advocacy for, 174, 181
  criticisms of, 174–75, 181, 183–85
  diachronic holism feature, 184
  emphasis of, 183
  Gedge's advocacy for, 181
  Lamarque on problems of, 175, 181–83, 184–85
  need for modifications of, 185–87
  oral life stories as core element, 178–79
  points made by proponents of, 178–79, 180–82, 183–84
  problems related to, 174–75
  relational structure of, 175, 178, 179, 183
  risks of disregarding first-person expressions, 175, 183–84, 186–87
  role in construction of a personal identity, 174, 175
  Schechtman's advocacy for, 181–82
  Zander-Schneider's example of, 179, 183

Facebook, 111–12, 113–14

false memories, 58
Felder, Ekkehard, 208–9
Ferenczi, Sándor, 96–97
fictional texts, 1–2. *See also* fictive stance
  benefits of, 1–2
  cross-fictionality theory, 156, 172
  dementia, external narratives,
    and, 181–82
  Theory of Mind and, 19
  use with dementia patients, 191
fictive stance
  advantages of adopting, 60–61
  challenge of adopting, 61
  comparison to "factual" character of
    narrative practices, 47
  comparison to Solution-Focused Brief
    Therapy, 62–63
  description, 59–60
  effectiveness, 62–63
  positive contribution to
    dementia, 191
  scope challenge and, 61
  self-governance and, 45, 52–53, 61
First Nations indigenous culture
    (Canada), 36–37, 38–39, 40
  Alcoholism, substance abuse and, 35–
    36, 37
  commonality of "dream
    narratives," 36–37
  negative impact of
    colonialism, 38, 40, 38
  suicidality and, 38
first-person delusions (Zelt's "The Messiah
    Quest"), 21–28
  belief in "the (magical, poetical,
    fantastical) code," 25–26, 27, 29–30
  comments by clinicians/
    therapists, 23, 28
  delusional logic, 27
  delusions of grandeur, 25–26, 27–28
  delusions of reference, 25–26
  framing of mother-infant relations as
    "telepathy," 24–25
  lauding of Zelt's contribution, 25
  onset/unfolding of delusions, 29–30
  paranoid delusions, 26–27
  sensitivity to nonverbal
    communication, 26

Zelt's choice of third person
    narrative, 23
first-person narratives, 155–56, 160–61,
    166, 175, 183–84, 186–87. *See also*
    autobiographical narratives
Forney, Ellen, 257–58. See also *Marbles:
    Mania, Depression, Michelangelo, &
    Me* (Forney)
  on psychic relief through drawing, 260
  readerly dynamics in *Marbles*, 267–70
Foucault, Michel, 127–28, 141–42
Frances, Allen, 145
Frank, Arthur, 33–34, 258–59. See also *The
    Wounded Storyteller* (Frank)
Freud, Sigmund, 96–97, 108, 241–42
Friedrich, Johannes Baptista, 124–25
Fun Home: A Family Tragicomic
    (Bechdel), 259

Gardner, Jared, 260–61
Garland, Alex, 278–79
Gedge, Elisabeth Boetzkes, 174, 181
Geertz, Clifford, 39
genealogical archaeology
    (Foucault), 127–28
Genette, Gérard, 232, 258
Gerrans, Philip, 59
Ghaemi, S. Nassir, 125–27
Gloeckner, Phoebe, 260
Goffman, Erving, 25–26
Goldie, Peter, 59
Göstas, Wilhelmsson, 69–70
graphic medicine, 259, 263
graphic memoirs about mental illness,
    257–71. See also *In the Shadow
    of No Towers* (Spiegelman);
    *Marbles: Mania, Depression,
    Michelangelo, & Me* (Forney);
    When Anxiety Attacks (Koscik)
  auto-therapeutic effect/psychic relief
    through drawings, 257–58, 260–61
  cathartic purposes of, 270
  illness, narrative, and, 258–61
  nonnarrative configurations in,
    258, 261–70
  proliferation of, 270
  readerly dynamics in Forney's
    Marbles, 267–70

graphic memoirs about mental illness
(*cont.*)
relation to the graphic novel, 261
split between narrating "I" and
experiencing "I," 259–60
suitability for depicting mental
illness, 259
Gravelin, Claire R., 87–88
Green, Amanda, 9, 232. See also *My Alien
Self: My Journey Back to Me* (Green)
Green, Justin, 259
Green, Katie, 259, 260. See also *Lighter
Than My Shadow* (Green)
Lighter Than My Shadow (Green)
Gubrium, Jaber, 34
guided imagination exercises, 57–58

Hatfield, Charles, 262–63
Heinroth, Johann Christian
August, 124–25
Henschel, Gerhard, 110–11
Herrndorf, Wolfgang, 110–11
*The Hidden Prejudice: Mental Disability on
Trial* (Perlin), 235
Hill, Suzanne, 87–88
Hinting Task, 19–21
Hinting Test, 19
History of Madness (Foucault), 127–28
History of Sexuality (Foucault), 140
Hitchcock, Alfred, 285
The Hitchhiker's Guide to the Galaxy
(Adams), 274
Holstein, James, 34
homosexuality, 141–43
Horst, Rutger, 95–96
House Mother Normal (Johnson),
individual experiences/normative
categorizations of mental health,
pathology, 193–204
Alzheimer's Society warning against
normative comparisons, 194–95
assessment/introduction of dementia
patients, 194
cold, distancing categorization of
patients in, 195–96
contesting of cultural
conceptualizations of
"normality," 203

description/representations of
dementia, 8–9, 191, 193–94, 195,
198–99, 200–2, 203–4
interior monologues of characters, 191–
92, 194, 196–99, 200–2
Hunt, Melissa, 111–12
Husserl, Edmund, 281
Hutto, Daniel D., 155
Hyperbole and a Half (Brosh), 259
Hyvärinen, Matti, 171–72

identity theory. *See* personal identity
(personal identity theory);
philosophical identity theory
Ildirar, Sermin, 285
illness narratives, 32–42
classic studies of, 33–34
cultural fabric of life and, 41–42
dramas of life and, 35–38
genre description, 33–34
Gubrium's/Holstein's description of, 34
impact of cultural traditions on, 40
indigenous women, living on reserve,
cardiac problems, 32–33, 35–39, 40–42
role of cultural landscape in, 38–41
role of "zooming together" of time
levels, 37–38
Sontag on illness, 32
storytelling format in indigenous
communities, 39
Instagram, 111–12, 113–14
interior monologues
of characters in *House Mother Normal*,
191–92, 194, 196–99, 200–2
International Classification of Diseases
(ICD), 3
Interpretative Phenomenological Analysis
(IPA), 73
In the Shadow of No Towers (Spiegelman),
257–58, 259, 264–65, 267, 270–71

Jacob's Room (Woolf), 241–42
Janet, Pierre, 95–96
Jaspers, Karl, 126–27, 135–37, 139
Jensen, Thomas Wiben, 212–13
Johannisson, Karin, 140, 141–42
Johannson, Johann, 281–82
Johnson, B. S., 8–9

Johnson, Mark, 211–12, 214–15
Johnson, Samuel, 241–42
Joyce, James, 278

Kaminer, Debra, 95–96
Kane, Joseph, 199
Kierkegaard, Søren, 118
Klein, Melanie, 98–99, 241–42
Kleinman, Arthur, 33–34
Knausgård, Karl Ove, 110–11
Korhonen, Kuisma, 171
Koscik, Terian, 259, 265–67, 266f, 270–
    71. See also *When Anxiety Attacks*
    (Koscik)
Kourgiantakis, Toula, 80
Kraepelin, Emil, 136, 214
Krausser, Helmut, 110–11
Kuhn, Thomas, 127, 136
Kuleshov effect, 284–86
Kunzle, David, 262–63

Labov, William, 210–11, 213, 222, 224
Lakoff, George, 211–12, 214–15
Lamarque, Peter, 175, 181–83, 184–85
Larsen, Elizabeth, 275–76
Launer, John, 54
Lejeune, Philippe, 106–7
Levy, Eric, 275–76
Lewis, Bradley, 235
Lewis, Helen B., 231
Lewy body dementia, 195
life stories (life storying)
    Christian faith frame of
        reference, 158–59
    comparison to psychological continuity
        accounts, 178
    of dementia patients, 180, 181, 183
    external narration of, 174, 178–79,
        180, 183
    inconsistencies in, 29
    as "inner talk" in diaries, 109–10
    integration of trauma in, 98
    positioning in the analyses of, 154–57
    role of, in psychotherapeutic work, 100
    sensitivities of, 41–42
    in the Vitality 90+ research project,
        157–58
Lighter Than My Shadow (Green), 259

Limburg, Joanne, 9. See also *The Woman
    Who Thought Too Much* (Limburg)
    description of shame, 231–32
    link to obsessive-compulsive disorder
        (OCD), 231, 234, 238–39
    quotes of passages from feminist
        literature, 241–42
    The Woman Who Thought Too Much, 9,
        232, 234, 241–48
Lindsay, Rachel, 259. See also *RX: A
    Graphic Memoir* (Lindsay)
Linell, Per, 212–13
linguistic discourse analysis, 2–3, 207–12.
    See also depression, representations
    in German mass media; metaphors
    conversational narrative analysis, 210
    impact of conceptual metaphor theory,
        211–13, 214–15
    importance of metaphor for, 211–13
    as seen in German linguistics, 211–9
    selected examples: depression is a
        fall, 218–20
    selected examples: depression is a heavy
        burden, 215–18
    selected examples: depression is
        darkness, 220–21
Linthout, Willy, 259, 260. See also *Years of
    the Elephant* (Linthout)
listening by practitioners. *See also* teaching
    the art of listening
    active-listening approach, 71, 79
    components of effective listening, 69–70
    need for support and practice, 76
    role in making sense of client
        narratives, 69–70
    role in narratives, 3–4, 21, 30
literary diaries, 109–12
Loftus, Elizabeth, 58
Lyotard, Francois, 136–37

madness/mad behavior, 8, 123–48
    eighteenth-century psychic school
        perspective, 124–25
    Enlightenment era perspective, 124–25
    Hippocratic/Platonic perspectives, 124–
        25, 128–30
    influence of Judeo-Christian, Greek/
        Hellenistic ideologies, 124

Mantel, Hilary, 242–43
Marbles: Mania, Depression, Michelangelo, & Me (Forney), 257–58, 259, 260
importance of the front page, 267–69, 268f
nonnarrative configuration in, 258, 261–70
readerly dynamics in, 266f, 267–70
Marshall, Tara C., 87–88
masturbation, 128–30, 135–36, 141–42, 248–50
Maus I and II (Spiegelman), 259
McCloud, Scott, 262–63. See also *Understanding Comics: The Invisible Art* (McCloud)
McConnell, Doug
on the potential dangers of narrative therapy, 56–57
on the role of self-narratives in addiction recovery, 45–54, 55, 56–58, 61, 63
Sense-Maximizing Thesis of, 49
Medeiros, Kate de, 155–56
media
role in spreading knowledge of dementia, 190–91, 204
social media, 111–12, 113–14, 209
media discourse. *See also* depression, representations in German mass media
defined, 209–10
drivers of, 209
medical discourse in Germany, 209
narrative in mass media discourse, 210–11
medical categorization and normalization, 143–44, 190–204
Memento film, 278–79
memoirs of mental distress, 9
mental distress
autobiographies about, 232
challenges of, 2–3, 6
changing definitions of, 6
Engström's treatment of, 134–35
global experiences of, 2–3
role of silence in narratives about, 4–5, 232
mental health, WHO definition, 232–33

Mental Health Foundation, 190–91, 236
mental health/mental health care. *See also* teaching the art of listening
categorization and normalization of, 192–203
current emphasis on diagnoses, standardization, time-limited interventions, 70–71, 80–81
holistic care, 1–2
importance of narratology for, 4–6
need for creativity of practitioners, 69–70
need for strengthening the art of listening, 70–72
"The Messiah Quest" (Zelt). *See* first-person delusions (Zelt's "The Messiah Quest")
Metaphor and Meaning in Psychotherapy (Siegelman), 98
metaphors. *See also* metaphors for depression
of "centering," 115–16
conceptual metaphors, 211–13, 214–15
gate metaphor for pain, 212–13
in graphic medicine in relation to anorexia, 263
helpfulness for mentally ill persons, 223
importance for linguistic discourse analysis, 211–13
metaphorical space in *Arrival*, 283–84
recontextualization of, 212–13
terms for mental illness, 214–15
variance based on context, register, genre, 212–13
metaphors for depression (German mass media)
depression is a fall, 218–20
depression is a heavy burden, 215–18, 219
depression is a journey, 221
depression is a loss of control, 219
depression is darkness, 220–21
depression is weight, 215–16
#MeToo movement, 86–87
Mildorf, Jarmila, 156
Mills, Stephen, 89–90
Milner, Marion, 241–42

Morson, Gary Saul, 170. *See also* narrative temporalities model (Morson)
Mourning Diary (Barthes), 104, 109–11
Mukwege, Denis, 100–1
Murad, Nadia, 87
"Music for Airports" (Eno), 281
My Alien Self: My Journey Back to Me (Green), 9, 232, 248–52
  allusions to dark humiliating experiences, 237–38
  comparison to Limburg's memoir, 250–52
  depiction of consequences of withdrawal response, 236
  depiction of the medicalization of women's bodies, 238–39
  description of source information, 248
  experiences of humiliation, 249
  links to borderline personality disorder diagnosis (BPD), 248, 249–50
  link to obsessive-compulsive disorder (OCD), 238–39, 248
  passages in support of Tomkins's "optimistic" description of shame, 234
  transformational energy of, 239–40
  use of narrating "I," 248–51

Narcissistic Personality Inventory (NPI), 111–12
Narrative Discourse (Genette), 258
Narrative Exposure Therapy, 45
narrative interviews, 7
narrative medicine, 4, 39, 41, 45, 155, 261
narrative positioning theory, 153, 154, 156–57, 165, 168–69
narrative psychiatry, 1–2, 80–81
narratives/narrative method
  autobiographical narratives, 37, 61, 119–20, 154, 155–56, 171, 191, 237–38, 258
  conceptualizations of, 4–6
  definition/description, 36–37, 90–91, 154, 155
  discourse narratology/modes, 153–58
  distinction from other "talking cures," 46
  explanatory challenge, 53–56
  first-person narratives, 155–56, 160–61, 166, 175, 183–84, 186–87
  goal of, 46
  Loftus's concerns about, 58
  manipulation challenge, 57
  mental health and, 2–4
  philosophical challenges of, 47
  as a philosophical concept, 8
  positioning theory, 153, 154, 156–57, 165, 168–69
  Rosenberg's negative opinion of, 54–56
  scientific credibility of, 17
  Scope Challenge, 56–57, 61
  skeptical challenges of, 53–58
  Strawson's case against, 57
  third-person narratives, 22, 23, 59, 160–61
  use of re-authoring techniques, 46, 53, 57–58
  "zooming together" of time levels, 37–38
narrative social work, 1–2, 80–81
narrative temporalities model (Morson), 170
Nerlich, Brigitte, 211–12
neurocognitive disorder (NCD), mild/ major, 192–93
neurodegenerative diseases, 191, 192–94, 200. *See also* Alzheimer's disease; dementia/dementia patients; *House Mother Normal* (Johnson), individual experiences/normative categorizations of mental health, pathology
nonnarrative configurations, in mental health memoirs, 257–71
Norrick, Neal R., 210–11

obsessive-compulsive disorder (OCD), 238–39, 241–43, 248
Odyssey (Homer), 282–83
On Being Ill (Woolf), 200
On Our Own: Patient-Controlled Alternatives to the Mental Health System (Chamberlain), 235
open-ended approaches, 3, 39, 71, 72–73

Padua inventory, 241–42

Page, Tyler, 259. See also *Raised on Ritalin: A Personal Story of ADHD, Medication and Modern Psychiatry*
panic attacks, 108
PANSS. *See* Positive and Negative Syndrome Scale (PANSS)
Pathological Narcissism Inventory (PNI), 111–12
Perlin, Michael, 235
persecutory delusions, 18
    assessment of, 19–21
    consequences on social functioning, 18
    Hinting Test measure of ToM, 19
    interactions between variables, 19–20
    PANSS assessment of, 19
    Phalen's research/assessment tools/ findings, 18–21
    Social Functioning Scale assessment of, 19–20, 21
    Theory of Mind's moderation of, 18
personal identity (personal identity theory)
    construction of, in dementia sufferers, 174
    criticisms of, 181
    diachronic holism and, 180–81, 184, 185–86
    external narrative accounts of, 159, 177
    Locke's definition of, 175, 176–77
    narrative approaches, 175–79
    numerical identity, 175–76, 186–87
    qualitative identity, 175–76, 186–87
    Schechtman on, 177–78
    Schmidhuber on, 178
    Strawson's criticism of diachronic unity in, 185
person-centered interviews, 3–4
Peter, Anu Mary, 263
Petzold, Hilarion, 108–9
Phalen, Peter L., 18–21
Phelan, James, 191
philosophical identity theory, 181–82
Pinel, Philippe, 128–30
Plath, Sylvia, 241–42
poetry, 1–2
positioning theory, 153, 154, 156–57, 165, 168–69
Positive and Negative Syndrome Scale (PANSS), 19

post-traumatic stress disorder (PTSD)
    rape-related, 88–89
    terrorist-attack related, 264
Power Threat Meaning Framework (PTMF), 1–2, 70
practitioners. *See* clinicians/practitioners
Prayers and Meditations (Johnson), 241–42
The Presentation of Self in Everyday Life (Goffman), 25–26
Prud'homme-Cranford, Raïn, 40
Psychiatric Tales (Cunningham), 259
psychiatry/psychiatric diagnoses. See also *Diagnostic and Statistical Manual of Mental Disorders* (DSM-III)
    behavioral categories, 127–28, 129t
    biological, psychological, social perspectives, 125–26, 128–30
    biomedical *vs.* "enhancement" approach, 126–27
    biopsychosocial (BPS) model, 125–26, 135–37, 139–40, 144–45
    blind spots, 143–45
    challenges of narrative medicine to, 4
    cultural influences, 127
    current ontological positioning of, 125–26
    current paradigm of, 6
    development of treatment/effect on diagnosis, 138
    Engström's diagnostic categories, 127–32, 131t, 133–36, 142–43
    Enlightenment-era development of, 124–25
    framing of mother-infant relations, 24–25
    healthy morals/disordered immorality in, 139–40
    historical background, 123
    History of Sexuality (Foucault) and, 140
    internal debates about causes, 138–39
    interpretation role of psychiatrists, 139
    medicalization of sexuality (in diagnoses), 141–42
    morality narrative in, 142–43
    moral *vs.* care perspective, 142–43

narrative psychiatry, 81–82
narrative shifts in cause and
    cure, 136–37
need for purposeful structuring of
    knowledge, 146–47
norm-infused grand narratives, 123–
    24, 127
onset of diagnosis using DSM-III, 127
Pinel's/Reil's mapping of madness/
    mental disorder, 127–30
pre-1980s positivist medical
    perspective, 127
purpose of diagnoses, 144–45
risks of unreliability, 146
Sweden, historical background, 126–27
psychic disharmony, 124–25
psychic functions (psychic energy). *See
    also* graphic memoirs about mental
    illness
causes of psychic disorders, 128–30
complexity of experiences of mentally
    ill people, 214–16
consequences of deficiency of, 238
disharmony of, 124–25
Engström on imbalances of, 128–32,
    131*t*, 138–39
Frances's comment on psychic
    disorders, 145
intrapsychic patterns, 144–45
Jaspers's comment on, 136–37
Johannisson's thoughts on, 140
psychic relief in graphic memoirs about
    mental health, 257–71
psychological continuity accounts, 178
psychology
    importance of narrative in, 3–4
    paradigm shift to narrative
        psychology, 7
"Pull Yourself Together!" survey (Mental
    Health Foundation), 236
Punzi, Elisabeth, 72–73

qualia, 5–6
Qvarsell, Roger, 124–25

*Raised on Ritalin: A Personal Story of
    ADHD, Medication and Modern
    Psychiatry* (Page), 259

rape
    health/affective consequences, 88–89
    India/Great Britain, findings, 87–88
    link to sexual trauma-related tinnitus
        (case study), 91–95, 96–99
    rates data (U.S.), 86–87
    societal reactions, 87–88
    by a stranger *vs.* by an
        acquaintance, 87–88
    use as a strategy in armed conflicts, 87
    victim blaming (secondary
        victimization), 87–88
Rapoport, Judith L., 241–42, 246
re-authoring techniques
    benefits of, 53
    description, 53
    risk factors, 57–58
    uses of, 46
redemption script, 51
Reil, Johan Christian, 127–30
Richter, Max, 281–82, 283
Ricoeur, Paul, 258
Rimmon-Kenan, Shlomith, 258–59
risk factors
    of exposure to trauma, 282–83
    of guided imagination exercises, 57–58
    of installing false memories, 58
    of psychiatry, 146
    of re-authoring techniques, 57–58
    of use of the BPS model, 136–37
Rosenberg, Alexander, 54–56
Rush, Benjamin, 138
RX: A Graphic Memoir (Lindsay), 259

Sacks, Oliver, 33–34
Schechtman, Marya, 174, 177–79, 180–
    83, 184
Schizophrenia Bulletin, 22–23. *See also*
    "The Messiah Quest" (Zelt)
schizophrenia/schizoaffective disorder
    persecutory delusions in, 18–22
    Phalen's research/assessment tools/
        findings, 18–21
Schmidhuber, Martina, 178, 179, 186–87
scope challenge, 56–57, 61
Scott, Ridley, 279–80
Sebald, W. G., 277, 278
The Second Sex (Beauvoir), 241–42

Sedgwick, Eve Kosofsky, 233–34
Seiffge-Krenke, Inge, 108
self-governance, 45, 52–53, 61
self-harming (skin-picking) behavior, 242–43, 244–45
self-narration/self-narratives
   of elderly people, 8
   empowering methods of, 46
   evaluation process for plausibility of, 52–46
   importance of, 45–46
   influence of co-authoring partners, 50, 51–52, 53
   McConnell/Snoek/on the role of, in an addicted person's recovery, 45, 48–54
   need for special narrative strategies, tactics, 51
   outcomes of successful therapy, 53
   potential causes of failure, 50, 51, 52–53
   Schechtman on personal identity and, 177
   Spiegelman on the basis of, 98
   Spence on the contributions of, 95–96
Semino, Elena, 211–13
Sense-Maximizing Thesis (McConnell), 49
sexual violence (assault, abuse). See also rape
   causative for PTSD, 88–89
   impact on women coming forth, 100–1
   India/Great Britain, study and findings, 87–88
   Mukwege's vision of how to deal with, 100–1
   as a strategy in armed conflicts, 86–87
SFBT. See Solution-Focused Brief Therapy
shame. See also My Alien Self: My Journey Back to Me (Green); The Woman Who Thought Too Much (Limburg)
   definitions, 233–34, 235, 237–38, 246
   gender, mental illness, and, 238–40
   impact of writing about, on gender identity, 239–40
   Lewis's view of, 231
   Limburg's description of, 231–32
   questions asked about, 233
   of rape victims, 88–89

Sedgwick's performative concept of, 233–34
   spreading of, 233–34
   theoretical/narratological approaches to, 233–38
   Tomkins on the shame response, 233–34
   withdrawal response, 233–34, 235–36, 245, 247
   in women's mental distress autobiographies, 240–52
Snoek, Anke, 46, 47–53, 55, 56–58, 61, 63
Social Functioning Scale, 19–20, 21
social media, 111–12, 113–14, 209
Social Stories interventions, 46
social work, importance of narrative in, 3–4
Solution-Focused Brief Therapy (SFBT), 60, 62–63
somatic illness, 108
Sontag, Susan, 32
Spence, Donald, 95–96
Spiegelman, Art
   Breakdowns: Portrait of the Artist as a Young %$@&*!, 259
   Maus I and II, 259
   In the Shadow of No Towers, 257–58, 259, 264–65, 267, 270–71
Stolorow, Robert, 275–77
"Story of Your Life" (Chiang), 273
storytelling
   benefits for mental health, 155
   benefits for trauma victims, 90–91
   cross-fictionality and, 156
   fictive storytelling norms, 61–62
   on health and illness, 40, 41–42
   importance of collaborative work of interlocuters, 210
   in indigenous communities, 39
   narrative gerontology and, 153
   Norrick on conversational storytelling, 210–11
   Rosenberg on the perils of, 55–56
   varied stylistic devices in, 279–80
Strawson, Galen, 57, 175
Streeten, Nicola, 260
strokes (minor/major), 195
substance abuse
   diagnostic debates on, 141

DSM-5 and, 142–43
Engström's ideas on, 128–30, 135–36
in First Nations in Canada, 38
grand narrative of morality and, 142–43
Suhr, Melissa, 107–8
suicide/suicidality, 38
  Camu's writing on, 241–42
  depression and, 207, 235
  gender, mental illness, and, 239–40
  by Herrndorf, 110–11
  masturbation and, 141–42
  shame and, 235–36
  tinnitus and, 93–94
swine flu global pandemic, 2–3

teaching the art of listening (interview
    study), 45–82
  components of effective listening, 69–70
  discussion of study, 79–82
  interviews and analysis, 72–73
  limitations, 82
  methodological/ethical
    considerations, 74
  need for practitioner openness to
    client, 69–70
  open-ended approaches, 3, 39,
    71, 72–73
  results: avoiding foreclosure, 75–76
  results: balancing theory and
    practice, 76–77
  results: providing supportive teaching,
    learning activities, 77–78
  results: resisting temptation to "cure"
    clients, 78–79
Theory of Mind (ToM), 19–20, 21
third-person narratives, 22, 23,
    59, 160–61
Thomas, Alan, 199
time, phenomenology of (Husserl), 281
Time and Narrative (Ricoeur), 258
time-bending science-fiction films, 273–
    75, 278–79, 281–82, 284
The Time Machine (Wells), 278–79
tinnitus
  definition, 92
  frustration hypothesis of, 92
  trauma-induced tinnitus (case study),
    91–95, 96–99

ToM. See Theory of Mind (ToM)
Tomkins, Silvan, 233–34
trauma/traumatic events. See also Arrival
    (film); rape; sexual violence
  affective responses of victims, 88–89
  challenges in learning to treat, 78–79
  definitions, 89–90
  impact on mental health, 2–3,
    33, 69–70
  influence on memory
    (memories), 91–92
  puzzle films, time, and, 279–80
  sexual trauma-induced tinnitus (case
    study), 91–95, 96–99
  silencing of (case study), 86–101
  use of Narrative Exposure Therapy
    for, 46
  use of re-authoring techniques, 46
Trotter, Thomas, 138
Tschick (Herrndorf), 110–11
Twitter, 111–12
The Twofold Vibration (Federman), 277

Understanding Comics: The Invisible Art
    (McCloud), 262–63
United Kingdom. See Power Threat
    Meaning Framework
United Nations special rapporteur, 70

Van der Hart, Onno, 95–96
variable-centered research, 16, 29, 30
variables (psychological variables)
  delusional variables, 18–21
  description, 16
  group-level analysis of patterns, 17, 21
  lack of agency in, 17
  measures of, in persecutory
    delusions, 19–21
  relationships between variables, 17
  variable-centered research, 16–
    17, 29, 30
vascular dementia, 195
Venkatesan, Sathyaraj, 263
Villeneuve, Denis, 75, 273. See also
    Arrival (film)
Vitality 90+ research project (Tampere
    University, Finland), 157–58. See also
    elderly people, life narratives

Volkskrankheit (folk disease). *See* depression, representations in German mass media

Waletzky, Joshua, 210–11, 213, 222, 224
Westerhof, Gerben J., 155, 158–59
When Anxiety Attacks (Koscik), 259, 265–67, 266*f*, 270–71
Whitehead, Anne, 280, 281
Williams, Ian, 260, 261
Winnicott, Donald W., 89, 109–10
Wirth-Cauchon, Janet, 249–50
Wojciehowski, Hannah, 287
Wolk, Douglas, 262–63
The Woman Who Thought Too Much (Limburg), 9, 232, 241–48
  allusions to humiliating experiences, 237–38, 245
  arrangement of text/chapter headings, 241–42
  comparison to Green's memoir, 250–52
  depiction of consequences of withdrawal response, 236
  depiction of her self-harming (skin-picking) habit, 242–45
  depiction of hiding in shame, 246
  depiction of shame as a radical silence, 246–47
  depiction of the medicalization of women's bodies, 238–39
  link to obsessive-compulsive disorder (OCD), 238–39, 241–43

passages in support of Tomkins's "optimistic" description of shame, 234
  quotation of Beauvoir, 244
  quotation of Rapaport, 246
  quotations from feminist literature, 241–42
  quotations from the Padua inventory, 241–42
  transformational energy of, 239–40
  use of narrating "I," 242–43, 245–46
Womersley, Gail, 282–83
Woolf, Virginia, 241–42
  On Being Ill, 200
  Jacob's Room, 241–42
World Health Organization (WHO), 207, 232–33
The Wounded Storyteller (Frank), 258–59
writing. *See also* diaries/diary writing
  artistic *vs.* non-artistic, 108–9
  benefits to clients, 28, 104–5
  blogs/blogging, 110–11, 119–20, 259
  types of, 105

Yalom, Irvin D., 108–9
Years of the Elephant (Linthout), 259

Zander-Schneider, Gabriele, 179, 183
Zelt, David, 22–27. *See also* first-person delusions (Zelt's "The Messiah Quest")
Zimmer, Hans, 281